Headache

Series Editors
Paolo Martelletti
Rigmor Jensen

For further volumes:
http://www.springer.com/series/11801

Aksel Siva • Christian Lampl
Editors

Case-Based Diagnosis and Management of Headache Disorders

Springer

Editors
Aksel Siva
Cerrahpasa School of Medicine
Istanbul University
Istanbul
Turkey

Christian Lampl
Headache Medical Center Seilerstaette Linz
Hospital Sisters of Charity
Linz
Austria

ISBN 978-3-319-06885-5 ISBN 978-3-319-06886-2 (eBook)
DOI 10.1007/978-3-319-06886-2
Springer Cham Heidelberg Dordrecht London New York

Library of Congress Control Number: 2014948189

Printed on acid-free paper

Springer is part of Springer Science+Business Media (www.springer.com)

Foreword

Today the presentation of a new book on headache can be seen as the umpteenth editorial offer in an area of clinical medicine always rich of various productions, different for types and scientific weight.

This time, for the first time, a Scientific Society projected and moulded a wide and continuative editorial project, the *Headache Series*. Conceived within the *European Headache Federation*, it is an official product of the Federation itself and this represents an innovation already.

The chosen topics are up-to-date, and this introductive volume, brilliantly edited by Aksel Siva and Christian Lampl, is a vivid testimony of it. Consolidated clinical skills are essential in the treatment of pathologies like headache disorders: this volume offers an exhaustive overview on various clinical cases, written by prestigious signatures, and gives the physician that everyday faces this ubiquitous pathology a vision on these clinical problems strongly oriented to multidisciplinarity.

Springer will publish the *Headache Series* from this first volume onward. Anyone will be able to assimilate what they believe is important for the improvement of the clinical practice.

On behalf of the European Headache Federation we are proud to introduce the *Headache Series* presenting this volume. We thank all the Book Editors for the enormous effort lavished in this project that will allow the Federation to complete its educational offer, keeping (if not rising) its own standards of excellence.

The European Headache Federation also thanks the Publisher, stalwart of this initiative, and every Book Editor committed to the upcoming volumes, trusting that their leaderships in the field and their consolidated clinical-scientific experience might act as flying-wheel for a new deal on headache research in the next years.

Rome, Italy — Paolo Martelletti
København, Denmark — Rigmor Høiland Jensen

Preface

This first *Headache* Series book endorsed by the European Headache Federation provides the physician with a practical approach to the diagnosis, evaluation, and management of headache disorders based on lessons learned from real-life headache patients. Case-based learning has become a major educational offering at all levels. As editors, we have enjoyed the work with internationally well-known headache experts, presenting cases taken from their own practice and discussing the evaluation and management of each case step by step. Clinical cases still represent the best way for physicians to learn clinical medicine. The clearly structured chapters cover initial evaluation and diagnostic work-up, imaging, differential diagnosis, interpretation of findings of further work-up, treatment options and response as well as key points. In the management of headache it is vital that clinicians learn to recognize, in case context, the similarities of cases with cases seen in their clinical practice, because they learn by comparing them to the way of thinking of other experts in the field. A wide spectrum of headache types is covered, including both primary and secondary headache disorders. The reader will learn how to diagnose and manage different headache disorders directly from the clinical experience of experts. We have allowed the experts to present their cases in their own style, so that the readers will get the feel for each case. Further, all cases are organized around the new International Headache Society Classification of Headache disorders (ICDH III-beta, 2013).

Case-Based Diagnosis and Management of Headache Disorders will be of value for neurologists and a wide range of physicians – from those in other specialties to primary care givers.

Istanbul, Turkey
Vienna, Austria

Aksel Siva
Christian Lampl

Contents

Chapter 1
Migraine Without Aura

Christian Lampl

1.1 Case Description

A 39-year-old female was admitted to our headache outpatient center with a 1-month history of three headache attacks with nausea. She was very anxious about that because her mother died with a history of stroke a few months ago. She reported that the first attack of her headache was exploding, with a relatively sudden onset. This first attack lasted 6 h. She was not able to move because while walking, her headache got worse. Therefore, she stayed at home, had bed rest, and she had to put up the blackout curtains. After a short sleep, she felt a little better but was even more anxious, so she went to her GP the same day. After a general examination, the GP advised her to undergo a CT scan of the brain. She was admitted to the emergency hospital the next day. After examination of blood pressure and routine blood tests, all of them were normal and due to persisting moderate headache, she was given an infusion with 500 mg aspirin and 1 g metamizole. Headache suspended within the next 1–2 h, leaving her completely ran out. At home, she felt sleepy and slept for 12 h. The day after, the headache returned. Besides nausea, she was extremely hypersensitive to sound and light, anxious, and somewhat dizzy. Her husband, who is a lawyer, brought her to the next emergency hospital. Again, an MRI scan was performed—without any pathology. Thereafter, she was admitted to the neurological department where she underwent complete neurological status examination, electroencephalo graphy (EEG), and visual evoked potentials (VEP), all of them without any abnormality. After 2 days of hospitalization, she was dismissed with the

C. Lampl
Headache Medical Center Seilerstaette Linz, Hospital Sisters of Charity, Linz, Austria
e-mail: christian.lampl@bhs.at

A. Siva, C. Lampl (eds.), *Case-Based Diagnosis and Management of Headache Disorders*, Headache, DOI 10.1007/978-3-319-06886-2_1

diagnosis of migraine without aura. One week after, the third attack started with a severe pulsating headache, vertigo, nausea, and sensitivity to light and sound aggravated by walking or moving the head. Aspirin 330 mg did not relieve the pain. This attack nearly lasted 15 h.

1.2 Differential Diagnosis and How to Work Up This Kind of Patient

Although this is a typical case of migraine without aura, some points have to be raised: The first attack started rather fast with a sudden onset of exploding headache; although the patient herself did not observe any abnormality like hemihypesthesia, weakness of upper or lower extremities, visual and sensory disturbances, or any other pathological signs, the probability of an intracerebral pathology may be considered; the consulting physician has to perform a complete neurological examination and needs to rule out any pathological intracerebral event. In that particular case, after a normal neurological examination, a CT scan of the brain would be sufficient.

1.3 Diagnostic Workup of the Case

Migraine without aura is typically manifest by episodic disabling headache and concomitant symptoms. It easily can be diagnosed with an extensive exploration of history, signs, and symptoms. Especially in the absence of any abnormal neurological sign, with the broad description of the headache phase, the character, and the quality of the headache, the certainty of that particular kind of headache is high. If migraine without aura occurs for the first time, it is advised to perform, once, a CT scan of the brain. Migraine usually lasts hours to days; the average attack frequency is once a month. Migraine should be distinguished from tension type headache (TTH); however, TTH is often chronic and it is present more often than it is absent. The second differential diagnosis is cluster headache, which is relatively rare and causes recurrent unilateral headache with autonomic dysfunction. The third challenging differential diagnosis is medication overuse headache (MOH). This typically complicates migraine which is then transformed into a chronic daily headache similar to chronic TTH often with some migrainous features. The frequency and periodicity of migraine is important: migraine-like headache more than twice every week is unlikely to be migraine without aura alone, but it may be migraine without aura, complicated by MOH and/or TTH (Table 1.1).

Table 1.1 Definition of migraine without aura according to the ICHD 3-beta version

A. At least five attacks, 1 fulfilling criteria B–D
B. Headache attacks lasting 4–72 h (untreated or unsuccessfully treated)
C. Headache has at least two of the following four characteristics: 1. Unilateral location 2. Pulsating quality 3. Moderate or severe pain intensity 4. Aggravation by or causing avoidance of routine physical activity (e.g., walking or climbing stairs)
D. During headache at least one of the following: 1. Nausea and/or vomiting 2. Photophobia and phonophobia
E. Not better accounted for by another ICHD-3 diagnosis

ICHD International Classification of Headache Disorders

1.4 Summary of the Case

A 39-year-old female with a severe pulsating headache, vertigo, nausea, and sensitivity to light and sound aggravated by walking or moving was presented. These typical signs and symptoms of headache without any neurological findings and a normal CT scan of the brain lead us to the diagnosis of migraine without aura.

1.5 Brief General Information

One in ten people have migraine. As shown in our case, the patient's history is the essential diagnostic tool. From a pathophysiological point of view, spontaneous overactivity and abnormal amplification in pain and other, predominantly sensory, pathways in the brainstem may lead to migraine. Current opinion favors a primarily neural cause, involving feedback loops through innervation of cranial arteries in the trigeminovascular system. Ongoing research is studying the relevance of calcium channel abnormalities and peptides such as calcitonin gene-related peptide, which may be closer than 5-HT to the underlying cause.

Management of lifestyle can appear to be very helpful, though evidence is largely anecdotal. Analgesics and antiemetics are effective for many migraine patients. Some of them prefer a nonsteroidal anti-inflammatory drug (NSAID), aspirin, or paracetamol. Triptans are only slightly more effective than simple analgesics with an antiemetic on the number needed to treat (NNT) basis. These data conceal substantial inter- and intra-patient variation. Ergot alkaloids may still have an occasional place in the acute management of migraine. Daily drug treatment to prevent migraine should be considered after acute treatment has been optimized, medication overuse abolished, lifestyle modification tried, and a migraine diary recorded for a month or three. Comorbid disease may suggest initial drug choice. It is unusual to offer prophylaxis for less than three attacks a month. Treatment should be titrated first for tolerability and then for efficacy.

Suggested Readings

1. Elrington G (2002) Migraine: diagnosis and management. J Neurol Neurosurg Psychiatry 72(Suppl II):ii10–ii15
2. Ferrari MD, Roon KI, Lipton RB et al (2001) Oral triptans (serotonin 5-$HT_{1B/1D}$ agonists) in acute migraine treatment: a meta-analysis of 53 trials. Lancet 358:1668–1675
3. Goadsby PJ (2006) Recent advances in the diagnosis and management of migraine. BMJ 332:25–29
4. Lipton RB, Scher AI, Kolodner K et al (2002) Migraine in the United States – epidemiology and patterns of health care use. Neurology 58:885–894
5. Olesen J, Friberg L, Olsen TS et al (1990) Timing and topography of cerebral blood flow, aura, and headache during migraine attacks. Ann Neurol 28:791–798
6. Silberstein SD (2004) Migraine pathophysiology and its clinical implications. Cephalalgia 24(Suppl 2):2–7
7. Silberstein SD (2004) Migraine. Lancet 363:381–391
8. Steiner TJ, MacGregor EA, Davies PTG. Guidelines for all doctors in the management of migraine and tension-type headache. Available at: http://www.bash.org.uk. Accessed 8 Sept 2001
9. Headache Classification Committee of the International Headache Society (HIS). The International Classification of Headache Disorders, 3rd edition (beta version) (2013) Cephalalgia 33(9):644–645

Chapter 2
Migraine with Typical Aura

Jes Olesen and Elena Lebedeva

This case involves migraine with typical aura and headache in addition to migraine with typical aura without headache and frequent episodic tension-type headache. The case emphasizes that multiple diagnoses are sometimes necessary. A precise diagnosis of aura requires specific questions. Both acute and prophylactic treatment must be carefully adjusted, which requires several visits. In this case, expert diagnosis and treatment led to a positive result, which is established in the majority of patients with typical aura.

2.1 Case Description

A 36-year-old man was referred to the Danish Headache Center (DHC), Department of Neurology, Glostrup Hospital, University of Copenhagen, by his general practitioner. He had previously been seen by a practicing neurologist, but the treatment response obtained was not satisfactory and he asked for referral to a higher level of the health care system in Denmark. DHC is a national center of excellence that receives patients from all over Denmark and from other countries who have been difficult to treat or have a rare headache disorder or in whom there is doubt regarding the diagnosis.

J. Olesen, MD, DMSc (✉)
Department of Neurology, Danish Headache Centre, University of Copenhagen, Glostrup Hospital, Ndr. Ringvej 57, Glostrup 2600, Denmark
e-mail: jes.olesen@regionh.dk

E. Lebedeva, MD, PhD
Department of Urgent Neurology, The Urals State Medical Academy, Pepina street 3, Ekaterinburg 620219, Russia

A. Siva, C. Lampl (eds.), *Case-Based Diagnosis and Management of Headache Disorders*, Headache, DOI 10.1007/978-3-319-06886-2_2

2.2 Family History

The patient's mother and one of her sisters, and possibly also the grandfather (who was deceased), suffered from migraine of uncertain type,.

2.3 History of Previous Illness

No previous hospitalizations were reported by the patient, who had recurrent rhinitis diagnosed as pollen allergy and treated with nasal spray. He had no arterial hypertension, asthma, diabetes, or any other chronic diseases.

2.4 History of Present Illness

The patient distinguished between three different types of headache. Some headaches were mild, bilateral, pressing, and induced by stress, and responded to plain analgesics. He experienced such headaches approximately four times a month but they were not bothersome. His main problem was attacks of neurological symptoms followed by severe headaches, occurring about twice a month. These attacks had already begun in childhood, at which time they were rare. About 5 years previously the attack frequency began to slowly increase to the level of the current frequency, which had been present for approximately 2 years. Recently the attacks had become so severe that he was losing 2 days of work every month. These attacks were similar in nature from time to time, varying mainly in severity, with some occurring after vigorous exercise or after exposure to bright light, but the majority of attacks had no obvious cause. The patient described blurring of vision lateral to the point of fixation, which then expanded slowly and developed a serrated edge. As it moved from the central field of vision toward the periphery it enlarged further, and he would notice additionally a blind spot where he was unable to see anything. For example, when he looked at faces, half of the face would sometimes not be visible. Usually this was on the right side but sometimes would also be on the left. The edge was yellow-white and flickering, with no other colors. It took approximately 20 min until all the visual disturbances had disappeared. In some of the attacks he described sensory symptoms usually starting toward the end of the visual disturbance or slightly earlier, which usually began in the fingers of the right hand and moved slowly up the arm to the elbow. He then experienced a tingling sensation in the right side of the chin spreading slowly across the face and into the right half of the tongue. On very rare occasions, and usually when the sensory disturbances affected his tongue, he would also have problems with speech which became slurred, and he would find it difficult to produce the correct words and sentences. The sensory symptoms lasted approximately half an hour. In most of these episodes a severe headache would follow the neurological disturbances, but in some others the headache was only modest, and in a few he would have visual disturbances without any headache. The headache was invariably half-sided but the patient was uncertain as to whether it was on the right or left. He tended to think that it was on the same side (right) as the neurological disturbances. The headache began approximately 20 min after the visual disturbances had disappeared, at a time when he would still experience the sensory and/or speech problems. The pain was severe, throbbing, and aggravated by physical activity. He also experienced nausea and, sometimes, vomiting, and was hypersensitive to light and sound. He was unable to function during attacks, and had to retire to bed in a dark and cool room. The duration of pain was 12–24 h. As treatment he had taken paracetamol and aspirin, without effect. The neurologist had prescribed sumatriptan tablets 50 mg, which he took as soon as the neurological disturbances began, but they had only a minor effect. The neurologist had also prescribed prophylactic treatment with propranolol, which in fact did reduce the attack frequency somewhat, but the patient gained weight and his libido decreased. He had therefore given up to taking sumatriptan.

2.5 Current Medication

The patient treated his attacks with plain analgesics and bed rest, without much success. No other medication was being taken.

2.6 Examinations

Physical and neurological examinations were normal. Laboratory evaluation was limited to normal routine blood tests, as no other tests were considered necessary.

2.7 Diagnosis

Formally speaking, this patient had three different headache diagnoses: frequent episodic tension-type headache, migraine with typical aura with headache, and migraine with typical aura without headache [1]. His dominant problem was migraine with typical aura followed by migraine headache. The only atypical feature of his migraine attacks was that he reported headache on the same side as the aura symptoms. He was asked to prospectively record the laterality of his headaches, and at a repeat visit he indicated that the headaches were actually contralateral to the aura symptoms. This patient had two important therapeutic needs. First, he required a better treatment for each attack, and second, he needed effective prophylactic treatment.

2.8 Acute Treatment

The patient took sumatriptan at the onset of the aura. It has been clearly documented that triptans are not effective when taken during the aura phase [2], and must not be taken until the headache sets in. He first tried to take sumatriptan later in the attack, but it was still not effective enough. Subsequently he tried rizatriptan tablets, with better effect. However, because he retched the tablet on several occasions we added a metoclopramide suppository, which he was instructed to take at the onset of the aura so that it had an effect when he later took the triptan. This approach provided a better response, but the patient still had a problem when he suffered attacks at his work because it took too long for him to recover. Finally, we prescribed sumatriptan 6 mg as an autoinjector and also added fast-acting diclofenac tablets, the latter to be taken together with the metoclopramide suppository at the onset of aura. This combination finally solved the problem, so that he would be fully functional 1 h after the onset of the aura symptoms and could remain almost fully functional in his workplace.

2.9 Prophylactic Treatment

We prefer the antihypertensive drugs lisinopril and candesartan because they have almost no side effects. Consequently we prescribed lisinopril 20 mg each night, but this led to a dry, irritative cough, which is a known side effect of lisinopril. The patient was thus switched to candesartan 16 mg each night, which was well tolerated but did not have a major effect on the attack frequency. We obviously tried these prophylactics in parallel with the optimization of his attack treatment as already described. We then switched to the class of antiepileptic drugs, starting with topiramate, increasing the dose gradually as recommended. Topiramate did reduce the attack frequency significantly, but at 50 mg twice daily the patient found it difficult to concentrate and he became forgetful. His cognitive disturbances did not disappear; consequently he was switched to sodium valproate 500 mg slow-release each evening, increasing after 1 week to 1,000 mg each evening. This reduced the attack frequency to one per month and was well tolerated. The patient was maintained on this treatment for 1 year, after which treatment was reduced by half for 2 months. There was no change in attack frequency. The medication was successfully discontinued and the attack frequency remained stable at one attack per month over the next 6 months, after which he was discharged. The patient's family physician was instructed to reinstate valproate treatment if the attack frequency at a later point in time was noted to increase. The attack treatment discussed herein remained highly effective, and the patient continued to take it for the remaining monthly attacks.

2.10 Discussion

This case was characterized by a typical symptomatology fulfilling all diagnostic criteria of the International Classification of Headache Disorders (ICHD-3beta) [1]. In such cases it is not necessary to perform scanning or other laboratory tests; in fact this may sometimes be counterproductive, because scanning often shows a small cyst or some other small abnormality, including white matter hyperintensities, on magnetic resonance imaging [3]. Such findings are difficult to explain to the patient and often scare patients, and may require even more tests. Half of all migraine patients with aura have exclusively visual auras, but about half also have other symptoms during attacks [4]. This was the case in the present patient, who quite often had sensory disturbances in addition to the visual disturbances. Moreover, he suffered rare attacks of aura that induced aphasia. It is noteworthy that he never had any weakness in the extremities. Such weakness suggests hemiplegic migraine, which differs in many respects from migraine with typical aura. The genetic background is different, and hemiplegic patients are not sensitive to the migraine-provoking agents nitroglycerin and calcitonin gene-related peptide [5, 6]. The aura of hemiplegic migraine may be more long lasting and, curiously, the attack frequency is usually low. The tension-type headache in this patient is also typical. Patients with frequent migraine attacks almost all have milder headaches, phenomenologically being tension-type headaches. It is unknown, however, whether these are in fact very mild migraine attacks or whether they have a different pathophysiology. Some patients say that these tension-type headaches respond to triptans, and others that they do not but that they respond to aspirin. In some cases they disappear on prophylactic migraine treatment, whereas in others only the typical migraine attacks are reduced. With regard to prophylactic treatment, the literature mostly consists of randomized, double-blind, controlled trials in a mixture of patients with and without aura. The use of such agents is completely dominated by patients who have migraine without aura, because it is rare for migraine with aura to have a high enough frequency of attack to indicate prophylactic treatment [7]. A few studies have focused exclusively on migraine with aura. There is one positive study using metoprolol [8]. Interestingly the cortical spreading depression inhibitor, tonabersat, was highly effective in reducing the attack frequency of auras, but this agent has not been marketed for commercial reasons [7]. In basic terms, one applies the same principles when treating migraine with aura prophylactically as one applies when treating migraine without aura. Intuitively, antiepileptics would seem to be more effective for migraine with aura than, for example, antihypertensives, but this has never been proved and it is not our experience. This case illustrates that frequent visits and frequent adjustments of treatment may be necessary not only to adjust prophylactic treatment but also to adjust the treatment for each acute attack.

References

1. Headache Classification Committee of the International Headache Society (IHS) (2013) The International Classification of Headache Disorders, 3rd. edition (beta version). Cephalalgia 33:627–808
2. Bates D, Ashford E, Dawson R et al (1994) Subcutaneous sumatriptan during the migraine aura. Sumatriptan Aura Study Group. Neurology 44:1587–1592
3. Bashir A, Lipton RB, Ashina S et al (2013) Migraine and structural changes in the brain: a systematic review and meta-analysis. Neurology 81:1260–1268
4. Eriksen MK, Thomsen LL, Andersen I et al (2004) Clinical characteristics of 362 patients with familial migraine with aura. Cephalalgia 24:564–575
5. Hansen JM, Thomsen LL, Olesen J et al (2008) Familial hemiplegic migraine type 1 shows no hypersensitivity to nitric oxide. Cephalalgia 28:496–505
6. Hansen JM, Thomsen LL, Olesen J et al (2011) Calcitonin gene-related peptide does not cause migraine attacks in patients with familial hemiplegic migraine. Headache 51:544–553
7. Hauge AW, Asghar MS, Schytz HW et al (2009) Effects of tonabersat on migraine with aura: a randomised, double-blind, placebo-controlled crossover study. Lancet Neurol 8:718–723
8. Kangasniemi P, Andersen AR, Andersson PG et al (1987) Classic migraine: effective prophylaxis with metoprolol. Cephalalgia 7:231–238

Chapter 3
Aura Without Migraine

Miguel J.A. Láinez and Ana García-Casado

3.1 Case Description

A 72-year-old male patient was referred to us for evaluation of recurrent episodes of loss of vision on his left side. The history of the visual episodes started when he was 52 years old. The patient described precisely how he suddenly lost the vision in the central part of his eyes, and after 5 min perceived flickering, scintillating lights moving to the left part of his visual field (in a zigzag "C" shape), followed by a loss of vision in the inner part of the "C." The lights gradually moved to the periphery of the left visual field, and vision recovered gradually in the inner area. The total duration of the episode was 20–25 min, after which the vision was perfect again. In the first 10 years he experienced one or two episodes of this type per year. However, the frequency then increased to six to seven episodes per year; nimodipine was prescribed unsuccessfully, with no improvement in the frequency or duration of the episodes. Later still he was started on ticlopidine in the hope that this might reduce the number of episodes.

The patient was referred to our department 17 years after the visual disturbances began, following an increasing frequency of up to ten episodes per year distributed irregularly; in some months the patient had two or three episodes, which would be followed by a cessation of these attacks for another 2–3 months. The symptomatology of the episodes remained stable over the years; only occasionally did the patient experience the same phenomena in his right visual field. He reported no

M.J.A. Láinez (✉)
Department of Neurology, Hospital Clínico Universitario, Universidad Católica de Valencia, Avda Blaco Ibáñez. 17, Valencia 46010, Spain
e-mail: miguel.lainez@sen.es

A. García-Casado
Department of Neurology, Universidad Católica de Valencia, Avda Blaco Ibáñez. 17, Valencia 46010, Spain
e-mail: annitagc@msn.com

A. Siva, C. Lampl (eds.), *Case-Based Diagnosis and Management of Headache Disorders*, Headache, DOI 10.1007/978-3-319-06886-2_3

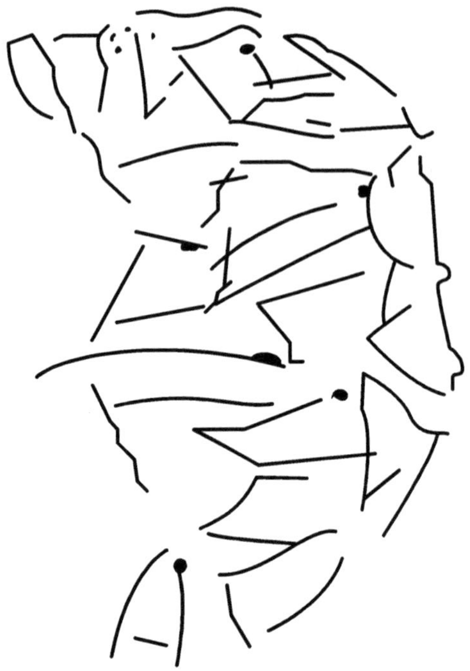

Fig. 3.1 Drawings made by the patient of the images seen during the episodes. Here the drawing represents the start of the episode in the central part

other associated neurological or general symptoms, and never had a headache during or after the visual symptoms.

The patient's neurological and neuro-ophthalmologic examinations were normal, as were the physical and neurovascular examinations. Blood pressure was 135/85 mmHg. He was referred to an internist while in his early 50s because of arterial hypertension, which was treated and regulated with lisinopril. He did not have any other significant medical problem requiring care afterward. The patient reported that he had never suffered headaches, nor had his parents (who both died of old age), two brothers, and three children.

Over the years, the patient has been sketching various drawings of the images he sees during the episodes. Figure 3.1 corresponds to the start of the episode in the central part. Figure 3.2 represents the fortification spectra. In Fig. 3.3 one can appreciate how the lights moved from the central to periphery of the visual field at intervals of approximately 5 min.

3.2 Differential Diagnosis and How to Work Up This Type of Patient

This patient reports acute and recurrent episodes of transient neurological deficit. Given the age of the patient (i.e., >50 years), vascular etiology is the first to consider. The history of high blood pressure as a vascular risk factor is also in favor of this etiology.

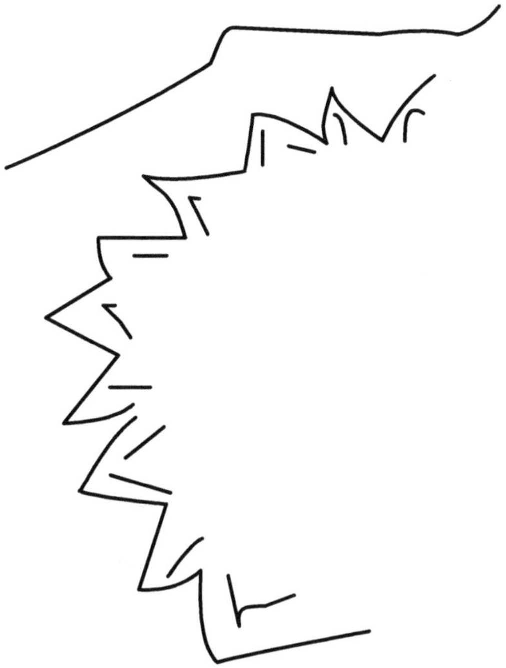

Fig. 3.2 The fortification spectra

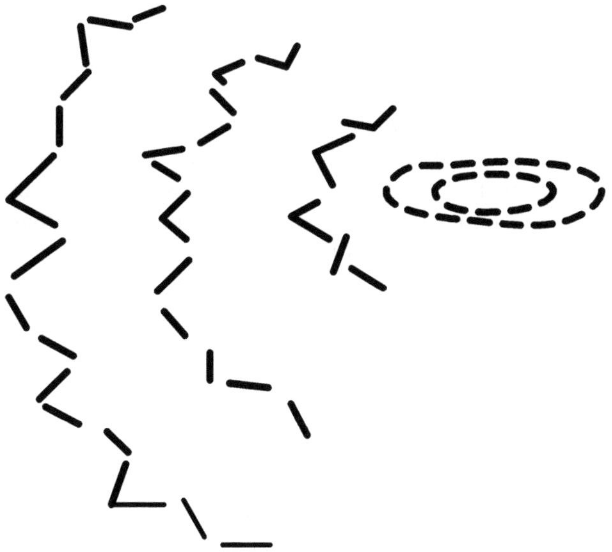

Fig. 3.3 Lights moving from the central to periphery of the visual field in intervals of around 5 min

The most common cause of sudden loss of vision in an older patient is amaurosis fugax, which is a sudden transient, partial, or total loss of vision of any cause; it comes from the Greek *amaurosis*, meaning dark and the Latin *fugax*, meaning fleeting. Although the term is related to vascular origin, it may be associated with a heterogeneous group of disorders. The origin can be vascular (embolic or hypoperfusion), ocular, neurological, or idiopathic. The clinician's goal must be to determine the underlying cause of the patient's transient visual disturbances.

In a historical series of 186 subjects reporting onset of a sudden visual deficit (not necessarily transient), the evaluation determined the underlying cause to be stroke or transient ischemic attack (24 %), ocular disease (17 %), transient monocular blindness (10 %), and migraine (14 %). The cause remained unknown in 22 %, with a miscellany of causes comprising the remaining 12 %.

In a more recent study of 337 prospectively studied patients with sudden, transient monocular loss of vision, 159 had a normal internal carotid artery (ICA) on the relevant side, 33 had a stenosis between 0 and 69 %, 100 had a stenosis of 70–99 %, and 45 had an ICA occlusion.

Some patterns of clinical presentation can suggest carotid disease, such as an altitudinal onset or disappearance of symptoms. A severe (70–99 %) stenosis has been associated with a duration of between 1 and 10 min, and with a speed of onset in seconds. ICA occlusion has been associated with attacks being provoked by bright light, an altitudinal onset, and the occurrence of more than ten attacks. The frequent repetition of these events in a short period of time could be suggestive of an impending brain infarct. Ischemic problems are usually associated with negative visual phenomena. On examination of the fundi the intravascular retinal emboli were visualized in some cases.

Age older than 50 years and the presence of vascular risk factors, such as hypertension, diabetes, or hypercholesterolemia, are also indicative of an ischemic origin of the problem.

Temporal arteritis, or giant cell arteritis, is another condition that can produce episodes of amaurosis fugax, especially in patients older than 60 years. This is a type of vasculitis whereby the vessels more often involved are the arteries of the scalp and head, especially the arteries over the temples. Giant cell arteritis can cause swelling and thickening of the small artery under the skin; the temporal artery becomes very sensitive and painful to palpation of the skull. The most common symptom is a headache around the temples or in another location, and general symptoms such as fatigue, loss of appetite, weight loss, or a flu-like feeling. Pain in the jaw with chewing is also common. The visual phenomenon is negative, and the duration of the clinical presentation is from weeks to a few months.

The list of "ocular" causes of amaurosis fugax is long. Blepharitis, dry eye syndrome, keratitis, glaucoma, optic disc drusen, vitreous detachment, retinal break, orbital or intraocular tumor, or vasospasm can produce these visual symptoms. The external signs of inflammation can help the diagnosis in blepharitis or keratitis.

The symptoms are monocular and the duration of the visual disturbances can be very brief (i.e., seconds), such as in retinal breaks or vitreous traction. The patients describe negative and positive symptoms, which can worsen with eye movements or when the patient is blinking or rubbing the eyes.

Visual disturbances of neurological origin may appear, derived from lesions from the optic nerve to the occipital lobe. Optic neuritis, papilledema, or increase in intracranial pressure can also produce amaurosis fugax.

Occipital and temporoparietal arteriovenous malformations can cause a variety of visual disturbances and headaches. The most typical symptoms are homonymous visual disturbances, headache, seizures, and hemorrhage. A symptomatic migraine with typical aura may be the only clinical manifestation.

Epilepsy, especially occipital seizures, usually begins with visual hallucinations such as flickering or colored lights, rapid blinking, or other symptoms such as eye movements, pallinopsia, or eye pain. The visual symptoms are usually complex, with metamorphoses and stereotyping, sometimes with associated headache. The initiation usually is acute and the duration short (minutes). Seizures are sometimes triggered by visual stimuli, such as seeing flashing lights or a repeating pattern.

Migraine aura is the name given to the many types of neurological symptoms that may occur just before or during a migraine headache. Said to be experienced by 20–25 % of individuals, aura is a fully reversible neurological syndrome, which can develop over 5 min and last for up to 2 h. Usually the aura is associated with headache, but in some cases is the only clinical manifestation.

Occasionally patients in the stroke population older than 40 years have unexplained transient focal neurological events in association with normal neuroimaging. Some authors describe late-life migraine accompaniments that are not uncommon in older populations. In this group the visual symptoms are the most frequent, and fulfill the criteria of migraine aura in a significant number of cases.

In performing the differential diagnosis, the most important tool is the clinical history. The way the episodes started, progression, presence of positive and negative symptoms, duration, worsening with movement, or possible precipitating factors give an initial indication of the etiology. It is also necessary to perform a full neurological examination (including fundi), cranial palpation, and neurovascular examination.

If an ocular origin is suspected, the patient should be referred to the ophthalmologist for a thorough examination. Laboratory testing must be part of the initial diagnostic workup: complete blood count and chemistry, erythrocyte sedimentation rate (ESR), and polymerase chain reaction (mandatory if temporal arteritis is suspect). If carotid disease is suspected a duplex examination is mandatory, and in some cases another neuroimaging procedure (magnetic resonance imaging (MRI) angiography or computed tomographic angiography) is required to evaluate the carotids and/or the brain (brain MRI). A cardiologic examination is essential if an embolic origin is suspected. An electroencephalogram (EEG) is necessary if epilepsy is considered to be the origin of the problem.

3.3 Diagnostic Workup of the Case

In this case the most important feature in establishing the diagnosis was the clinical history. As the patient recounted a history of stereotypical spells that described very well the fortification spectra, the origin of this visual phenomenon necessarily had to be the occipital cortex (right in the majority of episodes, although the patient referred also to episodes in the right visual field). The duration of the spells was typical for migraine aura, and the frequency (1–10 per year) and long history (17 years) was also in favor of migraine etiology.

The physical, neurological, and neurovascular examinations were unremarkable.

Given this history, ocular origin, temporal arteritis, and most of the neurological causes can be ruled out. Even the fact that the patient referred, in different episodes, to symptoms of both occipital lobes made unlikely the diagnosis of neurological conditions that normally present with unilateral episodes (e.g., arteriovenous malformation or occipital lobe epilepsy).

A history of such long duration also made a vascular origin unlikely. However, owing to the age of the patient and the history of high blood pressure, we decided to undertake a complete examination to rule out ischemic origin.

Laboratory testing, including complete blood count chemistry and ESR, were normal. The electrocardiogram and chest radiograph were also normal.

Brain MRI showed small lesions in the white matter and two small deep lacunar infarcts; both occipital lobes were completely normal. Echo Doppler of the carotid system showed only small plaques in the wall in both bifurcations without lumen compromise.

In the last months previous to his appointment the patient was experiencing two to three spells per month, and he asked us to provide a solution to reduce the episodes. Based on our previous experience, we prescribed lamotrigine slowly increasing to 100 mg per day. On follow-up consultation 3 months later, he reported one episode of visual spells after 15 days of lamotrigine treatment. We recommended stopping lamotrigine after 6 months, but the patient preferred to continue with treatment. On follow-up after 2 years of treatment, he described experiencing only two episodes of shorter duration during this period.

3.4 Summary of the Case

A 72-year-old man was referred for evaluation of recurrent episodes of loss of vision on his left side. He recounted a history of recurrent episodes of fortification spectra followed by scotoma in his left visual field (and very occasionally on the right); the duration of the spells was approximately 25 min and the initial frequency was very low (1–2 per year). The medical history of the patient was unremarkable, except for high blood pressure that was well controlled with lisinopril.

When the frequency of the episodes increased, at first nimodipine and later, ticlopidine were prescribed, without significant improvement. The patient was referred to our center 17 years after the start of the episodes following a progressive increase of the number of episodes. A detailed history allowed us to establish the diagnosis of typical aura without migraine. However, owing to the patient's age, a complete study was performed to rule out ischemic origin. Neuroimaging studies showed minimal changes typical for this age group. Lamotrigine was prescribed, which led to a significant reduction of the number of visual episodes

3.5 Definition According to the International Classification of Headache Disorders

According to the *International Classification of Headache Disorders*, 3rd edition (Cephalalgia 2013;33(9):629–808) (ICHD-3) the definition of typical aura without migraine is migraine with typical aura in which aura is neither accompanied nor followed by headache of any sort. These symptoms usually are a combination of positive and negative features. The development of the symptoms should be gradual; the duration should be less than 1 h and are not associated with headache.

To establish the diagnosis the patient should have at least two attacks of aura. These attacks should fulfill two conditions:

1. Aura in form of fully reversible visual, sensory and/or speech/language symptoms. Motor, brainstem, and retinal symptoms are not allowed
2. Two of these three conditions: (a) at least one aura symptom spreads gradually over more than 5 min, and/or two or more symptoms occur in succession; (b) each individual aura lasts from 5 to 60 min; (c) one aura symptom, at least, should be unilateral

According to the definition of aura without headache, headache is not present during aura nor does it follow aura within 60 min.

As in all the primary headaches, attacks cannot be attributed to another ICHD-3 diagnosis. In this case it is especially important to exclude transient ischemic attack.

3.6 Brief General Information

Aura is present in around 20 % of cases of migraine. It is usually associated with headache, but in some cases appears as the only clinical manifestation. A small number of patients, especially males, have exclusively typical aura without headache. In the few population studies performed, the prevalence of this problem is around 1 %. A more frequent occurrence, however, is when migraineurs with typical aura become older their headache may lose migraine characteristics or disappear completely, even though auras continue.

In a population study of 163 individuals who suffer migraine with aura, 62 had attacks of both migraine aura with headache and migraine aura without headache, and seven had exclusively attacks of migraine aura without headache (all visual). Visual aura is the most frequent symptom (99 %) followed by sensory (31 %), aphasic (18 %), and motor (6 %) aura. The typical visual aura starts as a flickering, uncolored, unilateral zig-zag line in the center of the visual field, which gradually progresses toward the periphery, often leaving a scotoma. Typical migrainous visual symptoms include both positive (scintillations, fortification spectra, photopsia) and negative (scotoma, hemianopsia) visual features, often presenting as a transient scintillating hemianopic visual disturbance. The usual duration is 25–30 min.

The most probable explanation for the aura is the cortical spreading depression described by Leao and confirmed in migraine patients. Changes in regional cerebral blood flow are the consequence of the cortical wave of depression that usually starts posteriorly and spreads anteriorly, and is usually above the ischemic threshold.

Key Points

- Visual aura is the most frequent symptom of migraine aura.
- In patients with recurrent episodes of transient neurological deficit, especially if older than 50 years, the vascular etiology is the first to consider.
- To perform the differential diagnosis, the most important tool is the clinical history. We also perform a full neurological examination (including fundi), cranial palpation, and neurovascular examination.
- A detailed description of the mode of presentation of the episodes allows diagnosis in a high percentage of cases.
- Laboratory testing, neuroimaging, EEG, or cardiologic examination should be ordered based on the clinical suspicion.
- Lamotrigine is potentially useful in preventing migraine aura.

Suggested Reading

1. Costa C1, Tozzi A, Rainero I et al (2013) Cortical spreading depression as a target for anti-migraine agents. J Headache Pain 14:62
2. Current management of amaurosis fugax. The Amaurosis Fugax Study Group. Stroke. 1990;21:201–208.
3. Cutrer FM, Huerter K (2007) Migraine aura. Neurologist 13:118–125
4. Dalkara T1, Zervas NT, Moskowitz MA (2006) From spreading depression to the trigeminovascular system. Neurol Sci 27(Suppl 2):S86–S90
5. Donders RC, Dutch TMB Study Group (2001) Clinical features of transient monocular blindness and the likelihood of atherosclerotic lesions of the internal carotid artery. J Neurol Neurosurg Psychiatry 71(2):247
6. Fisher CM (1980) Late-life migraine accompaniments as a cause of unexplained transient ischemic attacks. Can J Neurol Sci 7(1):9
7. Hurwitz BJ, Heyman A, Wilkinson WE et al (1985) Comparison of amaurosis fugax and transient cerebral ischemia: a prospective clinical and arteriographic study. Ann Neurol 18:698–704
8. Kupersmith MJ, Vargas ME, Yashar A et al (1996) Occipital arteriovenous malformations: visual disturbances and presentation. Neurology 46:953–957

9. Lavallée PC, Cabrejo L, Labreuche J et al (2013) Spectrum of transient visual symptoms in a transient ischemic attack cohort. Stroke 44:3312–3317
10. Luo RJ, Liu SR, Li XM et al (2010) Fifty-eight cases of ocular ischemic diseases caused by carotid artery stenosis. Chin Med J (Engl) 123:2662–2665
11. Pascual J, Caminero AB, Mateos V et al (2004) Preventing disturbing migraine aura with lamotrigine: an open study. Headache 44:1024–1028
12. Russell MB, Olesen J (1996) A nosographic analysis of the migraine aura in a general population. Brain 119:355–361
13. Wang M (2013) Cortical spreading depression and calcitonin gene-related peptide: a brief review of current progress. Neuropeptides 47(6):463–466
14. Wijman CA, Wolf PA, Kase CS et al (1998) Migrainous visual accompaniments are not rare in late life: the Framingham Study. Stroke 29:1539–1543
15. Zhang X, Levy D, Noseda R et al (2010) Activation of meningeal nociceptors by cortical spreading depression: implications for migraine with aura. J Neurosci 30:8807–8814

Chapter 4
Hemiplegic Migraine

Anders Hougaard and Messoud Ashina

4.1 Case Description

A 30-year-old woman was admitted to the hospital with suspicion of an acute stroke due to left-sided hemiplegia and right-sided headache. In the ambulance on the way to the hospital, the symptoms gradually disappeared. When asked about her symptoms, she told that she initially had visual disturbances in the form of right-sided flickering lights on the right side of her visual field, where after she gradually had lost all strength in the right side of her body. Fifteen minutes after onset of hemiplegia, the patient developed a severe headache in the left side of the frontal part of the head. The headache was reported as pulsating, the patient became increasingly nauseous and started vomiting, and she further developed hypersensitivity towards lights and sounds.

On arrival to the hospital, she reported that her vision and her strength in her right arm and leg had returned to normal. However, she still described a subtle tingling sensation in the right side of her body, in the right side of her face, and in the right side of her tongue. She still had severe, pulsating headache, photophobia, and phonophobia. She rated the headache 9 on a 0–10 visual analogue scale. The patient had no previous history of stroke or family history of stroke. She is otherwise healthy, does not smoke, rarely drinks alcohol, and exercises regularly.

Her father had previously suffered from the same type of attacks. She had experienced similar episodes before since she was 12 years old, but this was the most severe, which is why she called for an ambulance. Sometimes she would not have an attack for more than 6 months, but during the last 8 weeks, since she was fired from her job, she had attacks one to two times per week. Her GP had told her that

A. Hougaard, MD • M. Ashina, MD, PhD, DMSc (✉)
Danish Headache Center and Department of Neurology, Faculty of Health and Medical Sciences, Glostrup Hospital, University of Copenhagen, Nordre Ringvej, Glostrup DK-2600, Denmark
e-mail: ahougaard@dadlnet.dk; ashina@dadlnet.dk

A. Siva, C. Lampl (eds.), *Case-Based Diagnosis and Management of Headache Disorders*, Headache, DOI 10.1007/978-3-319-06886-2_4

she might suffer from migraine and had advised her to take sumatriptan as soon as possible when an attack started. She had tried this but did not feel that the medication worked. In between attacks she would have a mild, left-sided headache, which is why she had now started taking paracetamol and ibuprofen on a daily basis.

4.2 Differential Diagnosis and How to Work Up This Kind of Patient

The most important differential diagnoses of hemiplegic migraine in the acute phase are stroke and transient ischemic attack (TIA). As is the case for hemiplegic migraine, the symptoms of TIA are fully reversible, and neuroimaging often reveals no abnormalities. A characteristic feature of migraine aura symptoms is the gradual spread of symptoms, usually over 5–20 min. In contrast, cerebrovascular ischemic events usually develop within seconds. Migraine aura often involves positive symptoms such as visual perception of flickering lights, colors, and shapes and sensory symptoms with paresthesia, which is rarely the case for vascular events.

It may be difficult to distinguish hemiplegic migraine from migraine with sensory aura, because patients often describe numbness, which may cause inability to grasp or lift objects, as loss of strength. Todd paralysis following an epileptic seizure may also mimic a hemiplegic migraine attack but is often associated with loss of consciousness and postictal confusion.

In some cases hemiplegic migraine patients present with fever and decreased level of consciousness, making differentiation from CNS infections difficult. A rare differential diagnosis is the syndrome of transient headache with neurological deficits and cerebrospinal fluid lymphocytosis (HaNDL). CSF lymphocytosis and often increased protein levels is characteristic of HaNDL but is sometimes seen in hemiplegic migraine as well. Unlike hemiplegic migraine, HaNDL resolves spontaneously within 3 months.

Between attacks, most patients with hemiplegic migraine have a normal neurological examination, while some patients with familiar hemiplegic migraine type 1 have gaze-evoked nystagmus, ataxia, or dysarthria. During attacks, motor and sensory symptoms most often affect the upper rather than the lower limbs. Cerebral MRI should be performed in every new case of hemiplegic migraine and in the case of changes of the patient's usual symptoms, attack frequency, or attack severity. CT and MRI examinations rarely show abnormalities outside of attacks, but cerebellar atrophy has been described in familiar hemiplegic migraine type 1. Transient neuroimaging abnormalities have been reported in a few cases in the form of perfusion changes and contrast enhancement. Imaging in the ictal phase is rarely possible due to the unpredictable nature and relatively short duration of the attacks. However, detection of cerebral blood flow (CBF) changes could potentially be applied for diagnostic purposes in some cases. CBF is known to decrease during the aura phase. This hypoperfusion persists when the aura symptoms are gone and into the headache phase. After a few hours, hypoperfusion changes into marked hyperperfusion, persisting for more than 10 h from the point of attack. CBF measurements, e.g., using single-photon emission tomography (SPECT) following an attack and again in the interictal phase, could thus aid in verifying the diagnosis.

A thorough family history is important in order to distinguish familial from sporadic hemiplegic migraine. Genetic testing for mutations of the three genes that are known to cause familial hemiplegic migraine can be helpful in diagnosing the condition, but since hemiplegic migraine is a clinical diagnosis, it is not excluded by negative genetic test result.

4.3 Diagnostic Workup of the Case

On neurological examination the patient had normal vision and strength of the limbs, but she had a subtle decrease of sensibility in the right side of the face in first and second trigeminal branch areas on the right side. Her pericranial muscles were sore at the left side. She underwent an acute CT scan, which was normal.

Her sensory symptoms and headache gradually subsided within 6 h. In the emergency room she was treated with metoclopramide 20 mg, paracetamol 1 g, and diazepam 5 mg. The patient was recommended not to take sumatriptan in the event of future attacks. The use of triptans for hemiplegic migraine is controversial and generally discouraged because of a suspected risk of inducing ischemic events (see below).

The family history revealed that her father had experienced very similar episodes since an early age. The patient had four siblings on her father's side. The youngest who was 12 years old was beginning to develop similar symptoms.

When discharged from the hospital, she received a diagnostic headache diary for prospective description of a subsequent attack. She was seen in the outpatient clinic 3 months later, having described a single attack of hemiplegic migraine with aura in the form of gradually developing visual and sensory symptoms with positive as well as negative features. She described expressive aphasia and gradually developing hemiplegia most pronounced in her arm, causing her to be unable to move the arm. The headache and associated symptoms had all the characteristic features of migraine.

4.4 Summary of the Case

A 30-year-old with a severe case of sequential visual disturbances, sensory disturbances, hemiplegia, and headache was admitted to the ER. Her symptoms subsided, and during neurological examination she had normal vision and strength and only subtle unilateral hypesthesia, and she had a normal cerebral CT. She still complained of severe unilateral headache with accompanying photophobia, phonophobia, and nausea. She had experienced similar episodes before and she had first-degree relatives with the same type of attacks. Based on the features of her headache and prodromes, familial history, examination, and neuroimaging, she was diagnosed with familial hemiplegic migraine.

4.5 Definition of Hemiplegic Migraine

According to "The International Classification of Headache Disorders, 3rd edition (beta version)" [Cephalalgia 2013; 33(9)629–808], hemiplegic is defined by the same clinical features as migraine with aura but including motor weakness. Motor weakness in fact characterizes most attacks, even though the term "hemiplegic" implies paralysis. The aura consists of gradually developing and fully reversible visual, sensory, or aphasic symptoms as well as decreased strength. These symptoms are usually unilateral.

While typical aura symptoms last less than 60 min, motor symptoms may persist up to 72 h, and in some cases they may last for weeks. The symptoms are usually followed by a pulsating, unilateral, severe headache accompanied by hypersensitivity towards lights and sounds, lasting up to 72 h. The symptoms should not be better described by any other condition or any other headache diagnosis.

In the case of familial hemiplegic migraine, at least one first- or second-degree relative fulfills the diagnostic criteria. Familial hemiplegic migraine is further subdivided into three different genetic subtypes: FHM1 with a mutation on the CACNA1A gene, FHM2 with an ATP1A2 gene mutation, and FHM3 following SCN1A gene mutation. Familial hemiplegic migraine may occur with no mutations of these genes.

4.6 Brief General Information

Hemiplegic migraine (HM) is a rare subtype of migraine with aura, characterized by transient motor weakness during attacks. The diagnosis is clinical, based on the International Classification of Headache Disorders criteria (see above).

HM is subdivided into two main types: familial (FHM) and sporadic hemiplegic migraine (SHM). In the general population the prevalence of HM is estimated at 0.01 %, with sporadic and familial forms occurring at approximately the same prevalence. The average age of onset is around 17 years of age. The attack frequency is usually much lower than the non-hemiplegic migraine types with an average of three attacks per year. Patient-reported triggers of HM include stress, lights, too little or too much sleep, physical exertion, and mild head trauma.

The underlying cause of hemiplegic migraine aura is most likely cortical spreading depression, a wave of neuronal and glial depolarization that spreads across the cerebral cortex, giving rise to the gradually developing, sequential symptoms. The mechanisms of the following headache are not fully clear. Animal models of migraine have suggested that cortical spreading depression alters blood–brain barrier permeability allowing pain mediators to reach perivascular nociceptors, causing activation of peripheral trigeminal afferents and the release of vasoactive neuropeptides such as calcitonin-gene related peptide (CGRP), thereby generating migraine headache. Human studies support the involvement of neuronal activation at deep brain structures, sensitization of sensory nerve fibers, and dilatation of deep cerebral arteries in migraine. Firm evidence of blood–brain barrier abruption in humans during migraine is lacking, but case reports of MRI gadolinium enhancement following hemiplegic migraine exist.

Interestingly, while intravenous infusion of nitric oxide and CGRP effectively triggers migraine in patients with non-HM migraine, these substances are unable to provoke HM.

FHM has an autosomal dominant inheritance. Three genes have been identified (CACNA1A, ATP1A2, and SCN1A) but more are likely to be involved. Clinically, attacks of the three subtypes cannot be distinguished. Some patients have more severe attacks accompanied by encephalopathy or coma. Patients with these symptoms are more likely to have a gene mutation.

Neuroimaging is important in order to exclude other diagnoses. EEG and CSF analysis may also be useful for this purpose.

The treatment of HM generally follows the same principles as for non-hemiplegic migraine. Because the condition is very rare, no specific clinical trials for HM have been carried out. The use of triptans and ergots in the acute treatment of HM is controversial because of a theoretical risk of cerebral vasoconstriction. However, there is no scientific evidence of an increased risk of ischemic events for treatment of HM with triptans. Triptans are generally not effective when taken during the aura phase; rather, the efficacy is best when dosed early in the headache phase. Acute treatment with over-the-counter analgesics such as paracetamol (acetaminophen) and NSAIDs, preferably as effervescent tablets and in combination with gastric motility-increasing antiemetics, is effective in hemiplegic migraine. Anecdotal evidence suggests that ketamine and naloxone may be effective treatment of the aura symptoms. Prophylactic treatment can be considered when attack frequency exceeds two attacks per month or when severe attacks pose a great burden that requires reduction of severity and frequency. While beta-blockers are first choice for non-hemiplegic migraine, the use of these for HM is controversial since anecdotal evidence suggest that propranolol cause aura prolongation or ischemia in HM patients.

Options for prophylactic therapy include verapamil, flunarizine, lamotrigine, and acetazolamide. In a recent report, treatment with sodium valproate monotherapy or a combination of sodium valproate and lamotrigine showed a marked and sustained prophylactic effect.

Key Points

- Hemiplegic migraine (HM) is a rare disorder affecting 0.01 % of the general population.
- HM is differentiated from migraine with typical aura by the presence of motor weakness.
- Patients often describe sensory aura symptoms as loss of strength.
- Cases with first- or second-degree relatives are classified as familial HM; otherwise the diagnosis is sporadic HM.
- The diagnosis of FM is clinical, based on the reported symptoms, but investigations such as neuroimaging, EEG, and CSF analysis are important tools for excluding other conditions.
- The most important differential diagnoses of hemiplegic migraine in the acute phase are stroke and transient ischemic attack (TIA).
- Patients with HM can generally be treated with the same acute and prophylactic medications that are used for non-hemiplegic migraine, but the use of beta-blockers, triptans, and ergotamine remains controversial.

Suggested Reading

1. Artto V, Nissilä M, Wessman M et al (2007) Treatment of hemiplegic migraine with triptans. Eur J Neurol 14:1053
2. Athwal BS, Lennox GG (1996) Acetazolamide responsiveness in familial hemiplegic migraine. Ann Neurol 40:820
3. Berg MJ, Williams LS (1995) The transient syndrome of headache with neurologic deficits and CSF lymphocytosis. Neurology 45:1648
4. De Fusco M, Marconi R, Silvestri L et al (2003) Haploinsufficiency of ATP1A2 encoding the Na+/K + pump alpha2 subunit associated with familial hemiplegic migraine type 2. Nat Genet 33:192
5. De Vries B, Freilinger T, Vanmolkot KR et al (2007) Systematic analysis of three FHM genes in 39 sporadic patients with hemiplegic migraine. Neurology 69:2170
6. Dichgans M, Freilinger T, Eckstein G et al (2005) Mutation in the neuronal voltage-gated sodium channel SCN1A in familial hemiplegic migraine. Lancet 366:371
7. Dreier JP, Jurkat-Rott K, Petzold GC et al (2005) Opening of the blood–brain barrier preceding cortical edema in a severe attack of FHM type II. Neurology 64:2145
8. Ducros A, Denier C, Joutel A et al (2001) The clinical spectrum of familial hemiplegic migraine associated with mutations in a neuronal calcium channel. N Engl J Med 345:17
9. Gilbert GJ (1982) An occurrence of complicated migraine during propranolol therapy. Headache 22:81
10. Hansen JM, Hauge AW, Ashina M, Olesen J (2011) Trigger factors for familial hemiplegic migraine. Cephalalgia 31:1274
11. Hansen JM, Schytz HW, Larsen VA et al (2011) Hemiplegic migraine aura begins with cerebral hypoperfusion: imaging in the acute phase. Headache 51:1289
12. Hansen JM, Thomsen LL, Olesen J, Ashina M (2010) Coexisting typical migraine in familial hemiplegic migraine. Neurology 74(7):594–600
13. Hansen JM, Thomsen LL, Olesen J, Ashina M (2011) Calcitonin gene-related peptide does not cause migraine attacks in patients with familial hemiplegic migraine. Headache 51(4):544–553

14. Kaube H, Herzog J, Käufer T et al (2000) Aura in some patients with familial hemiplegic migraine can be stopped by intranasal ketamine. Neurology 55:139
15. Lampl C, Katsarava Z, Diener HC, Limmroth V (2005) Lamotrigine reduces migraine aura and migraine attacks in patients with migraine with aura. J Neurol Neurosurg Psychiatry 76:1730
16. Lindahl AJ, Allder S, Jefferson D et al (2002) Prolonged hemiplegic migraine associated with unilateral hyperperfusion on perfusion weighted magnetic resonance imaging. J Neurol Neurosurg Psychiatry 73:202
17. Mjåset C, Russell MB (2008) Intravenous nimodipine worsening prolonged attack of familial hemiplegic migraine. J Headache Pain 9:381
18. Mourand I, Menjot de Champfleur N, Carra-Dallière C et al (2012) Perfusion-weighted MR imaging in persistent hemiplegic migraine. Neuroradiology 54:255
19. Ophoff RA, Terwindt GM, Vergouwe MN et al (1996) Familial hemiplegic migraine and episodic ataxia type-2 are caused by mutations in the Ca2+ channel gene CACNL1A4. Cell 87:543
20. Pelzer N, Stam AH, Carpay JA, Vries BD, van den Maagdenberg AM, Ferrari MD et al (2014) Familial hemiplegic migraine treated by sodium valproate and lamotrigine. Cephalalgia [Epub ahead of print]
21. Pelzer N, Stam AH, Haan J, Ferrari MD, Terwindt GM (2012) Familial and sporadic hemiplegic migraine: diagnosis and treatment. Curr Treat Options Neurol 15(1):13–27
22. Razavi M, Razavi B, Fattal D et al (2000) Hemiplegic migraine induced by exertion. Arch Neurol 57:1363
23. Russell MB, Ducros A (2011) Sporadic and familial hemiplegic migraine: pathophysiological mechanisms, clinical characteristics, diagnosis, and management. Lancet Neurol 10:457
24. Thomsen LL, Kirchmann Eriksen M, Faerch Romer S (2002) An epidemiological survey of hemiplegic migraine. Cephalalgia 22:361
25. Thomsen LL, Olesen J (2004) Sporadic hemiplegic migraine. Cephalalgia 24:1016
26. Thomsen LL, Ostergaard E, Olesen J, Russell MB (2003) Evidence for a separate type of migraine with aura: sporadic hemiplegic migraine. Neurology 60:595

Chapter 5
Chronic Migraine Complicated by Medication Overuse Headache

Andrea Negro and Paolo Martelletti

5.1 Case Description

F.A. is a female 43-year-old lawyer, with a 30-year history of migraine. Her mother and her identical twin sister also suffered from migraine. Her mother, who died of brain cancer at 77 years, had suffered from migraine since her menopause, with low-frequency crisis. The temporal development of her migraine in comparison with that of her twin sister has been dichotomous.

Both experienced the onset of the first crisis at the menarche, and their disappearance during the pregnancy that they each carried to term, but the migraine progression in our patient was the same. At the age of 41 she experienced, concurrently with a subtotal hysterectomy with secondary depression, a rapid increase in her migraine crisis in terms of intensity first and frequency afterward, with fluctuating persistence of the crisis mixed with tension-type headache for up to about three-quarters of the month. Such chronicity has been interpreted, both by the patient and her physician, to be a consequence of her postpartum depression.

The complication of the pathology developing into chronic migraine has been chronicled through the overuse of a mixture of triptans, analgesics, and combination drugs containing butabarbital.

Such circumstances of self-medication seemed to be refractory to the usual and previously effective preventive therapies that her provincial consulting neurologist had successfully used to manage her clinical situation.

Each preventive drug used in the previous phase of episodic migraine and at the beginning of the chronic one was not more helpful, whereas the acute treatment demonstrated complete inefficacy, leading the patient to excessively consume acute

A. Negro • P. Martelletti (✉)
Department of Clinical and Molecular Medicine, Sapienza University of Rome and Regional Referral Headache Centre, Sant'Andrea Hospital, Rome, Italy
e-mail: paolo.martelletti@uniroma1.it

A. Siva, C. Lampl (eds.), *Case-Based Diagnosis and Management of Headache Disorders*, Headache, DOI 10.1007/978-3-319-06886-2_5

drugs. Over the years the patient experienced the onset of many drug-related side effects, such as weight gain (flunarizine, valproic acid, amitriptyline, propranolol, atenolol), cognitive disorders, loss of visual acuity (topiramate), and dyspnea on exertion (propranolol, atenolol).

She also experienced the onset of progressive diastolic hypertension, with a family history of such disease in her father, with no evidence in both renal function and renal ultrasound morphology. This has been suitably treated with amlodipine, 5 mg twice daily.

In the clinical history of this patient there have been two magnetic resonance imaging (MRI) examinations, the first at the age of 24 years when she experienced an exacerbation of her crisis immediately after the pregnancy, and the second 15 years later, carried out with contrast medium and angiography of the cerebral vessels, after overuse of medication ended in medication overuse headache (MOH).

Only through the second MRI has it been possible to detect the presence of white matter hyperintensities (WMHs) (Fig. 5.1), possibly related to the concomitant depression and the clinical situation of acute drug abuse.

The patient arrived at our Emergency Department (ED) suffering from headache not responding to analgesics and, despite not being positive on first neurological examination, for medicolegal reasons underwent a routine brain computed tomography (CT) scan, which was negative. At this point she was automatically transferred to the Regional Referral Headache Center of the same hospital. After 24 h she was registered as an ambulatory outpatient.

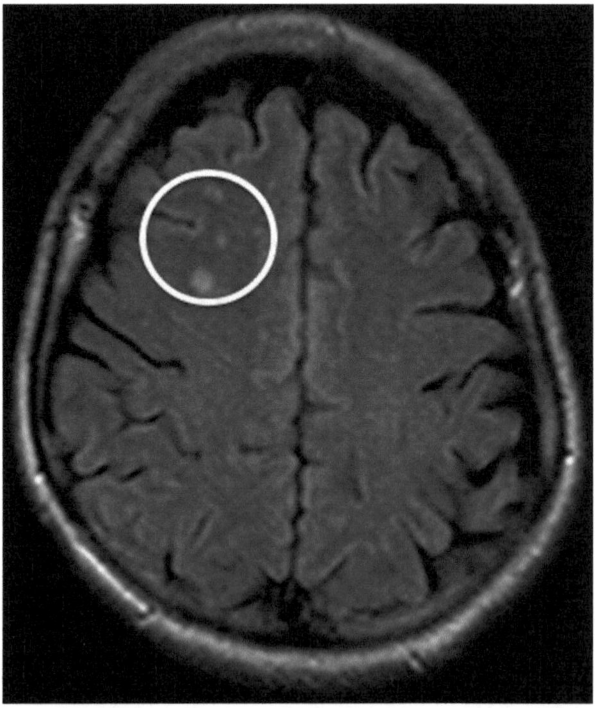

Fig. 5.1 Presence of WMHs as indicated by the *circle*

5.2 Differential Diagnosis and the Workup of a Chronic Migraine Patient

Chronic migraine represents the majority (40–60 %) of the clinical forms of headache observable in a third-level headache center. The prevalence of chronic migraine in the global population is approximately 2 %. Persons suffering from chronic migraine represent a subpopulation of patients with a high risk of disability profile, a high psychiatric comorbidity, and detrimental economic impact.

The recent headache classification from the International Headache Society (2013) defines chronic migraine as a form of migraine present in patients with a previous clinical history of migraine for more than 15 days per month. The clinical criteria for such disease are: at least 8 days per month with migraine characteristics, either registering the presence of aura or not, for at least 3 months.

The chronic migraine patient shows a widely variable developmental pattern from the episodic to the chronic form, with the alternation of phases of rapid increase in crisis frequency and stabilization, almost always leading to chronicity in a "Rossini Crescendo."

Emergency MRI is recommended only in cases of severe, rapid, and pharmacologically noncontrollable development of the pain, described as the worst pain ever suffered (known as "thunderclap headache"), associated with positivity at the neurological examination, and cognitive or neuro-ophthalmologic alterations. It is then possible to evaluate whether the exacerbation phase hides other life-threatening abnormalities in the craniocephalic area, such as subarachnoid hemorrhage, fissuring or breaking of a brain aneurysm, cerebral venous thrombosis, cervicocephalic arterial dissection, cerebral vasoconstriction syndrome, spontaneous intracranial hypotension, or other craniocephalic abnormalities. In patients with chronic migraine complicated by medication overuse, one should look for an underlying cause only in the case of true red flags, not in the more frequent cases of refractoriness to the usual acute-treatment drugs: access to the ED must be explained in detail and not be pushed by an unmotivated fear. It must be borne in mind that in Europe 2 % of the admissions to the ED are classified as headache, the majority of which are chronic migraines, but all of these patients, for evident medicolegal reasons, undergo brain CT scans.

On the other hand, there are many forms of chronic migraine that can be positively treated with the botulinum toxin therapeutic technique which, if applied early, offers the opportunity of de-chronicization from chronic migraine complicated by medication overuse. The treatment scheme has been coded by two large randomized controlled trials (PREEMPT1, PREEMPT2), and is based on quarterly sessions of infiltrations with OnabotulinumtoxinA, following a standardized injective paradigm based on the application of 155 U of OnabotulinumtoxinA in 31 sites, following the Fixed Doses Fixed Sites (FDFS) procedure. An additional 40 U can be injected unilaterally or bilaterally in three specific areas (neck/head) according to the Follow The Pain (FTP) procedure.

In the recent *International Classification of Headache Disorders 3 beta* (ICHD-3β), chronic migraine has been inserted in the main body of primary headaches and rightly, therefore, is part of the classification system. The secondariness of medication overuse or addiction to analgesics in this chronic migraine category has not yet been cleared, even though we now have therapeutic means aimed to treat these two strongly overlapping clinical situations. In any event, clinicians today have a well-defined diagnostic and therapeutic pattern for chronic migraine that can be of great help to both the headache expert and the family physician (see Sect. 5.4).

Early treatment of chronic migraine is preferred. Forms of chronic migraine that are treated too late develop, over the years, into multiple episodes of MOH despite the rehabilitation procedures of withdrawal from drug abuse, which offer a good platform for the beginning of OnabotulinumtoxinA therapy but at long-term follow-up inexorably develop into refractory chronic migraine; at this point a further mini-invasive treatment is requested, such as occipital or spinal neurostimulation.

5.3 Diagnostic Workup of the Case

The patient was admitted to the outpatient section of our Regional Referral Headache Center via the preferential online request made through the ED physician. The diagnosis of chronic migraine was readily reached based on the 2013 ICHD-3β criteria. This classification states that chronic migraine (ICHD-3 code 1.3) can be defined as a headache, both migraine and/or tension-type like, appearing for a 3-month period for more days than not on a monthly basis. Diagnosis must follow the criteria of migraine without aura (ICHD-3 code 1.1) or with aura (ICHD-3 code 1.2). During this 3-month observational period the number of migraine days must be more than 8 per month and the use of triptans or ergot derivatives, with derived benefit, must be deduced from the headache diary.

On the basis of the previous clinical diaries we also diagnosed MOH, the use of triptans and/or analgesics/anti-inflammatories being reported in 21 days per month. Therefore, the patient was sent to the Day Hospital section of our center, where she received the infusion procedure for drug withdrawal. On the first day of access we also carried out a standard routine biochemistry, electrocardiogram, and urinalysis, which provided standard results.

The dose of hydrocortisone sodium succinate, infused in a 120-min period, was progressively reduced from 1 g/500 mL NaCl on day 1 to 125 mg/500 mL NaCl on day 5, the day of her dismissal from hospital.

Arterial pressure (PA) was controlled every 30 min during the infusion.

The physician, supported by the psychologist, monitored daily the interruption of medications for migraine.

The psychologist carried out a series of psychological consults to maximize patient compliance to the therapy.

On the day of discharge the patient received treatment with OnabotulinumtoxinA 195 U, following the PREEMPT scheme (FDFS + FTP).

The treatment has been repeated quarterly since then, 195 U for the first two times and 155 U from the third time on, and after 30 months the patient reports a stable decrease of her migraine crisis (4–5 days of migraine per month) and with a much lower intensity, a complete responsiveness to triptans, and a quality of life that has definitely improved, our patient reporting: "I am so satisfied, it is excellent, like a new life."

The standard rehabilitation program provides an examination and a psychological consult every 3 months before receiving the infusion therapy. It all takes place in a reserved outpatient setting that can be booked only inside the hospital and at the expense of the National Health System, participating with a sum inferior to €200 per year to public health expenditure. The protocol provides that as soon as the patient durably (>3 months) reaches three migraine days she will be reassigned to the Ambulatory Outpatients Department of the Headache Center.

5.4 Summary of the Case

- A 43-year-old woman, suffering migraine without aura from the age of 13 years, after menarche. Family history of migraine. Frequency of migraine crisis stable between 3 and 5 days per month.
- Subtotal hysterectomy when she was 41 with a rapid chronicity of the crisis and transformation to chronic migraine complicated by medication overuse. Brain MRI indicates deep white matter lesions. Beck Depression Inventory score >24.
- When she accesses the ED, brain CT is negative. She is then assigned to the Headache Center.
- Detoxification procedure as day-hospital inpatient, psychological evaluation, treatment with OnabotulinumtoxinA on a 3-monthly basis for an actual follow-up of 30 months.
- Reduced frequency of migraine headache days (4–5/months) with mild intensity, easily resolved with triptan. Beck Depression Inventory score <24.

Suggested Reading

1. Classification Committee of the International Headache Society (2013) The International Classification of Headache Disorders, 3rd edition (beta version). Cephalalgia 33:629–808
2. Dodick DW, Turkel CC, DeGryse RE, Aurora SK, Silberstein SD, Lipton RB, Diener HC, Brin MF, PREEMPT Chronic Migraine Study Group (2010) OnabotulinumtoxinA for treatment of chronic migraine: pooled results from the double-blind, randomized, placebo-controlled phases of the PREEMPT clinical program. Headache 50:921–936
3. Farinelli I, Dionisi I, Martelletti P (2011) Rehabilitating chronic migraine complicated by medication overuse headaches: how can we prevent migraine relapse? Intern Emerg Med 6(1):23–28

4. Gentile G, Borro M, Lala N, Missori S, Simmaco M, Martelletti P (2010) Genetic polymorphisms related to efficacy and overuse of triptans in chronic migraine. J Headache Pain 11(5):431–435
5. Gentile G, Missori S, Borro M, Sebastianelli A, Simmaco M, Martelletti P (2010) Frequencies of genetic polymorphisms related to triptans metabolism in chronic migraine. J Headache Pain 11(2):151–156
6. Innamorati M, Pompili M, Fiorillo M, Lala N, Negro A, Del Bono SD, Lester D, Girardi P, Martelletti P (2013) Overattachment and perceived disability in chronic migraineurs. Clin Neurol Neurosurg 115(7):954–958
7. Lionetto L, Negro A, Palmisani S, Gentile G, Del Fiore MR, Mercieri M, Simmaco M, Smith T, Al-Kaisy A, Arcioni R, Martelletti P (2012) Emerging treatment for chronic migraine and refractory chronic migraine. Expert Opin Emerg Drugs 17(3):393–406
8. Martelletti P (2011) Dispute settlement understanding on the use of BOTOX® in chronic migraine. J Headache Pain 12:1–2
9. Martelletti P, Steiner TJ (eds) (2011) Handbook of headache. Practical management. Springer, Heidelberg/New York
10. Negro A, D'Alonzo L, Martelletti P (2010) Chronic migraine: comorbidities, risk factors, and rehabilitation. Intern Emerg Med 5(Suppl 1):S13–S19
11. Negro A, Martelletti P (2011) Chronic migraine plus medication overuse headache: two entities or not? J Headache Pain 12(6):593–601
12. Negro A, Rocchietti-March M, Fiorillo M, Martelletti P (2011) Chronic migraine: current concepts and ongoing treatments. Eur Rev Med Pharmacol Sci 5(12):1401–1420
13. Pompili M, Serafini G, Di Cosimo D, Dominici G, Innamorati M, Lester D, Forte A, Girardi N, De Filippis S, Tatarelli R, Martelletti P (2010) Psychiatric comorbidity and suicide risk in patients with chronic migraine. Neuropsychiatr Dis Treat 7(6):81–91

Chapter 6
Refractory Chronic Migraine Therapy with Botulinum Toxin A

Reto Agosti

6.1 Case Presentation

Case 1

Patient AB, a 33-year-old female, born in 1967, jeweler vendor, was seeking help in 2000 for her severe migraine without aura. The attacks occurred on 15–20 days per month typically between starts of her menstrual period and ovulation. She tried numerous migraine prophylactic substances such as propranolol, verapamil, and amitriptyline. Propranolol was used also for a chronic essential tachycardia around 110 bpm at untreated resting condition. With the combination of the above medications, the patient was able to maintain her part-time job. However, she used most of her leisure time to suffer or recover from her numerous migraine attacks and headache days. About 10–15 applications of sumatriptan were needed per month. In 2003, the use of Botox was finally approved by her health insurance and 100 units were applied for the first time in 2004. Already after 2 weeks headache days and migraine attacks began to diminish. Ever since the second treatment at a 3 month interval, her headache burden sank to a few mild attacks per month. Botox continued to suppress headaches and migraines now for 10 years. After the 4th treatment with Botox, she started to extend her treatment interval and is in need of Botox, now only every 6 months. Her quality of life has improved tremendously (Figs. 6.1, 6.2, and 6.3).

General introductory note: For reasons of simplicity, the term "Botox" is used in this chapter instead of onabotulinumtoxinA.

R. Agosti
Kopfwehzentrum Hirslanden Zürich – Headache Center,
Forchstrasse 424, Zollikon 8702, Switzerland
e-mail: reto.agosti@kopfwww.ch

A. Siva, C. Lampl (eds.), *Case-Based Diagnosis and Management of Headache Disorders*, Headache, DOI 10.1007/978-3-319-06886-2_6

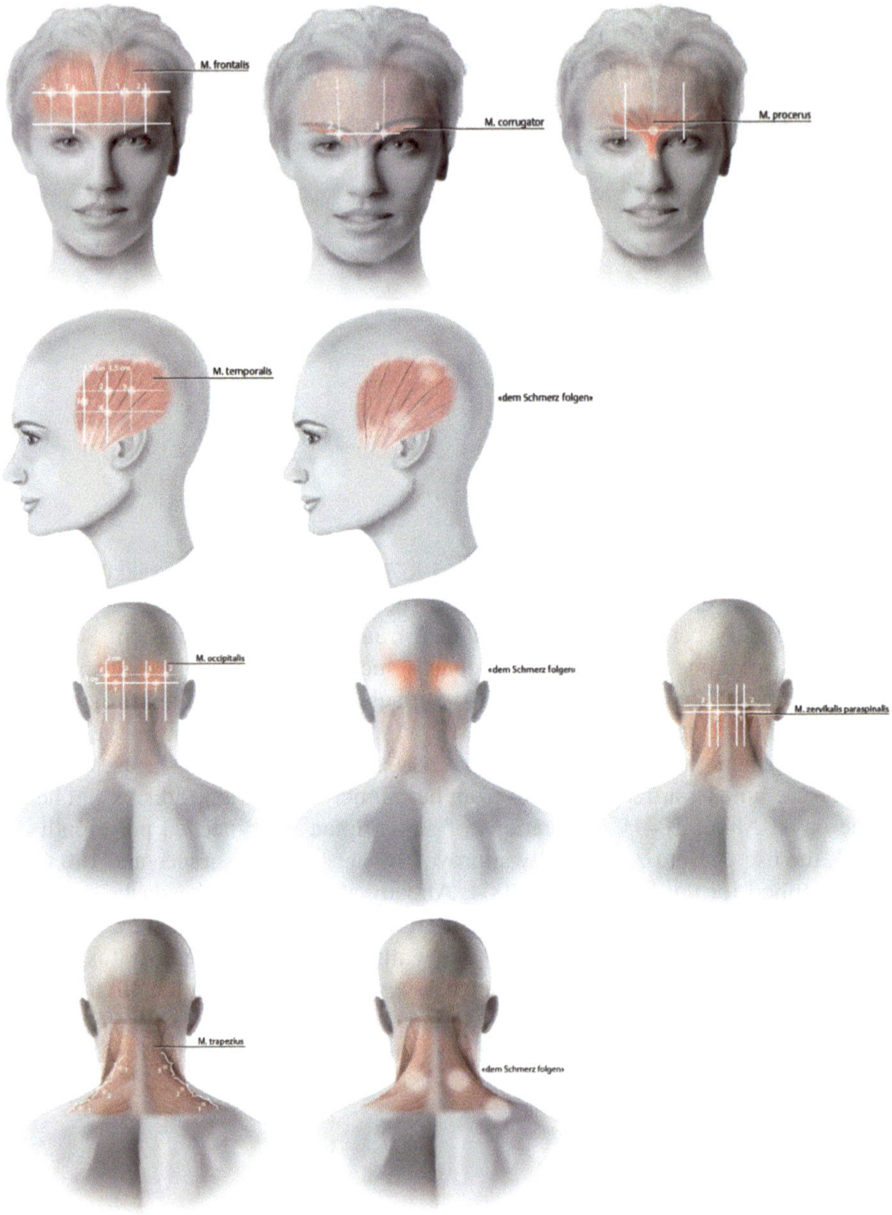

Fig. 6.1 Application of Botox (onabotulinumtoxinA) for chronic migraine according to the PREEMPT study protocol (155 IU "fixed dose, fixed site" and optional 40 IU "follow the pain") (Illustrations by Janine Heers)

Fig. 6.1 (continued)

Muscle	Left	Midline	Right
Frontalis	10		10
Procerus		5	
Corrugator	5		5
Temporalis	20		20
Occipitalis	15		15
Rectus superior	10		15
Trapezius	15		15

Illustration: Janine Heers

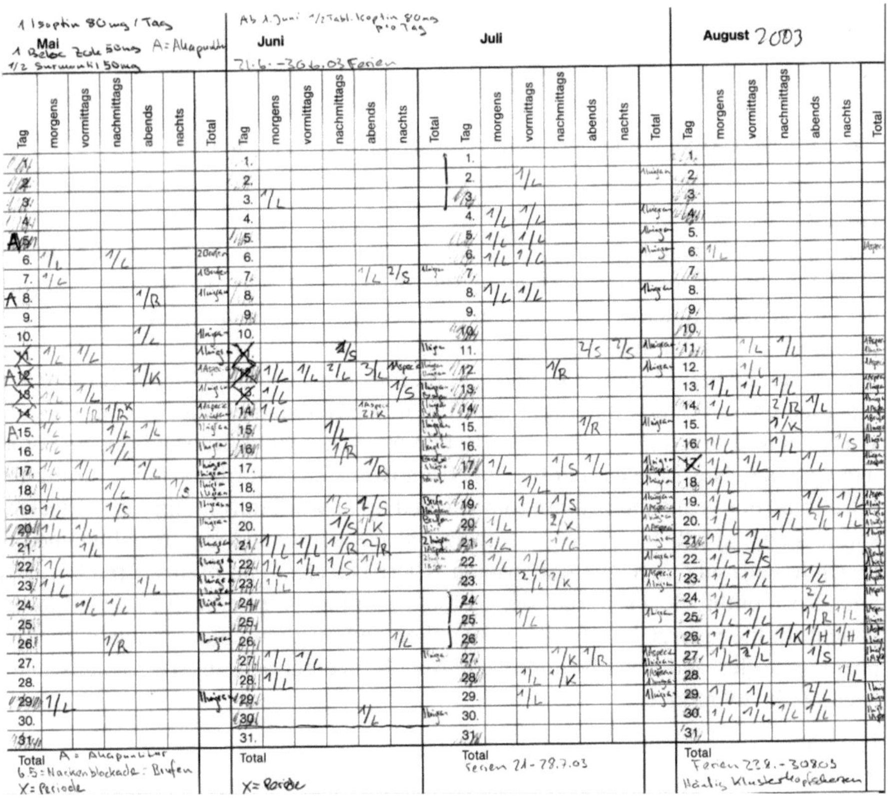

Fig. 6.2 Patient AB: headache diary before Botox treatment

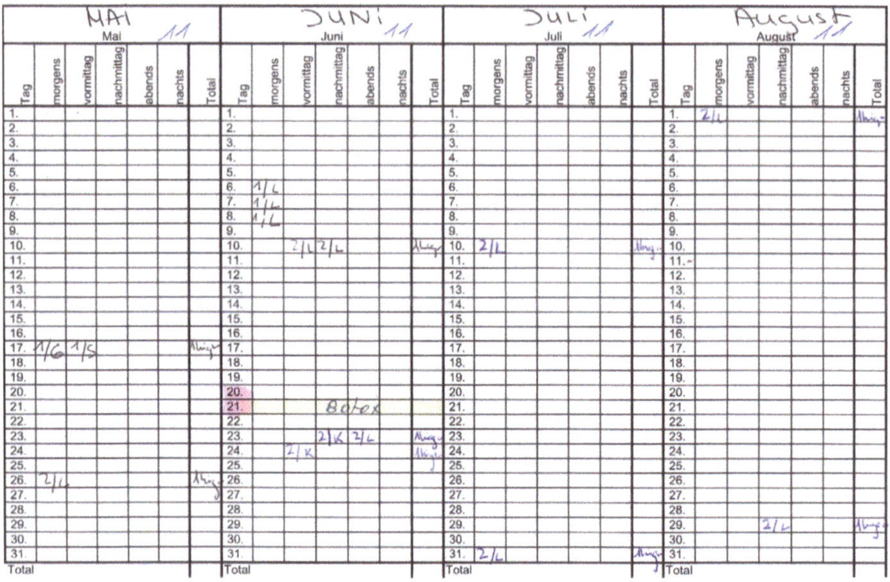

Fig. 6.3 Patient AB: Botox long-term efficacy (e.g., May to August 2011)

Case 2

Patient EG, a female born in 1960, chief dental hygienist, was started on Botox in 2004 for chronic migraine with numerous disabling attacks per month. Typically her husband had to leave his work and pick her up at her practice due to inability to continue her work or make the way home by herself. In addition to that, her husband had to pick up their daughter from day care. Injections were initiated according to a modified phase II study paradigm with 100 units. Her skin is causing extreme pain sensation to every single injection – despite pretreatment with local lidocaine ointment and ice. Nevertheless her benefits from Botox are "worth the pain" during the injections. For years she had not to be picked up at work during migraine attacks a single time. Attacks have been occurring less frequently and less disabling and are treatable with subcutaneous sumatriptan. There is a clear end of dose effect usually after 2.5 months. So far a total of 36 Botox treatments have been provided to the patient. In the year 2013, 155 IU was applied and residual tender points in the trapezius muscles additionally improved. Attack medications, mostly triptans, have been markedly reduced.

Case 3

Patient JF, a female patient born 1967, accountant, was suffering from severe chronic migraine with and without auras and severe depression for which she had in-house treatment two times. Botox was applied every 3 months since 2007, totally 25 times. Both her migraines and her depressions did improve, and since the beginning of Botox treatment, she did not require further hospitalization for severe depressions. Antidepressant medications were continued during Botox treatments until today. Under 155 IE according to the phase III Research Evaluating Migraine Prophylaxis Therapy (PREEMPT) protocol, her migraine condition further improved.

6.2 Differential Diagnosis and How to Work Up This Kind of Patient

Once diagnosis of a migraine is made (including imaging studies to rule out secondary headaches, criterion E of ICHD 1.1 or 1.2), no further diagnostic workup is needed before initiating a treatment with Botox. However, for Botox treatment of migraine, a diagnosis of "chronic migraine" (CM) is required according to the PREEMPT protocols. The most reliable tool is a patient headache diary in which the headache days can be distinguished between days with migraine and days with non-migraine headaches. Neurological exam may reveal tender points in those pericranial muscles that may receive additional dosages according to the "follow the pain" paradigm (temporalis, occipitalis, and trapezius muscles). Oral anticoagulation needs to be asked although full anticoagulation is not an absolute contraindication.

6.3 Diagnostic Workup of the Cases

Diagnoses were made according to the ICHD classification of 1988 and 2004. All patients had at least one MRI. They were all normal.

6.4 Summary of the Cases

All three cases fulfilled the criteria of chronic migraine, temporarily also of MOH. Suffering was very high and quality of life very low.

The success of Botox treatment was subjective and reported as reduction in frequency of headaches but a number of other improvements including severe episodes of depression in one case. However headache diaries provide a very useful semi-objective measure of suffering and success.

All patients try to extend the interval of Botox treatments, with success in one case but no success in the other two cases. All cases of chronic migraine changed into episodic migraine before receiving further treatments. The criterion for further treatments is usually the end of dose effect, i.e., increasing migraine frequencies while planning further treatments.

Typically patients in clinical practice will continue or start on migraine/headache prophylactic medications. There are no interactions known with any of the commonly used substances.

Botox against chronic migraine is extremely well tolerated and has numerous advantages over daily preventive medication intake.

6.5 Brief General Information

The treatment of chronic medication-resistant migraine is complicated and demanding both for the physicians and for the patients. Most CM cases bear also an overuse of attack medications (see Chap. 11 for diagnostic considerations). In this case reduction or cessation of attack medication is necessary. Treatment of CM is practically always based on medical treatment in combination with complementary approaches. Basically all preventive medications used to treat high-frequency (but still episodic) migraines are used. However, if a CM patient is seeking help from a headache specialist, many medical treatments have already been applied – without appropriate success or untolerable side effects.

Botox was introduced as a medical treatment in the 1970s for the treatment of strabismus. Botox fulfilled the two most important characteristics of an intramuscular ocular treatment: efficacy in a minimal amount and lasting effect as long as possible. Botox was consequently used to treat many different conditions characterized by muscular overactivity. In the late 1990s, William Binder in wrinkle study serendipitously discovered that by treating hyperactive facial lines in some persons, migraine improved as well. Several preliminary Botox migraine studies were made with quite conflicting results. The phase II program (only episodic migraine was included) revealed no superiority of Botox over placebo. However, it paved the ground for the phase III PREEMPT studies which showed a positive effect of 155 unit Botox over placebo. These studies lead to registration for Botox against chronic migraine by FDA (USA) and EMA in most European countries.

Botox bears several advantages over oral migraine preventive treatments: no oral intake, no known systemic interactions, perfect compliance, minimal effort (average treatment of every 3 months vs daily medication intake), and very high tolerability. Disadvantages are occasional minor and transient aesthetic changes in the face and occasional transient aches and pains in the neck. Some patients express high fears of injections or of the "poison" such that they will not try Botox. Efficacy is in the range of 50 % reduction in frequency but a number of other improvements, e.g., better efficacy of attack medications, reduced fear of the next attacks, or even psychological improvements.

Botox has been used against migraine at Hirslanden Headache Centre in Zurich since 2003 in over 1,000 patients. Originally 100 IU was applied and some patients are now switched to the PREEMPT protocol. However a number of patients with satisfying response are still treated with 100 IU. Efficacy remained high in most of the good responders. Typically patients try to extend the treatment interval beyond the typical 3 months and reschedule when they experience worsening of their migraines. Some patients for scheduling Botox treatments on demand resulting in irregular intervals. In case of very low or missing improvements, Botox treatment will be self-limiting to one or two cycles, thus limiting also the relatively high costs of this treatment option.

Botulinum toxin is so far the only medical treatment somewhat specific for the treatment of chronic migraine.

Key Points

- Botox is the only approved medical treatment against chronic migraine.
- Efficacy is in the range of 50 % (reduction of attack frequency by 50 %), and in approximately 10 %, practically all attacks are prevented. Long-term experience since the late 1990s and early 2000s shows persistent efficacy (over 30 treatment cycles in my personal experience).
- Botox is applied approximately every 3 months. All patients try to extend the interval. In the case that Botox treatment is not effective, the treatment will be ceased after one to three treatments – and overall costs will be limited automatically.
- The PREEMPT protocol (155 IU fixed dose, fixed site and optional 40 IU follow the pain) is clinically safe and useful.
- Safety and tolerability are very high. Some aesthetic considerations are sometimes made by patients concerning their face and some patients may complain of neck aches temporarily.
- With successful Botox treatment, savings can be made on attack treatments, urgent medical care, neurological consultations, and prophylactic treatment – in many cases weighing out substantially the previous costs caused by the patients' migraines before initiating treatment with Botox.

Suggested Reading

1. Antonucci F, Rossi C, Gianfranceschi L et al (2008) Long-distance retrograde effects of botulinum neurotoxin A. J Neurosci 28:3689–3696
2. Ashkenazi A (2010) Botulinum toxin type A for chronic migraine. Curr Neurol Neurosci Rep 10:140–146
3. Aurora SK, Dodick DW, Turkel CC et al (2010) OnabotulinumtoxinA for treatment of chronic migraine: results from the double-blind, randomized, placebo-controlled phase of the PREEMPT 1 trial. Cephalalgia 30:793–803
4. Aurora SK, Gawel M, Brandes JL et al (2007) Botulinum toxin type a prophylactic treatment of episodic migraine: a randomized, double-blind, placebo-controlled exploratory study. Headache 47:486–499

5. Binder WJ, Brin MF, Blitzer A et al (2000) Botulinum toxin type A (BOTOX) for treatment of migraine headaches: an open-label study. Otolaryngol Head Neck Surg 123:669–676
6. Blumenfeld A, Silberstein SD, Dodick DW et al (2010) Method of injection of onabotulinumtoxinA for chronic migraine: a safe, well-tolerated, and effective treatment paradigm based on the PREEMPT clinical program. Headache 50:1406–1418
7. Brin MF (1997) Botulinum toxin: chemistry, pharmacology, toxicity, and immunology. Muscle Nerve Suppl 6:S146–S168
8. Bumb A, Wetzel S, Agosti R (2013) Patients profiling for Botox® (onabotulinumtoxin A) treatment for migraine: a look at white matter lesions in the MRI as a potential marker. Springerplus 2:377
9. Cui M, Khanijou S, Rubino J et al (2004) Subcutaneous administration of botulinum toxin A reduces formalin-induced pain. Pain 107:125–133
10. Diener HC, Dodick DW, Aurora SK et al (2010) OnabotulinumtoxinA for treatment of chronic migraine: results from the double-blind, randomized, placebo-controlled phase of the PREEMPT 2 trial. Cephalalgia 30:804–814
11. Dodick DW, Mauskop A, Elkind AH et al (2005) Botulinum toxin type A for the prophylaxis of chronic daily headache: subgroup analysis of patients not receiving other prophylactic medications: a randomized double-blind, placebo-controlled study. Headache 45:315–324
12. Dodick DW, Turkel CC, Degryse RE et al (2010) OnabotulinumtoxinA for treatment of chronic migraine: pooled results from the double-blind, randomized, placebo-controlled phases of the PREEMPT clinical program. Headache 50:921–936
13. Dolly O (2003) Synaptic transmission: inhibition of neurotransmitter release by botulinum toxins. Headache 43(Suppl 1):S16–S24
14. Dowson AJ, Kilminster SG, Salt R (2008) Clinical profile of botulinum toxin A in patients with chronic headaches and cervical dystonia: a prospective, open-label, longitudinal study conducted in a naturalistic clinical practice setting. Drugs R D 9:147–158
15. Durham PL, Cady R, Cady R (2004) Regulation of calcitonin gene-related peptide secretion from trigeminal nerve cells by botulinum toxin type A: implications for migraine therapy. Headache 44:35–42
16. Eross EJ, Gladstone JP, Lewis S et al (2005) Duration of migraine is a predictor for response to botulinum toxin type A. Headache 45:308–314
17. Evers S, Vollmer-Haase J, Schwaag S et al (2004) Botulinum toxin A in the prophylactic treatment of migraine – a randomized, double-blind, placebo-controlled study. Cephalalgia 24: 838–843
18. FDA approves Botox to treat chronic migraine (2013) Available at: http://www.fda.gov/NewsEvents/Newsroom/PressAnnouncements/ucm229782.htm. Accessed 11 May 2013
19. Headache Classification Subcommittee of the International Headache Society (2004) The international classification of headache disorders: 2nd edition. Cephalalgia 24(Suppl 1):9–160
20. Jackson JL, Kuriyama A, Hayashino Y (2012) Botulinum toxin A for prophylactic treatment of migraine and tension headaches in adults: a meta-analysis. JAMA 307:1736–1745
21. Mathew NT, Frishberg BM, Gawel M et al (2005) Botulinum toxin type A (BOTOX) for the prophylactic treatment of chronic daily headache: a randomized, double-blind, placebo-controlled trial. Headache 45:293–307
22. McMahon HT, Foran P, Dolly JO et al (1992) Tetanus toxin and botulinum toxins type A and B inhibit glutamate, gamma-aminobutyric acid, aspartate, and met-enkephalin release from synaptosomes. Clues to the locus of action. J Biol Chem 267:21338–21343
23. Ondo WG, Gollomp S, Galvez-Jimenez N (2005) A pilot study of botulinum toxin A for headache in cervical dystonia. Headache 45:1073–1077
24. Ondo WG, Vuong KD, Derman HS (2004) Botulinum toxin A for chronic daily headache: a randomized, placebo-controlled, parallel design study. Cephalalgia 24:60–65
25. Ranoux D, Attal N, Morain F et al (2008) Botulinum toxin type A induces direct analgesic effects in chronic neuropathic pain. Ann Neurol 64:274–283

26. Relja M, Poole AC, Schoenen J et al (2007) A multicentre, double-blind, randomized, placebo-controlled, parallel group study of multiple treatments of botulinum toxin type A (BoNTA) for the prophylaxis of episodic migraine headaches. Cephalalgia 27:492–503
27. Shapiro RL, Hatheway C, Swerdlow DL (1998) Botulism in the United States: a clinical and epidemiologic review. Ann Intern Med 129:221–228
28. Silberstein S, Mathew N, Saper J et al (2000) Botulinum toxin type A as a migraine preventive treatment. For the BOTOX Migraine Clinical Research Group. Headache 40:445–450
29. Silberstein SD, Stark SR, Lucas SM et al (2005) Botulinum toxin type A for the prophylactic treatment of chronic daily headache: a randomized, double-blind, placebo-controlled trial. Mayo Clin Proc 80:1126–1137
30. Smuts JA, Schultz D, Barnard A (2004) Mechanism of action of botulinum toxin type A in migraine prevention: a pilot study. Headache 44:801–805
31. Turton K, Chaddock JA, Acharya KR (2002) Botulinum and tetanus neurotoxins: structure, function and therapeutic utility. Trends Biochem Sci 27:552–558
32. Winner PK, Sadowsky CH, Martinez WC et al (2012) Concurrent onabotulinumtoxinA treatment of cervical dystonia and concomitant migraine. Headache 52:1219–1225
33. Wollmer MA, De Boer C, Kalaka N et al (2012) Facing depression with botulinum toxin: a randomized controlled trial. J Psychiatr Res 46:574–581

Chapter 7
Complicated Migraine

Mark Obermann

7.1 Case Description

A 23-year-old medical student presents to the emergency room with moderate to severe right-sided headache over the past 5 days. She reports that nausea and vomiting, as well as phono- and photophobia, accompanied the headache initially. The pain is always present but fluctuates in pain intensity from moderate to severe. It always stays in the described location. Mechanical allodynia has developed over the right scalp over the past couple of days. She also reports that she experienced a gradual onset of visual field disturbances that developed into a right-sided hemianopia over several minutes and slowly resolved over 60 min, with a small residual visual field defect in the left lower quadrant. In parallel to the amelioration of her visual symptoms, she describes slow-onset sensory loss and paresthesia starting with her right hand and progressing to the whole arm within 10–15 min. She also experiences difficulties finding the right words and feels that people seem to misunderstand certain words she is saying. The mild aphasia and sensory symptoms did not resolve and are still present after 7 days on presentation in the emergency room. Her usual migraine attack frequency is once per month, but she never experienced aura before. Her mother suffers from migraine with typical aura, and she has no siblings. Her past medical history is otherwise unremarkable; she has never been to a hospital before and takes no drugs. She is a nonsmoker and does take oral contraception, however.

M. Obermann
Department of Neurology, University of Duisburg-Essen,
Essen, Germany
e-mail: mark.obermann@uni-due.de

A. Siva, C. Lampl (eds.), *Case-Based Diagnosis and Management of Headache Disorders*, Headache, DOI 10.1007/978-3-319-06886-2_7

7.2 Differential Diagnosis and How to Work Up Such a Patient?

The differential diagnoses that have to be considered in this case are those for migraine with typical aura and its complications, acute headache including stroke, intracerebral hemorrhage, subarachnoid hemorrhage, thunderclap headache, reversible cerebral vasoconstriction syndrome, posterior reversible encephalopathy syndrome, arterial dissection, sinus thrombosis, arteriovenous malformations, leptomeningeal angiomatosis (i.e., Sturge-Weber syndrome), and meningitis.

The key to the correct diagnosis of this patient is the differentiation of a typical aura with other causes of focal neurological deficits. The unusually long aura with otherwise typical migraine onset should prompt further investigations. A typical aura lasts between 5 min and 1 h, as our patients' visual aura did. It can be followed by another aura symptom which then can last for another 60 min and so on. More than three aura symptoms, i.e., visual, somatosensory, and aphasia, have rarely been reported and would therefore also have to be considered quite unusual. Motor symptoms are uncommon and can last longer than 60 min, and the new International Classification of Headache Disorders (ICHD-3 beta) suggests to regard migraine patients with motor deficits as hemiplegic migraine. In migraine with multiple aura symptoms, visual aura is often the first symptom, followed by somatosensory aura and aphasia. The aura usually has a gradual onset with symptoms developing over several minutes, reaching a steady plateau, and then slowly resolving. Sudden onset is unusual and indicative of cerebral ischemia or hemorrhage. Cerebral computer tomography (CCT) scan should be performed with CT angiography (CTA) to rule out cerebral hemorrhage and other vascular pathology. CSF analysis should be used to definitely rule out subarachnoid hemorrhage, when CCT is negative. However, CT is often not sensitive enough to detect smaller ischemic lesions. Magnetic resonance imaging should be performed where available. As our patient was outside any reasonable time frame for systemic or local antithrombolytic therapy, MRI was considered dispensable in the subacute phase and was then reconsidered after the first treatment attempts were unsuccessful. MRI is important to differentiate migrainous stroke from a rare condition termed persistent aura without infarcts.

7.3 Diagnostic Workup of the Case

Neurological examination revealed right visual field hemianopia, mild expressive aphasia, and hypoesthesia of the right arm, as well as moderate mechanical allodynia over the right temporal and parietal scalp. CCT with CTA was performed, but did not show any signs of acute cerebral infarct, subarachnoid hemorrhage, aneurysm, tumor, sinus thrombosis, or other intracranial pathology. Transcranial ultrasound did not show any signs of cerebral vasoconstriction, cerebral vessel stenosis, or dissection. Cerebrospinal fluid analysis was normal. Arterial blood pressure was

120/80 mmHg, heart rate was 84/min., and temperature was normal with 37.2° C. Routine blood work including CBC, ESR, CRP, and standard biochemistry, as well as thyroid function was unremarkable.

She was treated with 1,000 mg intravenous (IV) acetylsalicylic acid and 10 mg metoclopramide IV that considerably improved the headache for several hours but did not resolve the neurological deficits. Pain started to worsen again; she was treated with prednisolone 250 mg IV and diagnosed with status migrainosus and persistent migraine aura.

She continued to receive prednisolone 250 mg IV over 3 days, and the headache gradually resolved. The other symptoms slowly improved over the next 2 weeks. There were no residual neurological deficits on follow-up examination 3 weeks later. Magnetic resonance imaging (MRI) was performed 3 weeks after symptom onset and showed cortical laminar necrosis in the left occipital lobe consistent with migrainous infarction (Fig. 7.1).

7.4 Summary of the Case

This 23-year-old student suffered from migrainous infarction following her first migraine with aura attack. She hesitated to seek medical attention, because as a medical student she was well aware of her migraine and suspected this to be her first migraine with typical aura that she knew well from her mother. The persistence of symptoms made her realize that this may not be a typical migraine attack after all and present to the emergency room. Neurological examination revealed hemianopia, hypoesthesia of the right arm, and mild expressive aphasia. CCT scan was unremarkable and symptoms were classified as status migrainosus but remained refractory to specific treatment attempts. MRI in the post-acute phase revealed laminar necrosis indicative of migrainous infarction. The neurological symptoms gradually improved, and she was discharged from the hospital 3 weeks after symptom onset without any residual neurological deficit.

7.5 Definition of Complications of Migraine

Five complications of migraine are recognized by the ICHD-3 beta (Table 7.1): status migrainosus, persistent aura without infarction, migrainous infarction, migraine aura-triggered seizure, and in the appendix migraine aura status. The complication should be coded in addition to the underlying migraine subtype.

Status migrainosus is defined as debilitating migraine attack that lasts more than 72 h but has otherwise all the typical characteristics of a migraine attack with or without aura. Remissions of up to 12 h related to medication or sleep are accepted. Status migrainosus can last several weeks (mean 4.8 weeks; range 3–10), and patients with aura are more likely to develop status migrainosus. Precipitating factors can be stress and anxiety, menstruation, and lack of sleep.

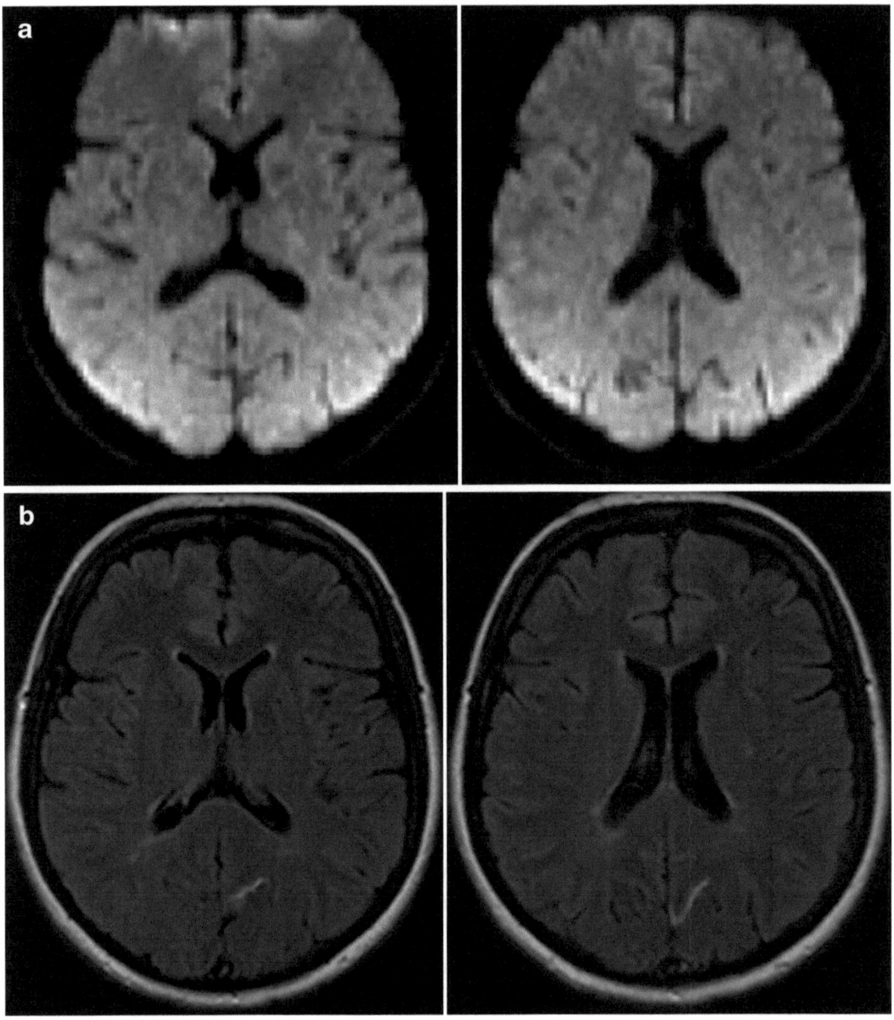

Fig. 7.1 (**a**) Diffusion-weighted image (DWI) 3 weeks after symptom onset does not show acute signs of ischemia anymore, (**b**) small laminar necrosis in the occipital cortex suggests migrainous infarction in fluid-attenuated inversion recovery (FLAIR) sequence

Migrainous infarction is defined as one or more migraine aura symptoms associated with an ischemic cerebral lesion on neuroimaging in the appropriate brain area. Usually, patients are younger women and demonstrate typical aura symptoms that last over 60 min. Lesions are mostly located in the posterior circulation. The migrainous infarct has to develop in the course of a migraine attack; otherwise, it is considered an ischemic stroke of other cause and has to be worked up accordingly. Migraine patients with aura have a twofold risk of ischemic stroke, but these strokes are not necessarily migrainous infarctions. The mechanisms associated with higher stroke risk remain unclear.

Table 7.1 Complications of migraine

Status migrainosus	Debilitating migraine attack that lasts more than 72 h Remissions of up to 12 h related to medication or sleep are accepted Status migrainosus can last several weeks Precipitating factors are stress/anxiety, menstruation, and lack of sleep
Persistent aura without infarction	Aura symptoms that last over 1 week without evidence of infarction on neuroimaging
Migrainous infarction	One or more migraine aura symptoms associated with an ischemic cerebral lesion on neuroimaging Infarct develops in the course of the migraine attack Aura symptoms last over 60 min Lesions mostly located in the posterior circulation Younger women are often affected
Migraine aura-triggered seizure	Occurs within 1 h after or during a migraine with aura attack
Migraine aura status	Multiple auras (at least 2) occurring per day for more than 3 days in patients with migraine with aura

Persistent aura without infarction is characterized by aura symptoms that last over 1 week without evidence of infarction on neuroimaging. Symptomatic causes for the persistent aura need careful diagnostic workup. Aura symptoms that last longer than 1 h, but less than 1 week, should be regarded as probable migraine with aura and not necessarily persistent migraine aura. This gap in the classification is subject to debate.

Persistent aura without infarction has to be differentiated from migraine aura status that is defined as multiple auras (at least 2) occurring per day over more than 3 days in patients fulfilling the diagnostic criteria for migraine with aura. Headache does not necessarily have to accompany these aura symptoms.

Migraine aura-triggered seizure is rather self-explanatory and should occur within 1 h after or during a migraine attack. It is much more common that an epileptic seizure triggers a migraine attack, which is sometimes referred to as "migralepsy." Even though a migraine aura-triggered seizure is a very rare condition, it underlines the close relationship of these paroxysmal brain disorders.

7.6 Brief General Information

Migraine with aura affects between 3 and 5 % of the adult population in industrialized countries. It is usually a paroxysmal and benign disorder but occasionally poses complications with sometimes serious consequences. Complicated migraine is not a strictly defined term but was used in different context with different meaning and association. Migraine with aura itself was also referred to as complicated migraine.

Complicated migraine is also known as complex migraine or migraine accompagnée and included syndromes such as hemiplegic migraine, basilar artery migraine, ophthalmoplegic migraine, and retinal migraine. Many of these conditions are much better defined today, and the complications of migraine are specified in Chap. 1.4.1–1.4.4 of the ICHD-3 beta.

The true prevalence and incidence of the five characterized complications of migraine remains unknown, but currently available clinical evidence suggests that they are quite rare. Only 3 % of 8,821 patients treated in French tertiary headache centers over the past 11 years presented with status migrainosus or migraine aura status. Both conditions more commonly occur in patients with low frequent migraine with aura that have one or more precipitating factors such as stress and anxiety, menstruation, and lack of sleep. One third of patients report recurrence of these migraine complications with at least a second episode in their life. Migraine frequency and pain severity return to normal after the status is over.

Migrainous infarction is a rare but specific type of ischemic stroke developing during an attack of migraine with aura. Migraine with aura is a risk factor for ischemic stroke in women under the age of 45 years, particularly when combined with other risk factors such as smoking and oral contraceptives. Individuals with migraine with aura seem to have more white matter lesions and larger ischemic infarctions than control patients. However, only a minority of these strokes can be classified as migrainous infarction. Estimated incidence of migrainous infarction as high as 0.5–1.5 % of all strokes was suggested. The most common clinical presentation is homonymous visual field defect due to ischemia in the distribution of the posterior cerebral artery, but it may affect all vascular territories. The pathogenetic mechanisms responsible for migrainous infarction remain unresolved. It was suggested that insufficient regional blood flow following cortical spreading depression (CSD) in susceptible patients leads to the development of migrainous infarction. CSD is associated with alterations in vascular perfusion, with initial hyperemia followed by a longer period of reduced cerebral perfusion. In normal migraine auras this perfusion deficit is time limited, does not reach the ischemic threshold, and is associated with decreased neuronal metabolism. In migrainous infarction the ischemic threshold appears to be lowered thus leading to permanent cerebral damage and persistent neurological deficit. It was hypothesized that repeated vasoconstriction, migraine-induced platelet aggregation, and endothelial activation may lead to a higher susceptibility for ischemic events. In the diagnostic evaluation of suspected migrainous infarction, the reverse causality of ischemia-triggered migraine attacks must be considered as ischemia may trigger CSD resulting in a migraine attack. Out of 200 retrospectively reevaluated patients with the initial diagnosis migrainous infarction, only 40 fulfilled the ICHD-2 criteria. All others turned out to have other cardiac or vascular conditions more likely to be responsible for the stroke.

Suggested Reading

1. Agostoni E, Aliprandi A (2006) The complications of migraine with aura. Neurol Sci 27(Suppl 2): S91–S95
2. Arboix A, Gonzalez-Peris S, Grive E, Sanchez MJ, Comes E (2013) Cortical laminar necrosis related to migrainous cerebral infarction. World J Clin Cases 1:256–259
3. Beltramone M, Donnet A (2014) Status migrainosus and migraine aura status in a French tertiary-care center: an 11-year retrospective analysis. Cephalalgia 34(8):633–637
4. Headache Classification Committee of the International Headache, S. (2013) The International Classification of Headache Disorders, 3rd edition (beta version). Cephalalgia 33:629–808
5. Laurell K, Lundstrom E (2012) Migrainous infarction: aspects on risk factors and therapy. Curr Pain Headache Rep 16:255–260
6. Rothner AD (2002) Complicated migraine and migraine variants. Curr Pain Headache Rep 6:233–239

Chapter 8
Migraine with Aura: A CADASIL Case

Sanne van Sonsbeek, Joost Haan, and Michel D. Ferrari

8.1 Case Description

This patient was a 42-year-old man who had suffered from headache attacks since he was 24 years old. Most of the attacks started with a gray dot in the corner of the right visual field, increasing to a right hemianopsia within 20 min, which quickly disappeared. There never were left-sided visual disturbances. During some of the attacks there were right-sided paresthesias in the arm and face; once his wife noticed slurred speech. Left-sided throbbing headache normally occurred shortly after the disappearance of these symptoms, with some nausea and photophobia and lasting for 1 or 2 days. One or two tablets of paracetamol would sufficiently decrease the intensity of the pain and enable continuance of daily activities. Frequency of the attacks varied from only one per year to once per month. A diagnosis of migraine with aura was made, with no need for further analysis or adjustment of treatment.

Nevertheless, he now visited our outpatient clinic because in the last 2 months he noticed a change in frequency of the attacks and a change in the occurrence of the symptoms. The visual symptoms might occur up to four times per day, sometimes without headache. They were still strictly right sided, but lasted up to 2 h. Neurological examination showed no abnormalities, and his blood pressure was normal.

S. van Sonsbeek, MD
Department of Neurology, Rijnland Hospital Leiderdorp, Leiderdorp, The Netherlands

J. Haan, MD, PhD (✉)
Department of Neurology, Rijnland Hospital Leiderdorp, Leiderdorp, The Netherlands

Department of Neurology, Leiden University Medical Center, Leiden, The Netherlands
e-mail: j.haan@lumc.nl

M.D. Ferrari, MD, PhD
Department of Neurology, Leiden University Medical Center, Leiden, The Netherlands

A. Siva, C. Lampl (eds.), *Case-Based Diagnosis and Management of Headache Disorders*, Headache, DOI 10.1007/978-3-319-06886-2_8

8.2 Differential Diagnosis and How to Work Up This Type of Patient

The initial diagnosis was typical aura with migraine headache (International Classification of Headache Disorders; ICHD category 1.2.1). The aura consists of visual phenomena (enlarging scotoma in the left or right visual field) in 90 % of the cases, and in the remaining 10 % sensory, speech, or motor symptoms occur along with the visual symptoms. Typically, the aura symptoms slowly increase and last less than 60 min. In the case of multiple aura symptoms, the total duration of the aura can be proportionally longer, but none of the separate symptoms exceeds 60 min.

Neuroimaging is not needed to make a diagnosis of migraine in typical cases. Only when there are atypical symptoms, or abnormalities during neurological examination, must cerebral computed tomography or (preferably) magnetic resonance imaging (MRI) be considered. In population-based MRI studies of migraine patients, an increased prevalence of cerebral infarcts and white matter lesions was found, but this probably reflects more the underlying mechanism of migraine rather than its clinical importance.

In this patient, the symptoms had changed over the last 2 months. There were auras without headache and several auras per day, besides which the aura symptoms lasted longer than 60 min. In cases of prolonged aura and aura without headache, structural or vascular etiology must be considered. The same holds true for aura symptoms always occurring on the same side.

8.3 Diagnostic Workup of the Case

There were several alarm signals in this case to consider. First, a notable change occurred in the attack frequency. Migraine patients can experience periods with both more and fewer attacks, which is often explained by factors such as sleep deprivation, depression, overuse of analgesics or caffeine, or (in women) hormonal factors. Second, prolonged auras occurred. It is not known how often a structural abnormality is found in cases of atypical, prolonged auras. From clinical experience, however, it would seem that atypical aura symptoms (acute onset or prolonged aura) can in rare cases point to vasculopathies.

In this case it was also remarkable that the aura symptoms always occurred on the right side. Almost all patients with migraine with aura have a "preferred" side for the aura, but now and then experience symptoms on the other side. Aura symptoms always on the same side may indicate a (contralateral) structural lesion, such as an arteriovenous malformation or carotid dissection, and therefore warrant (cerebral) imaging.

An extended family history of the patient revealed that his older brother was diagnosed with multiple sclerosis (MS), as was a paternal aunt. The patient's father had suffered from ischemic strokes since the age of 45 years, for which no cause was found. At the age of 73 he was now severely demented, with pseudobulbar palsy and a right-sided hemiparesis. The paternal grandmother died at the age of 60 years, in a state of severe cognitive decline that had developed in a stepwise fashion over 10 years.

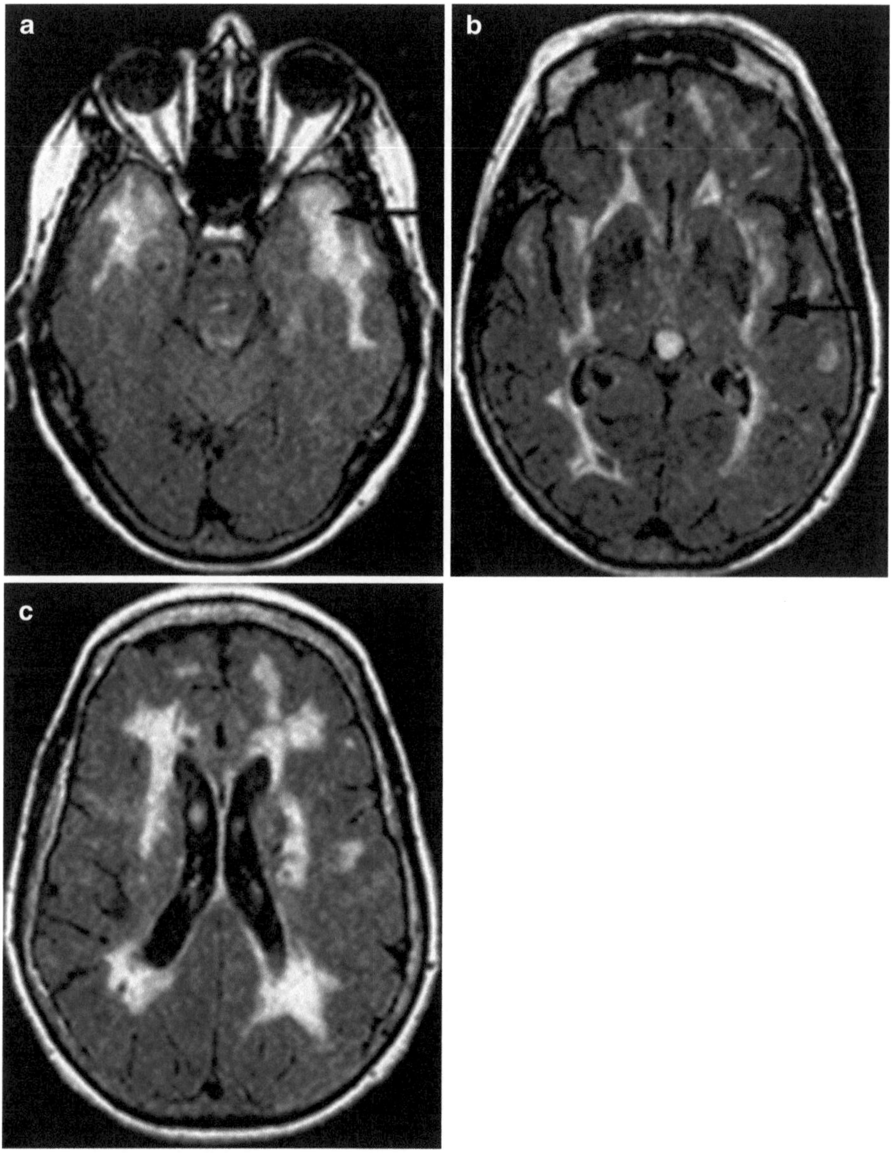

Fig. 8.1 Cerebral MRI scan showing extensive white matter hyperintensities (leukoencephalopathy) and multiple lacunar lesions. The white-matter hyperintensities were located periventricularly and in frontal, parietal, and temporal lobes of both hemispheres. There was also involvement of the external capsules (**a**) White matter lesions in the anterior temporal lobe (*arrow*), typical for CADASIL; (**b**) involvement of the external capsule (*arrow*); (**c**) extensive bilateral leukoencephalopathy with subcortical lacunar infarcts

A cerebral MRI scan was performed (Fig. 8.1), which showed extensive white matter hyperintensities (leukoencephalopathy) and multiple lacunar lesions. The white matter hyperintensities were located periventricularly and in frontal, parietal, and temporal lobes of both hemispheres. There was also involvement of the external capsules (Fig. 8.1). General laboratory screening (including blood chemistry and lipid spectrum) and additional hypercoagulability screening, as per usual in young stroke patients, did not reveal any abnormalities. Cardiac screening including a transesophageal echo did not show a source of cardiac embolism.

Based on the MRI findings of white matter hyperintensities one may consider MS, but the finding of lacunar lesions (at the age of 42) and the remarkable family history made this less likely. The family history raised the suspicion of CADASIL (cerebral autosomal dominant arteriopathy with subcortical infarcts and leukoencephalopathy). DNA analysis of the NOTCH3 gene, located on chromosome 19, indeed showed a mutation in exon 4 of this gene. Subsequent analysis showed that the brother and aunt (who were both thought to suffer from MS), in addition to the father of the patient, all carried the same mutation. On reconsideration, all affected family members were discovered to have a cerebral MRI appearance typical for CADASIL.

8.4 Summary of the Case

This 42-year-old man suffered from typical migraine attacks with (strictly unilateral) aura, but recently the frequency of the attacks had increased and atypical, prolonged visual auras had occurred. Structural and vascular causes had to be considered. An MRI scan showed lacunar lesions and extensive leukoencephalopathy. This typical image and the remarkable family history raised the suspicion of CADASIL, confirmed at DNA analysis by the NOTCH3 gene. Additional laboratory and cardiac screening ruled out other causes of (young) stroke.

8.5 CADASIL: Migraine, Stroke, Dementia, and More

CADASIL is a hereditary microangiopathy caused by mutations in the NOTCH3 gene on chromosome 19. Many different mutations in this gene have been found. The main features of CADASIL are ischemic episodes, cognitive deficits, migraine with aura, and mood disorders. The course of the disease can vary between families and between members of the same family.

Migraine affects 20–40 % of mutation carriers and often is the presenting symptom, with a mean age of onset in the mid-20s. Most CADASIL patients suffer from migraine with aura. The aura can vary from typical visual symptoms to extensive sensorimotor involvement, speech problems, and hemiplegia. Auras are often prolonged and atypical. CADASIL can also lead to sudden coma.

Of symptomatic individuals, 70–85 % experience (recurrent) ischemic episodes (transient ischemic attacks or strokes). After migraine, ischemic events are the most frequent presenting symptoms, with a reported mean age of onset of 41–49 years, ranging between 20 and beyond 60 years.

Cognitive deficits are also frequent in CADASIL and include attention deficits, mental slowness, and executive disorders. The cognitive decline is attributed to leukoencephalopathy and (multiple) lacunar infarctions. Cognitive disorders, however,

Table 8.1 Neuroimaging: MRI features of CADASIL

White matter signal hyperintensities (leukoencephalopathy) and lacunar lesions
Bilateral: almost symmetrically distributed within the white matter
Located at subcortical areas mostly in the frontal lobes, followed by the anterior temporal and parietal lobes, and external capsules
Presence of lacunar lesions mostly begins to appear in the fourth decade, besides which the deep white matter can also be present in the external and internal capsules, basal ganglia, thalamus, and brainstem
Lesion load and distribution significantly increases with age

can also be found before the onset of ischemic stroke. Most patients experience gradual cognitive deterioration, finally progressing to a subcortical dementia. In addition, 20–30 % of CADASIL patients suffer from psychiatric disorders, mostly mood disorders. Epileptic seizures, probably secondary to (multiple) strokes, have been reported in 5–10 % of patients.

Neuroimaging features of CADASIL (Table 8.1) include white matter signal hyperintensities (leukoencephalopathy) and lacunar lesions. In symptomatic patients, white matter hyperintensities are symmetrically distributed and are located in the periventricular and deep white matter. Within the white matter, lesions occur mostly in the frontal lobe, followed by the temporal and parietal lobes. Distinctive for young (20–30 years) and often asymptomatic mutation carriers is the presence of white matter abnormalities in the anterior temporal lobes, with the rest of the white matter unaffected (apart from periventricular caps). The presence of lacunar lesions increases significantly with age, and begins to appear in the fourth decade. These lesions are most frequently located in the deep white matter, but can also be present in the basal ganglia, thalamus, internal and external capsules, and brainstem.

8.6 Brief General Information

In patients presenting with atypical migraine aura or (lacunar) stroke at a young age without other cardiovascular risk factors, a detailed family history should be obtained. In cases of alarm symptoms in patients with migraine, an MRI scan should be included in the workup. CADASIL is a diagnosis that can be made on the clinical presentation in combination with family history and MRI. The detection of a mutation in the NOTCH3 gene on chromosome 19 confirms the diagnosis.

There are no treatment options for CADASIL. Some physicians prescribe salicylic acid or other anticoagulants, as is common practice in stroke prevention. Nevertheless, the effects of such agents on CADASIL patients are unclear. As one-third of patients with CADASIL show cerebral microbleeds on MRI, anticoagulants can even form a possible risk for cerebral hemorrhage.

Common sense dictates adequate management of cerebrovascular and lifestyle factors such as high blood pressure and cholesterolemia. However, not much is known about the effects of these interventions on the natural course of the disease in the long term.

Key Points for Patients with Migraine and Atypical or Prolonged Aura

- Atypical or prolonged aura must be specified and demands further analysis.
- In persistent aura, neuroimaging should always be in the workup.
- The differential diagnosis for headache and stroke is broad and includes giant cell arteritis, vasculitis, dural venous sinus thrombosis, arterial dissection, meningitis, reversible cerebral vasoconstriction syndrome, and many other diseases.
- A detailed family history and neuroimaging can give clues for the presence of hereditary diseases such as MELAS (mitochondrial encephalopathy, lactic acidosis, and stroke-like episodes) and CADASIL in migraine patients.

Suggested Reading

1. Adib-Samii P, Brice G, Martin RJ et al (2010) Clinical spectrum of CADASIL and the effect of cardiovascular risk factors on phenotype: study in 200 consecutively recruited individuals. Stroke 41:630–634
2. Chabriat H, Vahedi K, Iba-Zizen MT et al (1995) Clinical spectrum of CADASIL: a study of 7 families. Lancet 346:934–939
3. Chabriat H, Joutel A, Dichgans M et al (2009) CADASIL. Lancet Neurol 8:643–653
4. Headache Classification Committee of the International Headache Society (IHS) (2013) The International Classification of Headache Disorders (ICHD), 3rd edition (beta version). Cephalalgia 33:629–808
5. Levin M (2012) Resident and fellow section. Headache 52:687–693
6. Narayan SK, Gorman G, Kalaria RN et al (2012) The minimum prevalence of CADASIL in northeast England. Neurology 78:1025–1027
7. Palm-Meinders IH, Koppen H, Terwindt GM et al (2012) Structural brain changes in migraine. JAMA 308:1889–1897

Chapter 9
Syndrome of Transient Headache and Neurological Deficits with Cerebrospinal Fluid Lymphocytosis (HaNDL)

Julio Pascual and Nuria Riesco

9.1 Case Presentation

This 33-year-old teacher came to our emergency ward due to headache and speech difficulties. One hour earlier he had told his wife that he noticed headache, "I feel all my head pulsating darling". He took a paracetamol pill and went to bed. Twenty minutes later her wife found him agitated and with an incoherent and unintelligible speech. His wife called the emergency services and stroke code was activated. When he arrived he was conscious but tended to remain with his eyes closed and with his hands on his head. Global aphasia was evident and there seemed to be a slight motor weakness of his right extremities, where an indifferent plantar response was obtained. There were no apparent hemianopsia, meningeal signs, and abnormalities in the cranial nerves, including optic fundi, or in the neurovascular examination. Systemic examination was unremarkable, except for a slight axillary temperature elevation (37.6 °C). His blood pressure was 115/067 mmHg. Her wife explained us that 2 days earlier he had visited his GP due to an episode of pulsating headache, which lasted about 5 h and was accompanied by some feeling of numbness in his right hemibody. He was already asymptomatic and his physical exam was normal. His GP thought he had experienced a migraine attack with aura and gave an appointment for his neurologist specialist in 3 weeks.

He had no medical antecedents and took no medication. His wife said he had had some diarrhoea and general malaise 2 weeks earlier for about 2 days. Her mother had had, especially in her 30s, attacks of migraine both without aura and with typical aura. His father and two brothers were healthy and did not refer to a headache history.

J. Pascual, MD, PhD (✉) • N. Riesco
Neuroscience Area, Service of Neurology, University Hospital Central de Asturias and Ineuropa, La Corredoria s/n, 33011 Oviedo, Spain
e-mail: juliopascual@telefonica.net

A. Siva, C. Lampl (eds.), *Case-Based Diagnosis and Management of Headache Disorders*, Headache, DOI 10.1007/978-3-319-06886-2_9

9.2 Differential Diagnosis and How to Work Up This Kind of Patient

Even though the majority of patients consulting due to headache suffer from primary headaches, this patient came to our hospital due to an acute development of headache and symptoms and signs suggesting damage in cortical areas in his left hemisphere, which is one of the red flags on approaching a patient consulting due to head pain. What would be the diagnostic possibilities in this particular patient? A space-occupying lesion with an acute impairment, such as a haemorrhage within a neoplasm, would be the first diagnosis to be ruled out in terms of severity. When confronted with a patient with acute headache and remarkable focal signs, the first mandatory step is to obtain immediately a computerised tomography (CT) scan, preferably with and without contrast, to rule out a space-occupying lesion, which could justify his clinical picture. Thorax X-rays and urgent laboratory determinations are a mandatory first step in these patients.

The patient had no medical antecedent suggesting a neoplasm and came to our hospital as a stroke code. In fact, he had had an episode of right hemicorporal numbness which could be interpreted as a transient ischemic attack 2 days earlier. Therefore, if his admission CT scan is normal, the next immediate step would be to obtain an angio-CT of cranio-cervical vessels together with a diffusion-perfusion CT to rule out acute ischemic stroke. There are several clinical clues which do not support the possibility that acute ischemic stroke is the reason for our patient's clinical picture. First, headache was a very prominent symptom in this case, even in the first transient episode, and preceded the focal symptoms. Second, this is a young patient with no known medical antecedents. Angio-CT would also serve to rule out or confirm other diagnostic possibilities for this patient, "the syndrome of reversible cerebral vasoconstriction", which manifests as recurrent episodes of headache and a variety of focal symptoms.

This patient had a slight temperature elevation, headache, and prominent aphasia. Once a space-occupying lesion has been ruled out, it is also mandatory to exclude, by means of a lumbar puncture, a viral meningoencephalitis, mainly of herpetic origin. The opening cerebrospinal pressure, its aspect, the presence, type and number of cells, biochemistry, and microbiology must be studied.

Is migraine with aura a diagnostic option for this patient? Even though we cannot rule out 100 % of this possibility, there are several potent arguments, which do not support migraine with aura as his diagnosis. First, he did not have a history of previous headaches and most migraineurs have experienced their first migraine attacks well below age 30. The prevalence of migraine is so high, almost 20 % of the population, that we must be very careful on interpreting family antecedents. Just by chance, therefore, one out of five subjects in a given family will suffer from migraine attacks. Second, in this case there were no visual symptoms, which are noticed in more than 90 % of migraine auras. Also both prolonged aura duration and appearance after headache initiation are not typical of migraine with aura attacks. Finally, there are other aspects of the clinical history, such as gender or bilateral location of pain, which are not typical for migraine.

9.3 Diagnostic Workup of the Case

On admission his laboratory determinations, including biochemistry, haematology and clotting tests, ECG, thorax X-rays, and brain CT scan, were unremarkable. A cranio-cervical angio-CT and brain diffusion-perfusion imaging were also normal. A lumbar puncture was performed with the following immediate results: opening pressure 220 mm H_2O, glucose 60 mg/dl, protein 79 mg/dl, and 167 cells (98 % lymphocytes). Four hours after his arrival to our hospital, he became totally asymptomatic. Intravenous acyclovir was initiated. Brain MRI, angio-MRI, and an echocardiogram disclosed no abnormalities. A brain SPECT and an EEG, obtained 10 and 12 h after his arrival, showed decreased parietotemporal uptake in the left hemisphere and a generalised slowing over the left hemisphere, respectively. All cerebrospinal serologies and cultures were negative, including PCR herpes screening. Both SPECT and EEG results were within normal limits 2 days later. Acyclovir was stopped. He remained asymptomatic for 3 days, but after that period, he experienced two similar new episodes (in 1 week) of bilateral headache plus aphasia and right hemicorporal numbness and weakness lasting 6 h in one case and left hemicorporal numbness and weakness lasting 5 h in the other. A new lumbar tap 1 week after admission showed 278 cells (100 % lymphocytes), 87 mg/dl protein, normal glucose, and negative microbiological studies. The patient remained asymptomatic. A new lumbar tap, 2 months later, was within normal limits.

9.4 Summary of the Case

This otherwise healthy 33-year-old man came to our hospital due to two episodes in 48 h of bilateral headache and focal symptoms in his left hemisphere, both lasting several hours and resolving spontaneously. His interictal systemic and neurological exams were normal, except for the presence of a slight temperature elevation. A structural lesion was ruled out by the emergency CT scan. In addition, an evolving stroke or the syndrome of reversible vasoconstriction was also excluded by the normality of the cranial angio-CT and diffusion-perfusion studies. A lumbar tap found moderate lymphocytic pleocytosis with hyperproteinorrachia and normal glucose in a cerebrospinal fluid with increased pressure. All microbiological studies were negative, as well as cranial MRI and angio-MRI and echocardiogram, but both acute brain SPECT (Fig. 9.1) and EEG (Fig. 9.2) were suggestive of hypofunction of the left hemisphere. In spite of acyclovir treatment, he experienced a few days after admission two new reversible episodes of bilateral, pulsating headache and focal symptoms (in the right hemisphere in one occasion and in the left hemisphere in the last attack) lasting hours. After those episodes he remained asymptomatic and cerebrospinal fluid normalised in 2 months. This constellation of symptoms/signs and complementary studies is diagnostic of the syndrome of transient headache and neurological deficits with cerebrospinal fluid lymphocytosis (HaNDL).

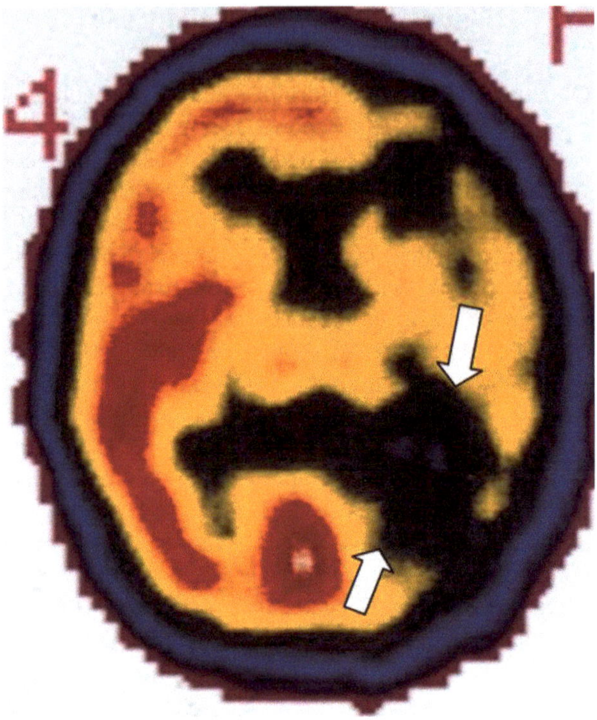

Fig. 9.1 Brain SPECT done the day after admission showing decreased radionuclide uptake in left hemisphere, predominantly in its posterior areas (*arrows*)

9.5 Definition of HaNDL

According to the "International Classification of Headache Disorders, 3rd edition (beta version)", the syndrome of HaNDL is described as migraine-like headache episodes accompanied by neurological deficit including hemicorporal paraesthesia and/or weakness and/or dysphasia, but positive visual symptoms only uncommonly, lasting >4 h. There is lymphocytic pleocytosis. The disorder resolves spontaneously within 3 months. As expected with all other set of criteria, this syndrome should not be better explained by any other ICDH-3 diagnosis.

9.6 Brief General Information

The clinical picture of HaNDL is of 1–12 discrete episodes of transient neurological deficits accompanied or followed by moderate to severe headache. Most of the episodes last several hours but some may last for more than 24 h. The neurological manifestations include sensory symptoms in about three quarters of cases, aphasia in two thirds, and motor deficits in a little over half. Migraine-aura-like visual symptoms are relatively uncommon (fewer than 20 % of cases). The syndrome is more common in males around 30 and resolves within 3 months without treatment.

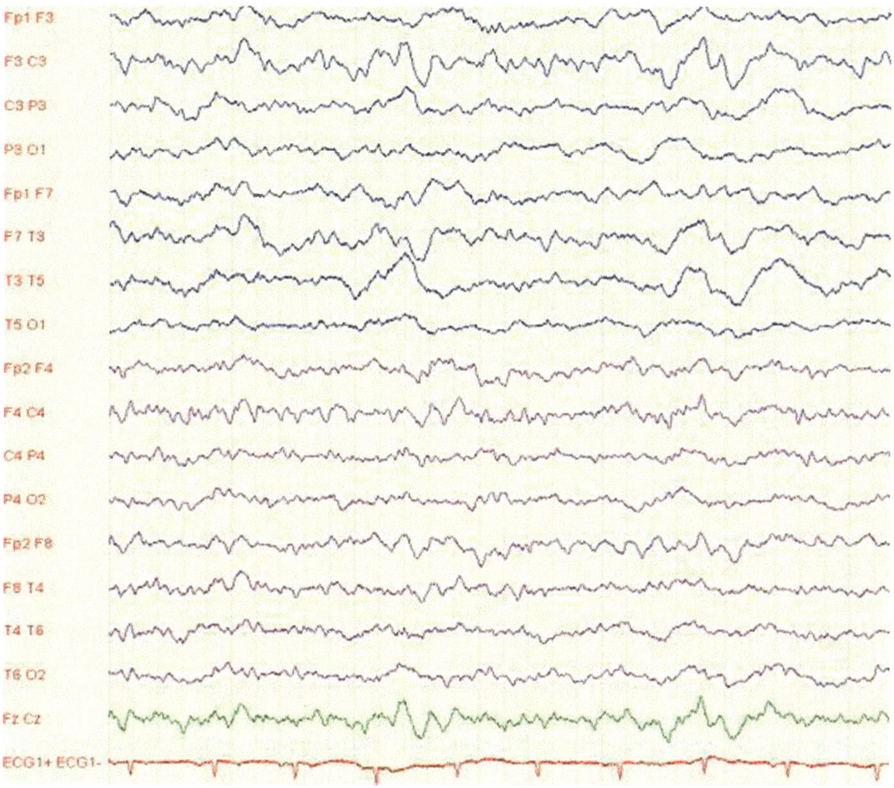

Fig. 9.2 EEG carried out 16 h showing generalised slowing over the left hemisphere

In addition to CSF lymphocytosis (up to 760 cells/µl), there are elevations of CSF total protein (up to 250 mg/dl) in >90 % of cases and of CSF pressure (up to 400 mm CSF) in more than 50 % of cases. Even though the aetiology of the syndrome is not known, the presence of a viral prodrome in at least one quarter of cases has raised the possibility of an autoimmune pathogenesis. A recent description of antibodies to a subunit of the T-type voltage-gated calcium channel CACNA1H in the sera of two patients with this disorder supports this view.

Increased cerebrospinal pressure is occasionally present. Routine CT and MRI scans (with or without intravenous contrast) and angiography are invariably normal when performed outside of an episode. Microbiological studies have been uniformly normal. EEG and SPECT scans may show focally abnormal areas consistent with the focal neurological deficits.

Most patients with this syndrome have no prior history of migraine. The clinician must consider other diagnoses that may share some of its clinical features, including hemiplegic migraine, neuroborreliosis, neurosyphilis, neurobrucellosis, mycoplasma, granulomatous and neoplastic arachnoiditis, encephalitis, and CNS vasculitis.

Key Points for the Diagnosis of HaNDL

- Men between 20 and 40 years of age
- "Viral" antecedent infection 2–3 weeks earlier
- Up to 12 episodes of moderate-severe bilateral headache accompanied by changing neurological deficits and occasionally some temperature elevation
- Most common: numbness + aphasia > hemiparesis lasting up to several days (mean 5 h)
- Total resolution within 3 months
- Cerebrospinal fluid: lymphocytosis with negative aetiological results
- Normal neuroimaging
- EEG: transient focal slowing
- SPECT: focal decreased uptake

Suggested Reading

1. Bartelson JD, Swanson JW, Whisnant JP (1981) A migrainous syndrome with cerebrospinal fluid lymphocytosis. Neurology 31:1257–1262
2. Berg MJ, Williams LS (1995) The transient syndrome of headache with neurologic deficits and CSF lymphocytosis. Neurology 45:1648–1654
3. Chapman KM, Szczygielski BI, Toth C et al (2003) Pseudomigraine and lymphocytic pleocytosis: calcium channelopathy? Clinical description of 10 cases and genetic analysis of the familial hemiplegic migraine gene CACNA1A. Headache 43:892–895
4. Gomez-Aranda F, Canadillas F, Marti-Massó JF et al (1997) Pseudomigraine with temporary neurological symptoms and lymphocytic pleocytosis: a report of 50 cases. Brain 120: 1105–1113
5. Guillan M, Alonso-Canovas A, González-Valcarcel J et al (2012) Stroke mimics treated with thrombolysis: further evidence on safety and distinctive clinical features. Cerebrovasc Dis 34:115–1120
6. Headache Classification Subcommittee of the International Headache Society (2013) The International Classification of Headache Disorders ICHD-III, beta version. Cephalalgia 33: 629–808
7. Kurtuncu M, Kaya D, Zuliani L et al (2013) CACNA1H antibodies associated with headache with neurological deficits and cerebrospinal fluid pleocytosis (HaNDL). Cephalalgia 32: 123–129
8. Pascual J, Valle N (2013) Pseudomigraine with lymphocytic pleocytosis. Curr Pain Headache Rep 7:224–228

Chapter 10
Migraine Patient with MRI Lesions

Peter S. Sandor and Andreas R. Gantenbein

10.1 Case Description

A 32-year-old chef having migraine without aura since the age of 22 suffered an epileptic tonic-clonic seizure a week before Christmas. He was brought to the emergency department, diagnosed with a low-grade glioma in the right parietal lobe and operated on the following day successfully. Pathology revealed grade II oligodendroglyoma. The postoperative imaging showed complete removal of the tumour, with some scar tissue at the place the craniotomy had been performed (Fig. 10.1).

Initially, his neurological examination was described to be unremarkable, but he strongly complained of severe migraine-type headaches, that, except for their intensity and daily occurrence, were very similar to the migraines he had experienced before the operation.

He also complained of difficulties falling asleep and it often took him until the early morning until he was able to get some rest.

About 2 months after the operation, he was referred to our specialized headache clinic. Until that time, he had not worked yet and his relationship to his girlfriend had become very difficult, as he had become a completely different person after the operation: without initiative, not sleeping, moderately depressed and about to lose his work due to these changes.

Thereafter, he was treated on monotherapy using valproate, topiramate and lamotrigine for control of both headaches with migrainous phenotype and epileptic discharges. As monotherapies were unsuccessful, combination treatments with

P.S. Sandor (✉)
ANNR Neurology RehaClinic, Im Ergel, Baden, Aargau 5404, Switzerland
e-mail: p.sandor@rehaclinic.ch, peter.s.sandor@gmail.com

A.R. Gantenbein
Department of Neurology RehaClinic, Quellenstrasse, Bad Zurzach, Aargau 5330, Switzerland
e-mail: a.gantenbein@rehaclinic.ch

A. Siva, C. Lampl (eds.), *Case-Based Diagnosis and Management of Headache Disorders*, Headache, DOI 10.1007/978-3-319-06886-2_10

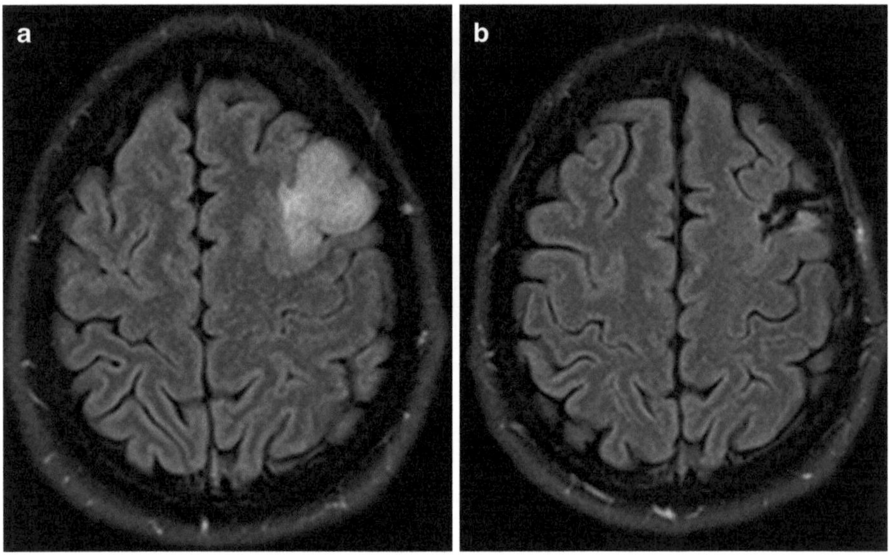

Fig. 10.1 T2-weighted MRI before (**a**) and 1 year after the operation (**b**) of a low-grade glioma. In the follow-up image, the craniotomy site and some degree of gliosis are to be seen

additional SNRIs (duloxetine, venlafaxine) were initiated, again, without clinically significant control of his headaches. All of the above treatments were tried in increasing dosages and at high doses for a sufficient length of time.

EEG, that was made every 3 months during the first year after referral, showed a breech rhythm, but was otherwise unremarkable. In one occasion, about 6 months after the operation, the patient came to the emergency unit complaining about excruciating migraine-type headaches, indicating that he was considering suicide. He was admitted to the medical department under neurological supervision, and the EEG showed mild slowing together with serial (up to 2 s) spike-wave complexes in the region of the operation site. Valproate serum levels were low, and, after having both corrected dosage and controlled for regular intake, resulting in therapeutic serum levels, the headaches returned to their previous levels of mostly moderate intensity.

One month after this, he presented routinely in the clinic complaining of a new symptom, which was a bizarre tremor of the legs resulting in difficulties walking, but without falls. He provided the information that he had finally lost both his work and his girlfriend. Another MRI and an EEG recording did not show any unexpected abnormality. His leg tremor was suspected to be of functional origin, which was confirmed by two other neurological colleagues having examined the patient at this occasion.

A psychiatrist was involved and diagnosed a pathological stress reaction with psychosomatic symptoms in addition to the neurological problems. The psychiatric opinion was that the chronic headaches with migrainous phenotype might well be of psychosomatic origin altogether, resulting from the difficulties to adapt to having been diagnosed with a brain tumour. Psychotherapy was initiated on an outpatient basis, without any benefit for 6 months. A subsequent psychosomatic hospitalization was discontinued by the treating psychiatrist because the patient had a tonic-clonic seizure that was diagnosed to be most probably functional in the neurological department where the patient had been brought to.

In the course of the disease, the patient was stabilized as far as his headache and sleep were concerned, but up to now, 2 years after his operation, has not returned to his previous life. He lives on a small invalidity pension and has started to work a few hours per week helping his successor as a chef in the same restaurant he had been prior to his operation.

10.2 Differevntial Diagnosis and How to Work Up This Kind of Patient

In this patient the differential diagnosis is complex; as for his headaches, his seizures and his behaviour, both somatic and functional might play a significant role.

The tumour is a somatic diagnosis and the exstirpation certainly might lead to *chronic post-craniotomy headaches*. Their classification according to the International Headache Society is possible without any phenotypic description, so migrainous features can well be accepted in this context. Thinking pathophysiologically, the headaches might be considered to be *chronic migraine*, triggered by the craniotomy based on previous episodic migraines. Classification following these pathophysiological considerations is not possible in the International Headache Society framework, but did influence the choice of prophylactic medication. There is a third possibility to account for at least the very strong headaches during repetitive epileptic discharges: *hemicrania epileptica*. As the onset of the excruciatingly strong headaches was not observed, a classification of these headaches cannot be made, but an epileptic origin of the exacerbation remains highly probable.

The role of *psychosomatic aspects* in this complex health problem is difficult to establish. It is reasonable to think that it might be considerable. However, concerning the headaches, there is sufficient evidence supporting a somatic origin that other causes are not necessary to explain the clinical picture. In the context of (peudo?-) seizures, this seems to be more complex.

10.3 Diagnostic Work-Up of the Case

In this patient, regular EEG recordings and MRI imaging but also blood tests including serum levels of antiepileptics/headache prophylactic substances complimented the rather frequent clinical appointments. The most important "diagnostic work-up" has been a good and trustful relationship accepting the complex and not merely neurological nature of the disorders.

10.4 Summary of the Case

This is a young episodic migraineur having been diagnosed with a low-grade glioma after a first epileptic seizure. After tumour extirpation, he suffered chronic, migraine-like post-craniotomy headache along with complex partly psychosomatic disturbances, and he was largely resistant to pharmacotherapy, but could be stabilized on a modest level.

10.5 Definition According to the International Classification of Headache Disorders (ICHD)

According to ICHD-II as well as ICHD-3 beta, the relevant diagnoses are episodic migraine without aura before the tumour and post-craniotomy headache and hemicrania epileptica in the clinical course of disease.

Key Points

- It seems to be key that most headaches can be pathophysiologically interpreted, facilitating a scientifically based approach concerning prophylaxis.
- Further, only very rarely, and certainly not in this case, can headaches convincingly be explained as of functional origin.
- The therapeutic relationship between headache specialist and patient seems to be important to result in – at least – some degree of improvement.

Suggested Reading

1. Cianchetti C, Pruna D, Ledda M (2013) Epileptic seizures and headache/migraine: a review of types of association and terminology. Seizure 22:679–685
2. De Gray LC, Matta BF (2005) Acute and chronic pain following craniotomy: a review. Anaesthesia 60:693–704
3. ICHD-3 beta. http://www.ihs-classification.org/_downloads/mixed/International-Headache-Classification-III-ICHD-III-2013-Beta.pdf
4. Kaur A, Selwa L, Fromes G, Ross D (2000) Persistent headache after supratentorial craniotomy. Neurosurgery 47:633–636
5. Rocha-Filho P, Gherpelli J, de Siqueira J, Rabello G (2010) Post-craniotomy headache: a proposed revision of IHS diagnostic criteria. Cephalalgia 30(5):560–566
6. Schankin CJ, Gall C, Straube A (2009) Headache syndromes after acoustic neuroma surgery and their implications for quality of life. Cephalalgia 29:760–771
7. Voigt K, Nagel A, Meyer B et al (2010) Towards positive diagnostic criteria: a systematic review of somatoform disorder diagnoses and suggestions for future classification. J Psychosom Res 68:403–414

Chapter 11
Migraine and Patent Foramen Ovale

Dagny Holle

11.1 Case Description

A 50-year-old shop assistant was admitted to my clinic from the cardiologist for neurological examination before planned patent foramen ovale (PFO) closure. The woman reported that she suffers from an episodic migraine since her 20s. Approximately four times a month, she has severe pulsating headache attacks accompanied by nausea, phono-, and photophobia. Pain is aggravated by routine physical activity and she prefers to lie down and sleep. Sometimes she sees flickering lights for approximately 15 min in terms of a visual aura before headache starts. When pain gets worse she takes ibuprofen which shows some beneficial effect. A prophylactic medication has never been tried.

The patient reported that she had a gastrointestinal infection a few weeks ago. She had to lie in bed for a few days and could not adequately eat and drink. When she tried to go to the toilet and rose up quite rapidly, she realized drowsiness and passed out. Her husband told that she slumped to the ground but regained consciousness within a few seconds. When she was brought to the emergency room, a low blood pressure was measured and the event was attributed to syncope. The further cardiologic diagnostic evaluation included transesophageal echogram (TEE) which showed a patent foramen ovale (PFO) but no further pathology. The PFO was medium in size showing a shunt during provocative maneuver (Valsalva) but not spontaneously. A cerebral MRI and EEG which showed no pathological findings had been performed, additionally.

When the patient was released, the cardiologist told her that no other reason for syncope was found than orthostatic dysregulation during gastrointestinal infection.

D. Holle
Department of Neurology, Westgerman Headache Center,
University Hospital Essen, Hufelandstr. 55, Essen, NRW 45127, Germany
e-mail: dagny.holle@uk-essen.de

A. Siva, C. Lampl (eds.), *Case-Based Diagnosis and Management of Headache Disorders*, Headache, DOI 10.1007/978-3-319-06886-2_11

Additionally, she was informed that she has a PFO "that is responsible for her migraine attacks." She was told that she "could be cured from the migraine by closure of the PFO."

The patient was quite excited about the chance never to suffer from a migraine attack again. She asked me about my opinion and was a little bit afraid of possible side effects of the intervention.

Her past medical and neurological history was unremarkable with the exception of a medically successful treated thyroid hypofunction. She told me that her sister and her daughters were also suffering from migraine attacks.

11.2 Differential Diagnosis and How to Work Up This Kind of a Patient

This patient suffers from an episodic migraine with visual aura according to the current IHS criteria. As she reports a typical clinical presentation and neurostatus was completely normal, no further differential diagnosis had to be pondered and no workup had to be done. A cerebral MRI had been already performed and did not show any pathology. However, cerebral imaging is not mandatory in these patients with clear migraine with aura.

11.3 Diagnostic Workup of the Case

No further diagnostic workup had to be done in this patient. When the patient ask about the likelihood of cessation of her migraine after PFO closure, I told her that based on the available study data the efficacy of this procedure has not been proven, yet. I recommended her to conduct a PFO closure only within a controlled clinical trial or to refrain from intervention. Anyway, the chance of complete cessation of migraine attacks would be very unlikely. The patient was afraid from possible side effects of the intervention and decided to cancel her appointment for PFO closure. The patient was informed about alternative evidence-based treatment options in episodic migraine with aura including acute and prophylactic treatment options. Despite drug treatment, nonmedical treatment options such as sport, relaxation techniques, and optimization of sleep behavior were discussed with the patient.

11.4 Summary of the Case

A 50-year-old shop assistant with a typical episodic migraine with visual aura was diagnosed by chance with a PFO. The cardiologist offered her to close the PFO and, hereby, cure the migraine. The patient was send to my neurology clinic for evaluation before intervention. As the patient had never had a proper acute or prophylactic treatment of her migraine, I informed her about the treatment options according to the current evidence-based guidelines. Up to now, clinical trials could not confirm the efficacy of this procedure in treatment of migraine. Furthermore, although PFO closure is a quite safe intervention, side effects, even serious ones, might occur. PFO closures for treatment of migraine should only be performed within clinical trials that will help to assess the efficacy of this procedure in the future. Based on this information, the patient decided to cancel her appointment for PFO closure.

11.5 Definition of Patent Foramen Ovale (PFO)

The foramen ovale is an important anatomic structure during fetal development. It is a small flap-like opening located in the interartrial septum of the heart that enables the blood to bypass the nonfunctional fetal lungs. When the pulmonary vascular resistance drops right after birth, the pressure in the right atrium decreases which leads to a closure of the foramen ovale. Sometimes, intra-atrial septa do not grow together and the foramen ovale stays open. This remnant opening between the right and the left atrium is called patent foramen ovale (PFO). Although the PFO might be structurally open, usually, the left atrial pressure exceeds right atrial pressure resulting in a functionally closed PFO. Under some circumstances, these closed PFOs can open up again, e.g., during Valsalva maneuver. During Valsalva, backflow to the heart is markedly reduced and right and left atrial pressure will decrease. After discontinuation of Valsalva, the venous return flow will increase leading to an increase of the pressure in the right atrium that then exceeds left atrial pressure, facilitating the blood flow from the right to the left atrium. Additionally, also spontaneous PFOs exist that do not need further maneuvers to unclose (Fig. 11.1).

11.6 Brief General Information

A PFO is present in about 25 % of the general population. Many epidemiological studies showed that there is an association between migraine and particularly large PFOs. Especially in patients with migraine with aura, a PFO was present in up to 60 % of patients in some studies. In this context an autosomal-dominant inheritance of migraine and PFO was suggested. Some observational studies suggested that a closure of the PFO may treat migraine. About 80 % of patients who underwent PFO closure for nonmigraine indications reported cessation or improvement of migraine attacks after PFO closure. However, these data were limited because of retrospective nonrandomized study designs and highly selected patients. Therefore, there was a need for a randomized controlled study to assess the effect of the PFO closure compared with a sham procedure in migraine treatment. A blinded study design is mandatory as a high placebo effect can be expected in migraine trials in general and in an interventional trial in particular. The MIST study (Migraine Intervention with

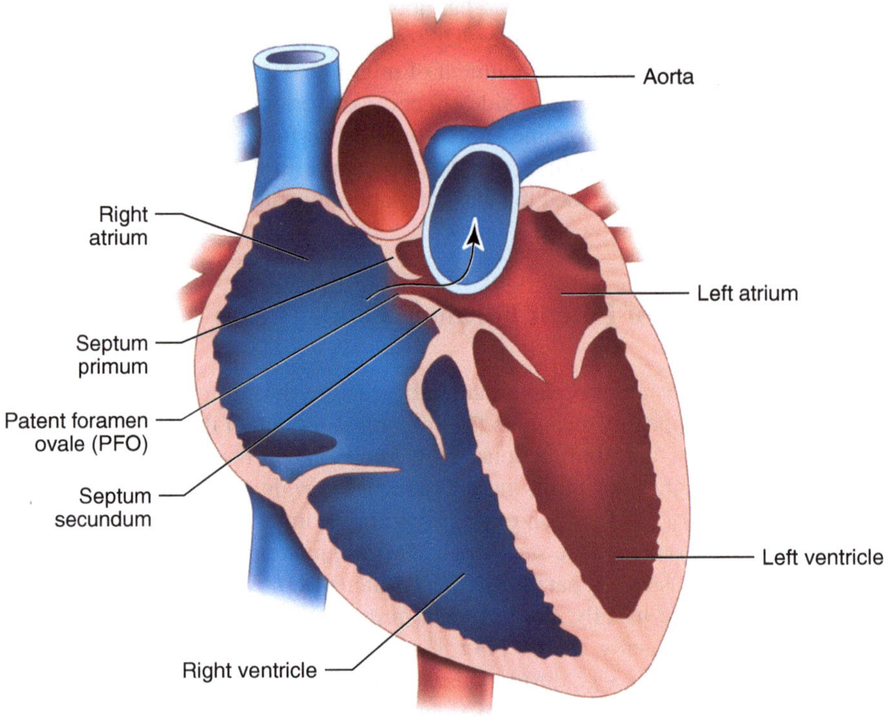

Fig. 11.1 Anatomy of the persistent patent foramen ovale (PFO). The PFO is an open flap that remains in some patients between the right and the left atrium of the heart. It allows the blood to bypass the lung and go directly from the body circulation to the brain

STARFlex® Technology) addressed this important question for the first time in a prospective randomized double-blind sham-controlled design. Patients with frequent migraine attacks and aura were included that had failed at least two classes of prophylactic medication. In total, 423 patients were screened for a PFO. In 38 % (163 patients) a moderate or large PFO could be diagnosed, confirming the high prevalence of right-to-left shunts in migraine patients with aura. The primary endpoint of complete cessation of migraine attacks was reached in 4 % of the patients in both intervention and sham intervention group which has no significant difference. The second endpoint was also not met as there was no significant difference regarding migraine frequency (Intervention: 3.23 ± 1.80 versus Sham procedure: 3.53 ± 2.13). In the context of the intervention, serious side effects were observed. One patient of the placebo group had an ischemic stroke. In conclusion, the MIST trial was not able to show the efficacy of PFO closure at least in the investigated patient population. Therefore, based on the currently available study data, PFO closure should not be performed for migraine treatment. A screening of migraine patients for a PFO is not necessary and useful as results do not change treatment recommendation but might worry some patients.

Key Points for Patients with PFO

- PFO is more prevalent in patients with migraine with aura.
- Migraine is not an indication to screen for a PFO.
- Up to now, routine PFO closure cannot be recommended for the treatment of migraine as the efficacy of this intervention has not been shown in a controlled trial.
- PFO closure as treatment of migraine should only be performed within the scope of a clinical trial.

Suggested Reading

1. Ailiani J (2014) Migraine and patent foramen ovale. Curr Neurol Neurosci Rep 14:426
2. Chambers J, Seed PT, Ridsdale L (2013) Association of migraine aura with patent foramen ovale and atrial septal aneurysms. Int J Cardiol 168:949–953
3. Davis D, Gregson J, Willeit P, Stephan B, Al-Shahi Salman R, Brayne C (2013) Patent foramen ovale, ischemic stroke and migraine: systematic review and stratified meta-analysis of association studies. Neuroepidemiology 40:56–67
4. Diener HC, Kurth T, Dodick D (2007) Patent foramen ovale and migraine. Curr Pain Headache Rep 11:236–240
5. Dowson A, Mullen MJ, Peatfield R et al (2008) Migraine intervention with STARFlex Technology (MIST) Trial. Circulation 117:1397–1404
6. Küper M, Rabe K, Holle D et al (2013) Prevalence of cardiac right left shunts in migraine: a population-based-control study. Neurol Sci 34(2):205–208
7. Post MC, Luermans LM, Plokker HWM, Budts W (2007) Patent foramen ovale and migraine. Cathete Cardiovasc Interv 69:9–14

Chapter 12
Refractory Chronic Migraine: Therapy with Combined Peripheral Neurostimulation

Roberto Arcioni and Paolo Martelletti

About 3 % of patients with episodic migraine each year trend toward a process of chronicity. These patients become refractory to prophylactic pharmacological therapy, leading to a high level of disability that affects their activities of daily living.

In 2003 Popeney published the first case series of 27 patients with refractory migraine who underwent occipital neurostimulation (ONS). After an 18-month follow-up, the results of this initial study were encouraging: 88 % of patients had a reduction in the number of attacks, and the intensity of headache was reduced by ≥50 %.

Anatomically, there is a functional relationship between the upper cervical sensitive afferents and the nucleus of the trigeminal nerve. This relationship has been demonstrated using animal models, from which the concept of the trigeminal cervical complex (TCC) was developed. The activation of the TTC is able to activate the parasympathetic autonomic response, which involves the sphenopalatine ganglion (SPG).

12.1 Case Description

The patient is a 49-year-old female shop assistant who has been under treatment at our center for about 10 years for progressive, difficult-to-treat migraine and tension-type headache localized to the occipital, left frontal, and left periorbital regions,

R. Arcioni
Pain Therapy Unit, Department of Medical, Surgical Science and Translational Medicine, Sapienza University of Rome, Sant'Andrea Hospital, Rome, Italy

P. Martelletti (✉)
Department of Clinical and Molecular Medicine, Regional Referral Headache Centre, Sapienza University of Rome, Sant'Andrea Hospital, Rome, Italy
e-mail: paolo.martelletti@uniroma1.it

A. Siva, C. Lampl (eds.), *Case-Based Diagnosis and Management of Headache Disorders*, Headache, DOI 10.1007/978-3-319-06886-2_12

with no coexisting painful diseases in anamnesis. During these years she has been treated prophylactically with anticonvulsants, tricyclic antidepressants, calcium channel blockers, and onabotulinumtoxin A.

She also has a history of uncontrolled use of drugs for acute migraine ranging throughout all of the pharmacological classes, such as acetaminophen, nonsteroidal anti-inflammatories, triptans, ergot derivatives, and drugs containing barbiturate combinations. Moreover, via "doctor shopping" she obtained opioids on prescription, which she tried without therapeutic success. She has since stopped using this wrong and harmful therapeutic approach.

For this reason she has fallen into a state of medication-overuse headache (MOH), which has been treated with seven repeated detoxification procedures, unresponsive to corticosteroids.

Visits to the emergency department became more frequent, with an increasing number of absences from work, and with a psychopathological profile clearly more oriented toward suicidal intent.

12.2 Differential Diagnosis

The absence of secondary pathology underlying the clinical diagnosis of chronic migraine followed by refractory chronic migraine was excluded twice, using magnetic resonance imaging, in November 2009 and then in December 2011.

12.3 Surgical Management

Considering the refractoriness to pharmacological therapy, it was decided in February 2012 to refer the patient for peripheral neurostimulation treatment.

Both ONS and supraorbital nerve stimulation (SONS) were the object of discussion regarding the therapeutic decision. As the current evidence base at the time reported the ONS to be the best interventional treatment for refractory chronic migraine with or without MOH, we decided to proceed with ONS, reserving the possibility to use SONS later.

In the 4 weeks before implant, the average self-reporting pain intensity was 5/6 on the Numeric Rating 11–point Scale (NRS), with 56 crises lasting 5–6 h with NRS 9/10. The patient took 32 tablets of ibuprofen 400 mg, 12 tablets of rizatriptan 10 mg, and 10 tablets of acetaminophen 500 mg/codeine 300 mg.

In April 2012, the patient was submitted to a workup in preparation for ONS.

She was first referred for psychological assessment to evaluate the psychosocial risk factors, after which colonization by methicillin-resistant *Staphylococcus aureus* was excluded by nasal swabbing.

The patient was placed in the prone position. After infiltration with local anesthetic, a midline access was chosen to avoid the occipital arteries and greater occipital nerve injury (5–28 mm lateral to midline). A vertical incision was made, extending approximately 4 cm caudal from a point 1 cm below the occipital protuberance. A subcutaneous pocket was fashioned by a lateral blunt dissection, exposing the fascia for anchoring.

A curved Tuohy needle, with a plastic stylet for easy removal, was advanced laterally 6–7 cm off midline, in a subcutaneous plane under ultrasound guidance to place the lead just above the fascia to a depth of approximately 0.8–1.2 cm.

One quadripolar lead (Pisces Quad Model 3487A-45; Medtronic, Inc, Minneapolis, MN, USA) was placed on each side and then anchored to the fascia of the lateral pocket by a plastic anchor and 2-0 nonabsorbable suture. To prevent lead migration, a strain loop was positioned in the occipital pocket.

Extensions were then tunneled and externalized to be connected to an external pulse generator.

The patient reported a significant reduction in the frequency and severity of her headaches during the 2-week trial period, and proceeded to permanent implantation under local anesthesia. Two extensions were tunneled down and connected to an implantable pulse generator (IPG) (Restore Ultra Model 3; Medtronic, Inc).

At 6-month follow-up, the patient's headache symptoms and prestimulator medications were significantly reduced.

In December 2012 the patient required an urgent visit because of worsening symptoms. In the previous month the symptoms had returned to the levels of the preimplantation period.

We tested different stimulation programs to change the polarity of contacts, rate, and pulse width, but with no therapeutic effect, so we decided to implant an additional electrode.

In January 2013 the patient underwent a new surgical procedure to activate the trigeminovascular complex, which is able to activate the parasympathetic autonomic response that involves the SPG. A left supraorbital eight-pole lead (Model 3778; Medtronic, Inc) was placed under local anesthesia and sedation.

The lead was positioned subcutaneously under ultrasound guidance, tangentially to the superciliary arch. It was tunneled under the skin above the ear to the occipital region and then to the IPG.

The occipital four-pole leads were both programmed (0−, 1−, 2−, 3+), with an amplitude of 1.6 V (right lead) and 1.4 V (left lead), pulse width of 110 ms, and frequency of 40 Hz. The eight-pole supraorbital lead was programmed (0+, 1+, 2−, 5+, 7−) with an amplitude of 1,2 V, pulse width of 90 ms, and frequency of 60 Hz.

At 6-month follow-up after supraorbital implant, the patient's headache symptoms and the intake of medication were significantly reduced. The average pain score was NRS 2/4, with 11 crises lasting 5–6 h with NRS 6/7. She took 2 tablets of ibuprofen 400 mg and 2 tablets of rizatriptan 10 mg.

At 12-month follow-up the patient's headache symptoms and medication regimen were stable to an extent comparable with the previous control.

12.4 Review

The positive outcome of this case confirms the results from Slavin, Reed, Linder, and Datta, whereby the ONS combined with SONS produced a synergistic effect.

In 2009 Reed published the first report on the use of combined ONS-SONS for chronic migraine. Promising results were reported in the series of seven patients, with six describing near complete resolution of the pain and associated neurological findings.

Linder first described the use of combined ONS-SONS in a group of adolescents, and reported very good results over the long term.

According to the Melzack and Wall theory of "gate control," the somatosensory neurostimulation of afferent fibers A and B stops the metameric nociceptive transmission. Therefore, the generally accepted clinical approach for the treatment of pain using neurostimulation is to produce a paresthesia in the same region where pain is perceived.

Despite this, previous studies have shown that ONS is able to modulate the pain even in regions metamerically discordant from C2/C3. For example, Schwedt, Magis, Dodick, Burns, Amin, and Asensio-Samper used ONS to treat frontal or supraorbital pain.

This particular analgesic effect of peripheral stimulation in the head is due to the particular and unique anatomy and physiology of the TCC, where all of the cephalic somatosensory afferents converge.

The combined neurostimulation, in particular from the occipital and trigeminal territory, synergistically activate the TCC.

Combined neurostimulation can be used for the management of refractory chronic migraine. In the case reported here, the patient was able to significantly reduce the intake of medications in addition to headache frequency and intensity. The efficacy of treatment was found to prevail at 12-month follow-up.

Key Points

- *Criteria for diagnosis of refractory chronic migraine*

  1. Diagnostic definition of chronic migraine following the International Classification of Headache Disorders 3 beta
  2. Unresponsive over time to preventive drugs including onabotulinumtoxinA
  3. Presence of MOH
  4. Unresponsive over time to the detoxification procedure for MOH

- *Multidisciplinary approach*
- The success of ONS depends on the close cooperation of the migraine physician, the psychologist, and the interventional pain physician.

1. The migraine physician makes the correct diagnosis, and states the indication for neurostimulation having established the ineffectiveness of medical therapy.
2. The psychologist assesses, by interview and the use of standardized measures, the mental health and social risk factors, in addition to the understanding of ONS by the patient and the expectations for the relief of pain.
3. The pain physician expert in neurostimulation performs the implant, minimizing the adverse events.

- *ONS adverse events*

1. Lead migration
2. Infection
3. Lack of efficacy
4. Lead malfunction
5. Battery malfunction
6. Pain at IPG
7. Lead skin erosion

Suggested Reading

1. Amin S, Buvanendran A, Park KS, Kroin JS, Moric M (2008) Peripheral nerve stimulator for the treatment of supraorbital neuralgia: a retrospective case series. Cephalalgia 28(4):355–359
2. Asensio-Samper JM, Villanueva VL, Pérez AV, López MD, Monsalve V, Moliner S, De Andrés J (2008) Peripheral neurostimulation in supraorbital neuralgia refractory to conventional therapy. Pain Pract 8(2):120–124
3. Bartsch T, Goadsby PJ (2003) Increased responses in trigeminocervical nociceptive neurons to cervical input after stimulation of the dura mater. Brain 126:1801–1813
4. Becser N, Bovim G, Sjaastad O (1998) Extracranial nerves in the posterior part of the head. Anatomic variations and their possible clinical significance. Spine 23(13):1435–1441
5. Burns B, Watkins L, Goadsby PJ (2009) Treatment of intractable chronic cluster headache by occipital nerve stimulation in 14 patients. Neurology 72:341–345
6. D'Amico D, Leone M, Grazzi L, Bussone G (2008) When should "chronic migraine" patients be considered "refractory" to pharmacological prophylaxis? Neurol Sci 29(Suppl 1):S55–S58
7. Datta S, Reed KL, Will KR (2011) Combined supraorbital and occipital nerve stimulation in failed surgical treatment of migraine: case report and review of the literature [abstract]. Presented at American Society of Intervention Pain Physicians 2012 Annual Meeting, Washington DC, Pain Physician, 2011
8. De Filippis S, Erbuto D, Gentili F, Innamorati M, Lester D, Tatarelli R, Martelletti P, Pompili M (2008) Mental turmoil, suicide risk, illness perception, and temperament, and their impact on quality of life in chronic daily headache. J Headache Pain 9(6):349–357
9. Deshpande KK, Wininger KL (2011) Feasibility of combined epicranial temporal and occipital neurostimulation: treatment of a challenging case of headache. Pain Physician 14:37–44, This is the first report on combined cephalic neurostimulation since our original article (45 above)
10. Dodick DWST, Trentman TL, Zimmerman RS, Hentz J (2007) Trigeminal autonomic cephalalgias: current and future treatment. Headache 47:981–986

11. Goadsby PJ, Knight YE, Hoskin KL (1997) Stimulation of the greater occipital nerve increases metabolic activity in the trigeminal nucleus caudalis and cervical dorsal horn of the cat. Pain 73:23–28
12. Goadsby PJ, Zagami AS (1991) Stimulation of the superior sagittal sinus increases metabolic activity and blood flow in certain regions of the brainstem and upper cervical spinal cord of the cat. Brain 114:1001–1011
13. Goadsby PJ, Hargreaves R (2008) Refractory migraine and chronic migraine: pathophysiological mechanisms. Headache 48(9):1399–1405
14. Hoskin KL, Zagami AS, Goadsby PJ (1999) Stimulation of the middle meningeal artery leads to Fos expression in the trigeminocervical nucleus: a comparative study of monkey and cat. J Anat 194:579–588
15. Linder S (2011) Combined occipital/supraorbital nerve stimulation for treatment of refractory headaches: initial adolescent experience (ages 12–17) [abstract]. Headache 51:47
16. Lionetto L, Negro A, Palmisani S, Gentile G, Del Fiore MR, Mercieri M, Simmaco M, Smith T, Al-Kaisy A, Arcioni R, Martelletti P (2012) Emerging treatment for chronic migraine and refractory chronic migraine. Expert Opin Emerg Drugs 17(3):393–406
17. Magis D, Allena M, Bolla M (2007) Occipital nerve stimulation for drug-resistant chronic cluster headache: a prospective pilot study. Lancet Neurol 6:314–321
18. Mammis A, Gudesblatt M, Mogilner AY (2011) Peripheral neurostimulation for the treatment of refractory cluster headache, long-term follow-up: case report. Neuromodulation 14:432–435
19. Martelletti P, Jensen RH, Antal A, Arcioni R, Brighina F, de Tommaso M, Franzini A, Fontaine D, Heiland M, Jürgens TP, Leone M, Magis D, Paemeleire K, Palmisani S, Paulus W, May A (2013) Neuromodulation of chronic headaches: position statement from the European Headache Federation. J Headache Pain 14(1):86
20. Narouze SN, Kapural L (2007) Supraorbital nerve electric stimulation for the treatment of intractable chronic cluster headache: a case report. Headache 47:1100–1102
21. Palmisani S, Al-Kaisy A, Arcioni R, Smith T, Negro A, Lambru G, Bandikatla V, Carson E, Martelletti P (2013) A six year retrospective review of occipital nerve stimulation practice–controversies and challenges of an emerging technique for treating refractory headache syndromes. J Headache Pain 14(1):67
22. Pompili M, Di Cosimo D, Innamorati M, Lester D, Tatarelli R, Martelletti P (2009) Psychiatric comorbidity in patients with chronic daily headache and migraine: a selective overview including personality traits and suicide risk. J Headache Pain 10(4):283–290
23. Popeney C, Alo K (2003) Peripheral neurostimulation for the treatment of chronic, disabling transformed migraine. Headache 43:369–375
24. Reed KL, Black SB, Banta CJ, Will KR (2010) Combined occipital and supraorbital neurostimulation for the treatment of chronic migraine headaches: initial experience. Cephalalgia 30:260–271
25. Reed KL, Will KR, Chapman J, Richter E (2011) Combined occipital and supraorbital neurostimulation for chronic migraine headaches: an extended case series [abstract]. Presented at 15th Congress of the International Headache Society, Berlin. Cephalalgia. pp 98–99
26. Schwedt TJ, Dodick DW, Trentman TL (2006) Occipital nerve stimulation for chronic cluster headache and hemicrania continua: pain relief and persistence of autonomic features. Cephalalgia 26:1025–1027
27. Schulman E, McGeeney BE (2013) Current concepts in refractory migraine. Curr Treat Options Neurol 15(1):40–55
28. Serafini G, Pompili M, Innamorati M, Gentile G, Borro M, Lamis DA, Lala N, Negro A, Simmaco M, Girardi P, Martelletti P (2012) Gene variants with suicidal risk in a sample of subjects with chronic migraine and affective temperamental dysregulation. Eur Rev Med Pharmacol Sci 16(10):1389–1398
29. Slavin KV, Colpan E, Munawar N, Wess C, Nersesyan H (2006) Trigeminal and occipital nerve stimulation for cranio-facial pain: a single-institution experience and review of the literature. Neurosurg Focus 21:1–5
30. Spencer SE, Sawyer WB, Wada H, Platt KB, Loewy AD (1990) CNS projections to the pterygopalatine para-sympathetic preganglionic neurons in the rat: a retrograde transneuronal viral cell body labeling study. Brain Res 534:149–169

Chapter 13
When Headache Becomes "Troublesome" in a Child: What May Be Behind Chronification of Pediatric Migraine?

Vincenzo Guidetti and Elisa Salvi

13.1 Case Description

L., a 12-year-old boy, was admitted because of worsening recurrent headaches. He described having three attacks a week for the past 3 months. Pain was located in the parietal area on one side; it was throbbing and would last about 4 h with photophobia and phonophobia, nausea, and, at times, vomiting. His parents mentioned that he would stop most of his daily activities during his headache attacks and that his mood became depressed. Headache attacks had started at the age of 7 years and were infrequent initially but had increased in frequency and duration in the past year. He had been admitted to a pediatric emergency department three times within the past year. L. had used a number of analgesics and triptans and was also given preventive therapies, all without result.

13.2 Collecting the Clinical History of the Family

The family consists of four persons: father, mother, and two children. The older sister was not present during the first observation. The posture and gesture of the parents was highly rigid, with the parents on both sides and the child in the center. During the history taking the mother continuously interrupted the doctor and, mainly, the child. The father read the newspaper throughout.

V. Guidetti (✉) • E. Salvi
Department of Pediatrics and Child and Adolescent Neuropsychiatry, "Sapienza" University of Rome, Via dei Sabelli 108, 00185 Rome, Italy
e-mail: vincenzo.guidetti@uniroma1.it

A. Siva, C. Lampl (eds.), *Case-Based Diagnosis and Management of Headache Disorders*, Headache, DOI 10.1007/978-3-319-06886-2_13

13.2.1 Family History

There was no significant medical or neurological family history other than the father's migraine-type headaches that he had experienced since he was 8 years old. Neither the mother nor the sister had any type of headache, including migraine.

13.2.2 Personal History

Pregnancy and delivery were normal: the patient's weight at birth was 3.1 kg; he was breast-fed appropriately; developmental milestones were normal; he achieved sphincter control at age 2.8 years; and he had regular sleep-wake rhythm. He had had most of the exanthematic illnesses such as smallpox, mumps, chickenpox, measles, rubella, and scarlet fever. At age 5 years he was admitted to the hospital for an appendectomy. The mother stressed the difficulties the child experienced on attending primary school, with an initially very high level of anxiety that obliged the family to introduce the child to the classroom progressively to avoid a high level of distress.

13.2.3 Examinations

The patient underwent a complete blood count, contrast nuclear magnetic resonance imaging, and electroencephalography, all of which were normal. All general and neurological examinations also were normal.

13.3 First Step: Talks with the Parents and the Child

We decided to speak with the parents and, in a separate setting, with the child.

13.3.1 The Father

Highly surprised at our approach, he spoke of himself for long periods, referring to a history of low levels of mood without any awareness of a possibility of depression, altered sleep-wake rhythm (he is a concierge), lack of concentration, and temper tantrums with a low level of impulse control.

13.3.2 *The Mother*

She was more willing to speak. She seemed to be uncompromising and indifferent to the situation of the child and, at the same time, angry with L. She considered the problem of her son mainly a "bother." In the last 6 months she had also been admitted with a generalized anxiety disorder.

Both of the parents emphasized the difficulties of the child in school, and held his teachers responsible for his difficulties and stress.

13.3.3 *The Child*

In the first talk the boy was shy, never looking at the interviewer with his eyes always staring at the floor. The doctor was obliged to almost force him to answer. The answers were monosyllabic.

After more than half an hour, He began to describe in a detailed way all of the single characteristics of his headache and to stress how he felt depressed. Gradually, he stated, he decided not to go out with friends because of a "lack of energy" and to break off with sports: "I am in a situation without a future, I really do not know how to get out of this." He was also worried about his poor school performance and the high number of school absences (7 in 1 month).

13.4 Second Step: Tests and Further Talks with the Child

At the end of the first step, an evaluation using psychometric tests was suggested in addition to three talks with the child. Parent training was suggested to the couple. No preventive therapy was decided upon.

13.4.1 *Test Results*

The SAFA Test [6] and the PSPS-Jr [12] were performed.

The first is a test to analyze the level of anxiety (A), depression (D), presence of eating disorders (ED), obsessive-compulsive disorder (O), somatization (S), phobias (PH), and hypochondria (H). The patient scored high levels of A, D, O, and S.

The PSPS-Jr rates all aspects connected to perfectionistic behavior. The patient scored values over the mean line.

13.4.2 The Three Talks with the Child

After the second talk the child began to be cooperative, revealing his worries and impotence regarding his father's behavior toward his wife and child, which tended to be violent both physically and psychologically.

This behavior is associated with a continuous devaluation of the child. In the previous 6 months his father changed his hours of work and spent more time at home, deeply worsening the situation.

13.5 Third Step: Psychotherapy, Parent Training, and Contact with the Teachers

A 1-week session of cognitive psychotherapy with the child was programmed, and parent training was proposed.

We also decided to contact his teachers.

13.5.1 Teacher Contact

The teachers pointed out the child's tendency of isolation, and emphasized the progressive withdrawal that became worse in the last year. His behavior was totally different with the only male teacher, when he would become highly aggressive and disturb all the activities of the group.

13.5.2 Parent Training

The attempt at parent training was unsuccessful, mainly because of the opposition of the father who, after a time, became very aggressive with the doctor and with his wife when she tried to analyze the couple's relationship and his behavior toward his relatives.

Despite the difficulty with the parents, some success was obtained through psychotherapy with the child.

13.5.3 Child Psychotherapy

Psychotherapy, lasting 1 year, has been focused on reduction of anxiety and depressive characteristics, increasing the self-esteem of the boy and modifying his behavior and migraine attacks through psychoeducational training (Theory of Mind) [2].

13.6 Follow-Up

Follow-up at 6 months: Migraine attacks were reduced to two attacks per month, reduction of depressive feeling and, mainly, reduction of pervasive perfectionist behavior. Self-esteem was improved, and school absences were also reduced to 2 days per month. School performances significantly improved.

Follow-up at 1 year: Migraines were reduced to one attack per month, most of the psychiatric problems were improved, and there were no more school absences.

The main problem at school is the permanent conflict with the male teacher, which is probably related to the oppositional behavior of the patient's father who continuously tries to interfere with his psychotherapy.

13.7 Comment

This child has a clinical condition characterized by migraine without aura, in comorbidity with depressive disorder, high levels of anxiety, and disruption of social activities (e.g., sports). He also presents perfectionist personality traits, low school performances, frequent absences from school, difficulties in relationships with male figures, low self-esteem and self-efficacy, maladaptive coping strategies, and frequent conflict with teachers.

Several studies have shown that children and adolescents with headache, in particular migraine, have worse outcomes in comparison with those without migraine. Quality of life and school attendance are decreased, and such children are more likely to have somatic symptoms (e.g., abdominal pain) in addition to anxiety and mood disorders, such as depression [9, 10].

Headache is the most frequent somatic disorder in children. Adolescents who suffer from migraine report high levels of anxiety, depression, and behavioral disorders [16]. Cahill and Cannon suggested a link between migraine, psychiatric disorders (overall anxiety and depression), personality traits, and stress [4]. Guidetti et al. [11] reported feelings of exclusion, insecurity, and repressed hostility in headache patients. It has been hypothesized that a dysregulation of a brain neurochemical system, principally the serotonergic system, could be responsible for the increase in the patient's vulnerability to anxiety and affective disorders in addition to migraine. Alternatively, it is possible that each disorder may increase the risk of the other [11]. Particular attention has been directed at the temporal relationship between the onset of the headache and changes in the patient's life (education first and harassment/violence after), such as the presence of psychological disorders in the clinical history of the parents (in this case the father suffered from migraine from the age of 8 and the mother was diagnosed with generalized anxiety in the last 6 months). The parental sensitivity, appropriate reciprocal social exchange, mutuality, synchrony, stimulation, positive attitude, and emotional support are related to secure attachment [3]. Maternal responsiveness and secure attachment in childhood lead to better social skills and mental health in children [15]. Insecure attachment, especially when it is disorganized, is correlated with an increase in behavioral problems over time [18]. The behavior of parents influences the pain levels reported by children. In experimental situations, the presence or absence of mothers and their level of anxiety changes the perceptual threshold of the painful stimuli in children (regardless of the presence of a painful disease and/or anxiety in children) [13]. Therefore, communication and nonverbal behavior serve as signals of parental anxiety levels or concern, and aggravate the behavioral distress in children [5]. Evidence from animal models shows the importance not only of the amount of maternal care [7] but also the consistency of such care and exposure to new experiences in cognitive and social development, in addition to physical growth [1, 20]. A key mediator appears to be self-regulation of stress by the mother [19].

13.8 Vulnerability

The main vulnerability factor (current and lifetime) in L.'s history is his own family setting. A key role is played by the mother, whom L. describes as supervising, invasive, and rigid. All these maternal characteristics were enhanced as consequence of headache development in L. However, the mother has strongly supported psychotherapy for L., counteracting the strict opposition of his father.

Other important vulnerability factors are the psychological and physical abuses that both L. and his mother have suffered at the hand of the father. In the eyes of L., the mother figure is seen as unable to manage this context of domestic violence, and the boy has suffered because of his role as unarmed and defenseless spectator and victim. It is well known that a stable attachment in childhood to an adult caregiver is a central element in achieving healthy development, building self-effectiveness, reaching a valid level of self-esteem, and developing the basis of mature relationships [17]. Moreover, major depressive disorder and higher anxiety levels are important triggers in most severe migraine attacks in adolescence. In particular, Juang et al. [14] have shown that in adolescence headache is often related to childhood psychological and physical abuse. In general, being a victim of abuse in childhood and adolescence leads to short- and long-term consequences that include psychological and physical problems [8].

From this point of view, L.'s vulnerability to headache could be explained by the separation anxiety experienced in childhood and by his tendency to read and interpret any body signal in a catastrophic way. In this scenario, it is crucial to focus attention on the somatic component (migraine) of the condition despite psychological issues.

13.9 Conclusions

When a child or an adolescent presents with chronicity of headaches, and particularly in cases with migraine, it is compulsory to analyze the psychiatric comorbidity and the influence that lifestyle and environmental stressors might have on the process. Therapy does not consist of drugs alone!

References

1. Akers KG et al (2008) Social competitiveness and plasticity of neuroendocrine function in old age: influence of neonatal novelty exposure and maternal care reliability. PLoS One 3:e2840
2. Apperly IA (2012) What is "theory of mind"? Concepts, cognitive processes and individual differences. Q J Exp Psychol (Hove) 65(5):825–839
3. Bakermans-Kranenburg MJ et al (2003) The importance of shared environment in mother-infant attachment security: a behavioral genetic study. Child Dev 74(6):1769–1782
4. Cahill CM, Cannon M (2005) The longitudinal relationship between comorbid migraine and psychiatric disorder. Cephalalgia 25(11):1099–1100
5. Chambers CT, Craig KD, Bennett SM (2002) The impact of maternal behavior on children's pain experiences: an experimental analysis. J Pediatr Psychol 27:293–301
6. Cianchetti C, Sannio Fancello G (2001) Scale psichiatriche di valutazione per fanciulli e adolescenti (SAFA) Organizzazioni Speciali, Firenze
7. Francis D, Diorio J, Liu D, Meaney MJ (1999) Nongenomic transmission across generations of maternal behavior and stress responses in the rat. Science 286:1155–1158
8. Genizi J, Srugo I, Kerem NC (2014) Headache and physical and sexual abuse among Jewish and Arab adolescents in Israel. J Child Neurol 29:505–508
9. Guidetti V et al (2013) Headache and comorbidity in children and adolescent. J Headache Pain 14(1):79
10. Guidetti V, Galli F (1998) Evolution of headache in childhood and adolescence: an 8-years follow-up. Cephalalgia 18(7):449–454
11. Guidetti V et al (1998) Headache and psychiatric comorbidity: clinical aspects and outcome in an 8-years follow-up study. Cephalalgia 18:455–462
12. Hewitt PL et al (2003) The interpersonal expression of perfection: perfectionistic self-presentation and psychological distress. J Pers Soc Psychol 84(6),1303–1325
13. Hohmeister J et al (2006) Long-term alteration of pain sensitivity in school-aged children with early pain experiences. Pain 125:278–285
14. Juang KD et al (2004) Association between adolescent chronic daily headache and childhood adversity: a community-based study. Cephalalgia 24(1):54–59
15. Landry SH, Smith KE, Swank PR (2006) Responsive parenting: establishing early foundations for social, communication, and independent problem-solving skills. Dev Psychol 42(4):627–642
16. Masi G et al (2000) Somatic symptoms in children and adolescents referred for emotional and behavioral disorders. Psychiatry 63(2):140–149
17. Miller WB, Sable MR, Csizmadia A (2008) Pregnancy wantedness and child attachment security: is there a relationship? Matern Child Health J 12(4):478–487
18. Stams GJ, Juffer F, van IJzendoorn MH (2002) Maternal sensitivity, infant attachment, and temperament in early childhood predict adjustment in middle childhood: the case of adopted children and their biologically unrelated parents. Dev Psychol 38(5):806–821
19. Tang AC et al (2012) Maternal modulation of novelty effects on physical development. Proc Natl Acad Sci U S A 109:2120–2125
20. Tremblay A, Chaput JP (2012) Obesity: the allostatic load of weight loss dieting. [Research Support, Non-U.S. Gov't Review]. Physiol Behav 106:16–21

Chapter 14
Headache in the Pediatric Patient

Joanne Kacperski, Marielle A. Kabbouche, Hope L. O'Brien, and Andrew D. Hershey

14.1 Case Description

A 14-year-old, right-handed girl is brought to the neurology clinic by her mother for a history of recent worsening of her headaches. She reports that her headaches started at the age of 7 but have been increasing in frequency and severity over the last 4 months. Her headaches start with a prodrome described as feeling tired and with food cravings. She identifies several triggers including stress related to schoolwork, strong smells, and not getting enough sleep. Her headaches do not worsen around her periods. The headache starts with pain that is often frontal and/or bitemporal and builds in intensity within 30 min to a severity of 6 on a 0–10 pain scale which she rates as severe. The pain is characterized as throbbing and constant. Her headaches are accompanied by frequent nausea with occasional vomiting, phonophobia, photophobia, osmophobia, and fatigue. She also describes difficulty with concentration during her headaches. Her typical headache lasts 4 h, but she has had headaches lasting for 1–2 days. Her current headache frequency is about three headaches per week, or up to 17 headache days per month. She has been at this frequency for the past 4 months. Physical activity makes her headaches worse. She denies any history of head trauma. Her PedMIDAS score is 62. She has required visits to the emergency department for treatment of her headaches on several occasions. An MRI ordered by her primary care physician 4 months prior to presentation

---

J. Kacperski, MD (✉) • M.A. Kabbouche, MD • H.L. O'Brien, MD
A.D. Hershey, MD, PhD
Division of Neurology, Cincinnati Children's Hospital Medical Center,
3333 Burnet Avenue, MLC 2015, Cincinnati, OH 45229, USA

Department of Pediatrics, College of Medicine, University of Cincinnati,
Cincinnati, OH, USA
e-mail: joanne.kacperski@cchmc.org; marielle.kabbouce@cchmc.org;
hope.o'brien@cchmc.org; andrew.hershey@cchmc.org

A. Siva, C. Lampl (eds.), *Case-Based Diagnosis and Management of Headache Disorders*, Headache, DOI 10.1007/978-3-319-06886-2_14

was reported as normal. She treats her headaches with ibuprofen 400 mg. She often waits until the pain is severe before she treats, and often, she does not treat her headaches at all.

She is drinking approximately four glasses of fluid per day with caffeine up to 3 days per week. She no longer exercises since she quit playing soccer. She skips breakfast up to 5 days per week because she "does not have time in the mornings to eat," and she occasionally skips lunch. She gets 7 h of sleep per night and often gets less on the weekends when she stays up late with her friends. She has missed 8 days of school recently secondary to her headaches. Otherwise, between headaches, she reports that she feels normal and now comes in for evaluation.

All of her remaining review of systems were reviewed and were positive for a current headache rated as 7 out of 10 on a 0–10 point pain scale, but otherwise were negative.

Her past medical history is positive for depression. She also reports a history of car or motion sickness, sleeping difficulties, and feelings of low self-esteem. She follows with a psychiatrist once monthly who prescribes Celexa 20 mg daily. Otherwise, her birth history was normal. Developmental history was also described as normal. She has no known medication allergies. Her immunizations are up to date.

Family history is notable for migraine headaches in the mother, an older sister, maternal grandmother, and maternal aunt. Her mother also reports a history of visual aura with her headaches. The maternal grandfather has a history of tension-type headaches.

Socially, she lives with her mother, father, and 17-year-old sister. She is in the 9th grade. She is an "A/B" student. Her grades have gotten worse due to the headaches.

Her weight was 60.1 kg (65.5 percentile), height was 165.1 cm (61.8 percentile), BMI was 22.04 (62 percentile), blood pressure was 104/61, and heart rate was 73. Her general physical examination including skin, HEENT, extremities, lung, and cardiac and abdominal examination was normal with lungs clear to auscultation; heart had a regular rate and rhythm; and abdomen was soft and non-tender without organomegaly.

On neurological examination she was alert, attentive with normal mental status. Speech was fluent. Skull, spine, and meninges were normocephalic and atraumatic with a supple neck. Cranial nerves II through XII were normal with a normal fundoscopic examination including sharp disks, no papilledema, and normal fundus bilaterally. Motor examination was normal for tone and bulk with full strength throughout. Sensory examination was normal for light touch, temperature, vibration, and joint position sense. Finger-nose-finger, fine finger movements, and heel-knee-shin were normal. Deep tendon reflexes were symmetric and 2+ throughout with toes downgoing. Station and gait were normal including toe walking, heel walking, tandem walking, running, skipping, and one-legged standing, and there was no Romberg's sign.

She had a normal comprehensive headache examination. Neck was supple with normal rotation and normal trapezius muscle tightness. No bruits or palpitations were heard over carotid or jugular veins. There was a negative Muller sign with no pain on the neck bending with pressure and no signs of allergy or sinus symptoms.

14.2 Establishing the Diagnosis of Migraine

When a child presents with a complaint of headache, the evaluation requires a complete general health and neurological assessment, in addition to a comprehensive headache history. A thorough evaluation is necessary to make the correct headache diagnosis based on criteria established by the International Headache Classification of Headache Disorders 3rd edition (ICHD-III) which can help determine the appropriate treatment. The American Academy of Neurology has published a list of practice parameter guidelines to address treatment options.

The diagnosis of migraine in children and adolescents can be established through a headache history in the vast majority of patients. The clinician must remember that this history needs to be directed not only to the parent but also toward the child, as the parent often bases their answers on their own observations and experiences. Younger patients may need to have questions phrased at a more developmentally appropriate level.

The history should initially focus on headache pattern to elucidate whether or not the headaches are a chronic or episodic problem. The pattern may also identify whether or not a secondary underlying disorder is the cause of the headaches. One of the first components, and sometimes the most important, is to identify if the headaches are attributed to a secondary disorder. If a secondary disorder is suspected, then its treatment should result in headache resolution.

Specific questions can identify those at risk for headaches secondary to underlying pathology. Many times, a secondary headache disorder may be clear from an inciting event, such as a head trauma. Asking the patient how long they have had headaches can also help identify the difference between a primary and secondary headache disorder. If there is a long-standing history of headaches, such as in our patient, then the chance of a primary, recurrent headache is more likely. However, one must be wary of a new type of headache that has developed in a patient with a long-standing history of headaches, as this may indicate the possibility of an underlying, secondary etiology.

The clinician should aim to obtain a very detailed description of the headache. This should include the location of the pain, quality of the pain, severity of the pain, and any associated symptoms. Focal pain may be consistent with migraine, whereas a more diffuse description of pain may be consistent with tension-type headaches. Quality of pain may be difficult to describe, especially for the younger patient. This may also be true when describing the severity of the pain. A variety of tools are available to assess severity, and the most appropriate scale should be used based on the patient's developmental stage. Some may be able to describe the pain as mild, moderate, or severe or use a numerical scale of 0–10. Younger patients may find using the Faces Scale more helpful when describing their pain. When asking about associated symptoms, the clinician should not just focus upon the classic symptoms of migraine including nausea, vomiting, and light and sound sensitivities, as symptoms of other headache disorders or secondary headaches may be missed. For example, autonomic symptoms may indicate the presence of a trigeminal autonomic cephalgia. Focal neurological symptoms such as focal weakness or sensory or visual disturbance may indicate a mass lesion.

Frequency and duration of the headaches are important as these responses may alter treatment choices. For example, a child may describe few headaches, but these headaches may last several days at a time, which would prompt the clinician to focus on the appropriate use of acute and abortive therapies. However, some kids may have headaches of shorter duration, but that may be frequent. Such a presentation may warrant discussion about preventative therapies.

The frequency and duration of headaches may also aid in characterizing the impact the headaches have on the child's quality of life. The evaluation of a child with headaches should incorporate headache disability and quality of life assessments. The PedMIDAS (Pediatric Migraine Disability Assessment) has been tested and validated for ages 4–18, and it parallels the use of the adult MIDAS that Lipton and Stewart developed for adults age 20–50. These questions aim to determine how the headaches have impacted the child's performance in both the school and home settings and during social and sports functions. It provides a developmentally sensitive, reliable, and valid assessment of disability related to childhood and adolescent headaches. It may also act as a tool to assess the impact of migraines in children and to monitor response to treatment.

The history should also include a complete review of systems, past medical and surgical histories, previous traumas, serious illnesses, birth and developmental histories, as well as social and family histories. A detailed drug history including current medications and use of any drugs or alcohol should be obtained. The history can aid in identifying any comorbid conditions that may be contributing to headache frequency and that may also affect the child's response to treatment. It can also help in choosing an appropriate preventative therapy if one is warranted and aid in recognizing any potential secondary causes. A family history of headaches is common in patients with primary headaches disorders, and a detailed family history is needed to identify appropriate diagnosis.

Once a thorough history has been obtained, complete physical, neurological, and headache examinations should be performed. The examination can be the most sensitive indicator for the need for further diagnostic testing, and it should be tailored to identify those who require further investigation. In the majority of patients with a primary headache disorder, the examination should remain normal and an abnormality may indicate that a secondary headache is present. For example, head circumference should be obtained in young patients to assess for macrocephaly. When significantly enlarged, this may warrant further investigation to evaluate for hydrocephalus or other secondary causes. A skin examination may identify skin stigmata associated with neurocutaneous disorders such as neurofibromatosis. Incoordination or gait abnormalities may indicate a posterior fossa lesion. Evaluation for a cranial bruit may reveal an underlying vascular abnormality. A fundoscopic examination may demonstrate papilledema and evidence for elevated intracranial pressure as the cause of the child's headache.

14.3 Diagnostic Testing

The diagnosis of a primary headache disorder is a clinical diagnosis. Currently, there is a lack of consensus concerning the role of diagnostic testing. Investigations are not routinely indicated, but neuroimaging should be considered in children whose headaches do not meet the criteria for one of the primary headache syndromes and in those with an abnormal neurological examination. Other reasons to consider neuroimaging include the development of a subacute headache that is rapidly progressive in severity, new onset of a headache in an immunosuppressed patient, first or worst headache, or the presence of associated or systemic symptoms including fever or nuchal rigidity. Children with a space-occupying lesion may present with a new-onset headache (less than 1 month duration), abnormal neurological examination, gait abnormalities, seizures, headaches awakening the child from sleep, intractable vomiting, or confusion. Neuroimaging should also be considered in those children without a family history of primary headache disorders. A subcommittee of the American Academy of Neurology and the Practice Committee of the Child Neurology Society state that obtaining neuroimaging on a routine basis is not indicated in children with recurrent headaches and a normal neurological evaluation (Table 14.1).

When neuroimaging is warranted, an MRI is more sensitive in evaluating for a posterior fossa lesion, neoplastic disorders, vascular disorders, ischemia, and infection. A CT is highly sensitive in acute hemorrhage and is often ordered in the emergency room setting.

Historically, electroencephalograms were ordered in the diagnostic evaluation in children presenting with headache. An EEG is not recommended in the routine evaluation of a child with recurrent headaches because it is unlikely to improve the

Table 14.1 Summary of suggested guidelines for requesting neuroimaging in children and adolescents with headaches

1. Abnormal neurological examination
2. Recent headache of less than 6 months with a progressive course
3. Atypical presentation of headache Intractable vomiting, headache wakening the child from sleep, vertigo, mental status changes, confusion, or other focal neurological complaints
4. Any child less than 6 years of age
5. Absence of family history of a primary headache disorder
6. New type of headache in a patient with history of recurrent headaches
7. First or worst headache
8. Systemic symptoms and signs
9. Occipital headache

diagnostic yield in primary headache. In young children, however, atypical symptoms may be prominent, especially in children with periodic symptoms or migraine variants including the periodic syndromes of childhood. These syndromes, which are often precursors to migraine, can occur without an apparent headache and may make the clinician suspicious for an underlying seizure disorder. In such cases, the EEG is not warranted for the diagnosis of migraine, but to evaluate for a seizure disorder.

A lumbar puncture is also not routinely necessary when evaluating a child with headaches. However, clinical presentations such as those in which infection is present, there is a suspected increase in intracranial pressure such as in the presence of papilledema or there is a suspicion of a subarachnoid hemorrhage, all warrant a lumbar puncture.

Clinical laboratory testing is often not necessary in the evaluation of a primary headache disorder, unless a secondary cause is suspected such as an underlying anemia. It should be done prior to initiating some preventative headache therapies, as well as to monitor their toxicity and the patient's compliance with such medications during treatment.

14.4 Treatment: Abortive Therapy

Management of migraine headaches requires a tailored regimen of pharmacological and behavioral measures that consider both the child's headache burden and their level of disability. As published by the AAN practice parameter, abortive therapy should work fast and consistently and without headache recurrence and the need to use rescue medications, restore an individual's ability to function, and care for themselves without the need to utilize other resources be cost-effective and have minimal side effects. Acute treatment should also effectively stop all features of migraine, including the associated symptoms. Furthermore, acute medication should be properly dosed based on the child's weight. Children should be educated on the importance of treating early, even while in school, and ways to avoid the potential for medication overuse.

14.5 Treatment: Prophylaxis

Preventative medications should be limited to those children whose headaches occur with sufficient frequency or severity to warrant daily treatment. The goal of therapy should be directed at reducing headache frequency, reducing the progression to chronic daily headache, and decreasing associated pain and disability. Most clinicians require a minimum of 1 headache per week or three to four headaches per month to justify placing a child on a daily medication. Prophylaxis should also be considered if acute treatments are ineffective, not tolerated, contraindicated, or overused. Patients who report intensive and prolonged headaches (lasting > 48 h) should also be considered.

Children meriting prevention should be provided with appropriate education, thus enabling them to manage their disease and enhance personal control of their headaches. Clinicians should thoroughly discuss this long-term treatment plan so that families understand that the effort will be a long-term one and response will not be rapid, as the onset of improvement is often delayed in the pediatric patient. A typical goal of one to two headaches per month or fewer is recommended for a sustained period of 4–6 months. The doses of preventative agents must be titrated slowly to minimize side effects. Once an effective dose is reached, relief must be sustained for 2–3 months before considering an alternative medication. Once sustained relief is obtained, a plan to wean the child off the medication is also necessary. Both the clinician and family must establish a sense of functional disability before committing the child to a course of daily medication as therapy should also aim at the improvement of an overall quality of life.

Several classes of medications may be used for prophylaxis and include antidepressants, antiepileptics, antihistamines, and antihypertensives. The majority of these medications have been extensively prescribed for other conditions, including depression and other mood disorders, epilepsy, and other pain disorders, thus making their side effect profiles well described. When selecting an agent, one should take into account any comorbid conditions that may be present. Clear instructions should be given to families regarding the medication's mechanism of action, possible side effects, and the importance of not missing doses. Clear titration instructions should be provided. It is important to remind families that it may take time, often several weeks, for the preventative to become effective. Slow titration over a period of 4–12 weeks may be necessary to assure that the child tolerates the medication with minimal side effects. If a trend of improvement is seen, the dose is then adjusted for optimal control. Treatment should not be abandoned until it has been given an adequate trial of at least 6–8 weeks on the full dose unless there are intolerable side effects. When improvement is sustained and a satisfying response is achieved over a period of 4–6 months, then the child may be slowly weaned off of the medication.

14.6 Behavioral Measures

Lifestyle modifications are often discussed with patients, including maintenance of good sleep hygiene, defined as regular bedtimes and waking times with sufficient sleep time. Maintenance of a regular diet also appears to be important. Regarding dietary restrictions, the American Headache Society only limits caffeine intake and does not restrict any type of food unless a very specific food trigger is identified. A balanced diet is beneficial and patients should be encouraged to avoid skipping meals. Patients are also often counseled on the importance of keeping well hydrated as dehydration is commonly identified as a headache trigger.

14.7 Summary of the Case

In summary, this is a 15-year-old girl with a history of depression and a long-standing history of headaches which have been increasing in frequency over the last 4 months. The headaches are intermittent but frequent, frontal and bitemporal in location, and associated with nausea and occasional vomiting, photophobia, and phonophobia. They are throbbing and moderate to severe in intensity. The headaches last from 4 to 48 h and are so disabling that she was forced to quit soccer. Her PedMIDAS score is 62, indicating severe disability. She has a family history significant for primary headache disorders, including migraines and tension-type headaches. Her general physical, neurological, and headache examinations are normal. She has had an MRI which was also normal. With no red flags reported in the history, a family history of primary headache disorders, and a normal examination, an MRI was likely unnecessary. Her headaches meet the ICHD-III criteria for migraine without aura and chronic migraine. She was instructed to treat her headaches early with an NSAID, namely, ibuprofen 600 mg (10 mg/kg), at the onset of her headache with a sufficient amount of fluid, such as 32 oz of water or a sports drink. This could be repeated after 4 h of the headache had not resolved. To prevent overuse of her abortive therapy, she was instructed not to take the ibuprofen more than 2–3 days per week. Due to the frequency and disability of her headaches, preventative medications are warranted. Because of her history of comorbid depression and current treatment with an antidepressant, medications that fall within the class of tricyclic antidepressants (e.g., amitriptyline) should be avoided. The decision was made to treat her with topiramate, slowly increasing to a dose of 50 mg twice daily over a 4–6-week period. Multiple lifestyle modifications were prescribed including increasing her fluid intake to eight to ten glasses of fluid per day and abstaining from caffeine. She was encouraged to exercise and become active once again. The importance of eating three meals daily was discussed, in addition to a regular sleep schedule, striving for 8–9 h of sleep per night.

14.8 Definition of Migraine Without Aura and Chronic Migraine in Pediatric Patients

The specific diagnostic criteria for migraine in children are complex and rest on criteria similar to those used to diagnose migraine in adults. It is important, however, to appreciate several fundamental differences. These differences include the duration of attack, which is often far shorter than in an adult, and the location of the attack, which may be bilateral in many children. In adults, migraine headache is defined by the International Classification of Headache Disorders, 3rd Edition (beta version) [Cephalalgia 2013; 33(9)629–808] as an idiopathic, recurring headache disorder manifesting in attacks lasting 4–72 h. Typical characteristics of migraine headaches are often unilateral location, pulsating quality, moderate to severe intensity, aggravation by routine physical activity, and nausea and/or vomiting, photophobia, and phonophobia. However, difficulties may be encountered when making a diagnosis of migraine in the pediatric and adolescent age groups. These differences are addressed in the notes and comments section of the ICHD-III. For example, gastrointestinal complaints are more prominent, such as abdominal pain, nausea, and vomiting. Children also tend to experience headaches which are often shorter in duration, with attacks lasting from 2 to 72 h. The location is more likely to be bilateral and is often described as frontal or bitemporal, as opposed to the more common unilateral headaches seen in adult migraineurs. However, this unilaterality may emerge in adolescence. Because younger children may have difficulty understanding and describing the concepts of photophobia and phonophobia, these signs may need to be inferred by the parents on the basis of the child's actions.

Our patient also fulfills ICHD-III criteria for chronic migraine. Her headaches occur on 15 or more days per month for more than 3 months. Her headaches have migrainosus features on at least eight of those headache days. It is important to ask about the use of both over-the-counter and prescription pain medications because half of patients with chronic migraine are thought to overuse such medications and withdrawal of these medications may revert their headaches to an episodic headache pattern. Our patient reported rarely using such medications.

14.9 Brief General Information: Migraines in Children and Adolescents

Primary headache disorders are one of the most prevalent health problems worldwide. Studies to determine the prevalence of childhood headache have been investigated across pediatric age groups with variable estimates ranging from 3 % in school-age children to 20 % in adolescents. Multiple epidemiological studies have demonstrated the high incidence of headaches in this group, with migraine being the most disabling type. Prior to puberty, the prevalence of migraine is slightly higher in boys when compared to girls. The mean age of onset is 7 years for boys and 11 years for girls. However, data from the American Migraine Prevalence and Prevention study demonstrated that as children approach adolescence, the incidence and prevalence of migraine appear to increase more rapidly in girls when compared to their male counterparts.

Migraine can often become a chronic and disabling disorder with a substantial effect not only on the child's quality of life, but it may also contribute to school absenteeism and affect both peer and social interactions. When looking specifically at children, population studies have demonstrated that over 130,000 school days are missed every 2 weeks and three million bedridden days occur per month as a result of migraines. Some have also demonstrated that the negative impact of having migraines on a child's overall quality of life is similar to pediatric cancer, heart disease, and rheumatic disease. Because migraine headaches can commonly start in childhood and adolescence, early recognition and establishment of a treatment plan and implementation of lifestyle changes can alter disease progression and ultimately improve the child's quality of life.

Key Points When Evaluating a Child or Adolescent Presenting with Headache

- Always involve the child in the history-taking process and ask questions in a developmentally appropriate manner.
- Identify if the headaches can be attributable to a secondary disorder.
- If a secondary disorder is suspected, then its treatment should result in headache resolution.
- Obtain a very detailed description of the headaches, including frequency, quality, duration, and associated symptoms.
- Obtain detailed past medical, family, and psychosocial histories as this may aid in diagnosis and guide the clinician in treatment.
- The examination can be the most sensitive indicator for the need for further diagnostic testing, and it should be tailored to identify those who require further investigation.
- Investigations are not routinely indicated, but neuroimaging should be considered in children whose headaches do not meet the criteria for one of the primary headache syndromes and in those with an abnormal neurological examination.
- Management of migraine headaches requires a tailored regimen of pharmacological and behavioral measures that consider both the child's headache burden and level of disability.

Suggested Reading

1. Bonfert M, Straube A, Schroeder AS, Rellich FE, Heinen F (2013) Primary headache in children and adolescents: update on pharmacotherapy of migraine and tension-type headache. Neuropediatrics 44:3–19
2. Eidlitz-Markus T, Haimi-Cohen Y, Steier D, Zeharia A (2010) Effectiveness of nonpharmacologic treatment for migraine in young children. Headache 50:219–223
3. Headache Classification Subcommittee of the International Headache Society (2013) The International Classification of Headache Disorders, 3rd edition (beta version). Cephalalgia 33: 629–808
4. Hershey AD (2010) Current approaches to the diagnosis and management of pediatric migraine. Lancet Neurol 9:190–204
5. Hershey AD (2012) Pediatric headache: update on recent research. Headache 52(2):327–332
6. Hershey AD, Powers SW, Vockell AL, LeCates S, Kabbouche MA, Maynard MK (2001) PedMIDAS: development of a questionnaire to assess disability of migraines in children. Neurology 57(11):2034–2039
7. Hershey AD, Powers SW, Winner P, Kabbouche MA (2009) Pediatric headaches in clinical practice. John Wiley & Sons, Ltd., West Sussex
8. Jacobs H, Gladstein J (2012) Pediatric headache: a clinical review. Headache 52(2):333–339
9. Lewis D (2009) Pediatric migraine. Neurol Clin 27:481–501
10. Lewis D, Ashwal S, Hershey A, Hirtz D, Yonker M, Silberstein S (2004) Practice parameter: pharmacological treatment of migraine headache in children and adolescents: report of the

American Academy of Neurology Quality Standards Subcommittee and the Practice Committee of the Child Neurology Society. Neurology 63:2215–2224
11. O'Brien HL, Kabbouche MA, Hershey AD (2012) Treating pediatric migraine: an expert opinion. Expert Opin Pharmacother 13(7):959–966
12. Powers SW, Andrasik F (2005) Biobehavioral treatment, disability, and psychological effects of pediatric headache. Pediatr Ann 34(6):461–466
13. Silberstein SD (2000) Practice parameter: evidence-based guidelines for migraine headache (an evidence-based review). Neurology 55:754–762
14. Winner P, Hershey AD (2007) Epidemiology and diagnosis of migraine in children. Curr Pain Headache Rep 11:375–382

Chapter 15
Abdominal Pain Associated with Migraine

Aynur Özge

15.1 Case Description

A 17-year-old boy was referred with intractable headache and vomiting attacks. The history disclosed clear infantile colic attacks starting from the first months of the life to the 6 months of age. Repeated emergency room admissions and gastroenterological investigations could not show any reason. His family described several attacks of nonspecific abdominal pain, vomiting, and motion sickness without any known cause in the first 3 years of life. At the age of 3 years, he underwent a cranial magnetic resonance imaging (MRI) examination showing Dandy-Walker malformation like his mother, uncle, and grandmother. Afterwards, he showed normal motor and mental developments but had low quality of life because of the recurrent gastrointestinal disturbances like vomiting, abdominal pain, and bowel irritability. Further gastrointestinal investigations in different centers including five endoscopies did not show any potential cause of this situation. In the last 5 years, he developed recurrent headache attacks independent from these gastrointestinal disturbances. He had three to four attacks per month in average; mean attack duration was 2–3 h with generally throbbing quality, located on the forehead. He described the mean severity of the attacks as seven according to visual analog scale (VAS); they associated with light and noise sensitivity, rarely nausea but frequent vomiting, dizziness, and osmophobia, but he reported no aura. Attacks were generally provoked by hunting, heavy physical activity, and emotional distress. They relieved partially after sleeping and with early intake of nonsteroidal anti-inflammatory drugs. The patient and his family worries about these headache attacks and disturbed daily living activities. Sometimes headache attacks started during the midnight resulting in disturbed sleep

A. Özge, MD
Department of Neurology, Medical Faculty, Mersin University,
Çiftlikköy Kampüsü, Yenişehir-Mersin 33343, Turkey
e-mail: aynurozge@gmail.com, aynurozge@aynurozge.com

A. Siva, C. Lampl (eds.), *Case-Based Diagnosis and Management of Headache Disorders*, Headache, DOI 10.1007/978-3-319-06886-2_15

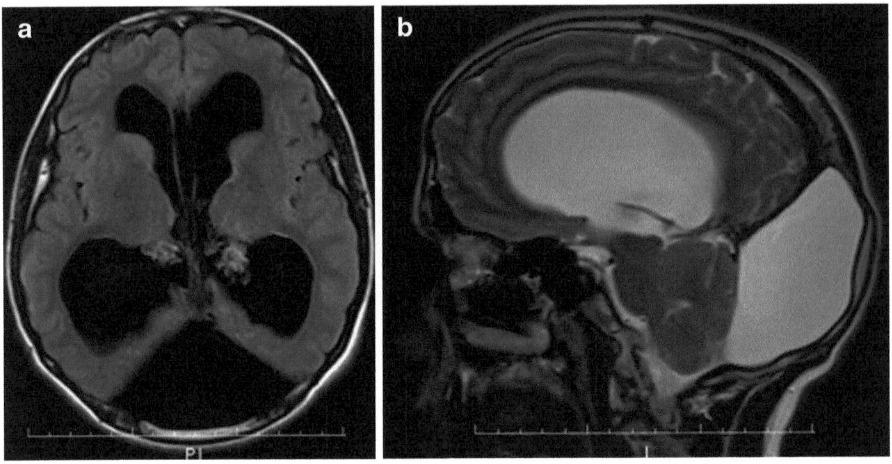

Fig. 15.1 (**a**, **b**) MRI scans showed Dandy-Walker malformation and thin corpus callosum

quality. Furthermore, frequent vocal tics aggravated social problems with friends in the last 2 years. His family history showed that his mother, aunt, and grandmother had headache disorders partially fulfilling migraine criteria on questioning. They want to learn the real cause of these problems and how to solve it.

15.2 Summary of the Available Investigations

Possible gastrointestinal causes of these attacks associated with intractable abdominal pain, vomiting, bowel problems, and spasms were investigated before. He also had three cranial and one cervical MRI investigations showing only Dandy-Walker malformation (see Fig. 15.1a (axial T1W) and 1b (sagittal T2W)) and thin corpus callosum, but not any potential cause of the described headache, sleep, and tic disorders. Moreover, he had three routine EEG recordings; all were evaluated as normal. Motor and mental examinations were within normal ranges. Neuropsychological evaluation disclosed generalized anxiety disorder and simple vocal tics not fulfilling the Tourette syndrome criteria according to DSM-V.

15.3 Diagnostic Workup of the Case

This patient was diagnosed with childhood/adolescent migraine associated with abdominal pain and simple tic disorder and anxiety disorder as comorbidity. He had tried valproic acid and propranolol as prophylactic managements before, along with several attack treatment options, but none of them were effective. We educated the family and the patient, explained the diagnosis, regulated his daily routines including sleep hygiene, and prescribed flunarizine and added topiramate afterwards. In the first years of follow-up he did well, but then during college period, he complained of severe attacks refractory to all medications, including triptans. We performed three successful great occipital nerve blocks with lidocaine accordingly. He also had specific psychotherapy for psychiatric disturbances and his symptoms relieved clearly. He had only one attack relieved with domperidone together with flurbiprofen without any recurrence in the last years.

15.4 Summary of the Case

A young boy with previous infantile colic and intractable unexplained gastrointestinal disturbances described migrainous headache attacks in the last 5 years. He had psychiatric (tic disorder and generalized anxiety disorder) and variant anatomical (Dandy-Walker malformation) comorbidities. Positive history of migraine and family history supported the diagnosis. Medical management of migraine followed by nerve blocks relieved not only his headache attacks but also all gastrointestinal disturbances, especially vomiting attacks. His quality of life improved and psychiatric comorbidities were also better.

15.5 Definition According to the International Classification of Headache Disorders (ICHD)

This case was diagnosed as "abdominal migraine" at first. According to ICHD-III beta, it was coded as 1.6.1.2. Recommended diagnostic criteria were as follows:

A. At least five attacks of abdominal pain, fulfilling criteria B–D
B. Pain has at least two of the following three characteristics:

   1. Midline location, periumbilical or poorly localized
   2. Dull or "just sore" quality
   3. Moderate or severe intensity

C. During attacks, at least two of the following:

   1. Anorexia
   2. Nausea
   3. Vomiting
   4. Pallor

D. Attacks last 2–72 h when untreated or unsuccessfully treated
E. Complete freedom from symptoms between attacks
F. Not attributed to another disorder

In the following period, the same case was diagnosed with migraine without aura. According to ICHD-III beta, this was coded as 1.1. Recommended diagnostic criteria were as follows;

A. At least five attacks fulfilling criteria B–D
B. Headache attacks lasting 4–72 h (untreated or unsuccessfully treated)[1]
C. Headache has at least two of the following four characteristics:

   1. Unilateral location
   2. Pulsating quality
   3. Moderate or severe pain intensity
   4. Aggravation by or causing avoidance of routine physical activity

D. During headache at least one of the following:

   1. Nausea and/or vomiting
   2. Photophobia and phonophobia

E. Not better accounted for by another ICHD-3 diagnosis

15.6 Brief General Information

15.6.1 Migraine

Migraine is among the most specific and important causes of headache disorders in all age groups. Totally, 10.4 % of the children and 18.6 % of the adolescents were diagnosed with migraine in Turkish population. Migraine equivalents are a group of periodic and paroxysmal neurological diseases. The prevalence of migraine equivalents in the literature varies between 1.8 and 4 %, reaching up to 9.8 % if we consider only the population of migrainous patients.

15.6.2 Infantile Colic

Infantile colic is a common cause of inconsolable crying during the first months of life. According to the criteria reported by Wessel, it is usually diagnosed by crying and fussing for more than 3 h per day, more than 3 days per week, and for more than 3 weeks in an otherwise healthy and well-fed infant. For children with migraine, the odds of having colic as an infant were increased, in contrast to other primary headache disorders.

[1] In children and adolescents (aged under 18 years), attacks may last 2–72 h.

15.6.3 Chronic Abdominal Pain

Chronic abdominal pain is common in children and adolescents. Generally "chronic abdominal pain" describes intermittent or constant abdominal pain (of functional or organic etiology) that has been present for at least 2 months. The term "chronic abdominal pain" encompasses "recurrent abdominal pain," classically defined by four criteria:

1. ≥3 episodes of abdominal pain
2. Pain sufficiently severe to affect activities
3. Episodes occur over a period of ≥3 months
4. No known organic cause

15.6.4 Recurrent Abdominal Pain (RAP)

Recurrent abdominal pain (RAP) is common in children, and the reported prevalence rates in population-based studies have varied between 6 and 15 %. Potentially identifiable causes of RAP include constipation, food or lactose intolerance, gastroesophageal reflux, peptic ulceration, duodenitis, Crohn's disease, urinary tract infections, and menstrual disorders. RAP disappears in about half the children, persists in a quarter, and is replaced by other painful symptoms (mainly headache) in the remaining quarter. Familial Mediterranean Fever (FMF) should also be included in the differential diagnosis of children with RAP, especially if they are from certain ethnic groups such as Turks, Jews, Armenians, or Arabs, in whom this hereditary inflammatory disease is more commonly seen.

15.6.5 Cyclic Vomiting Syndrome (CVS)

Cyclic vomiting syndrome (CVS) is recurrent episodic attacks of intense nausea and vomiting, usually stereotypical in the individual and with predictable timing of episodes. Attacks may be associated with pallor and lethargy. There is complete resolution of symptoms between attacks. CVS has been classified as a childhood periodic syndrome (CPS) or "migraine equivalent" that is commonly a precursor of migraine in the ICHD-II. CVS usually occurs between ages 4 and 10 years. In a meta-analysis, the prevalence of headache/migraine was 40.5 %, family history of migraines was 27.8 %, history of anxiety or depression was reported in 26.7 %, and travel sickness in 28.3 %.

15.6.6 Abdominal Migraine (AM)

Abdominal migraine (AM) is an idiopathic disorder seen mainly in children as recurrent attacks of moderate to severe midline abdominal pain, associated with vasomotor symptoms, nausea and vomiting, lasting 2–72 h and normalization between episodes. Headache does not occur during these episodes. Children with abdominal migraine had demographic and social characteristics similar to those of children with migraine. Most children with abdominal migraine will develop migraine headache later in life. In young children the presence of headache is often overlooked and underdiagnosed.

AM represents 4–15 % of pediatric gastroenterology patients followed up for idiopathic recurrent abdominal pain. This entity is more common in those with a family history of migraine headaches, appears between the ages of 3 and 10 years old, and rarely persists into adulthood.

If we take into account all these shared symptoms, such as comorbidities, triggers, and responses to treatment, it is becoming more obvious that infantile colic, CVS, and AM are important causes of RAP syndromes, and they are probably not separate entities from adult migraine but a part of the same migraine spectrum.

15.6.7 Dandy-Walker Syndrome

Dandy-Walker syndrome is a congenital brain malformation involving the cerebellum and the fluid-filled spaces around it. The key features of this syndrome are an enlargement of the fourth ventricle, a partial or complete absence of the area of the brain between the two cerebellar hemispheres, and cyst formation near the lowest part of the skull. Migraine-like headache attacks or abdominal pains are not among the known symptoms of this disorder and a causal relationship could not be established. We thought that this was a confusing comorbidity of our migraine patient.

Key Points

Sometimes a patient had many confounding features but the real cause was only a simple one like demonstrated in this case. Previous infantile colic, cyclic vomiting, and recurrent abdominal pain attacks are migraine equivalents. Some features could be confusing like Dandy-Walker abnormality or associated psychiatric disturbances like generalized anxiety disorders. However, like tic disorders, there are several problems such as anxiety disorders were reported with high prevalence as migraine comorbidity. In this case specific migraine management, including preventive medication, supported with interventional procedures like GON blockage and completing with education of the patients and parents are effective for solving the problem.

Suggested Reading

1. Abu-Arafeh I, Russell G (1995) Prevalence and clinical features of abdominal migraine compared with those of migraine headache. Arch Dis Child 72:413–417
2. American Academy of Pediatrics Subcommittee on Chronic Abdominal Pain (2005) Chronic abdominal pain in children. Pediatrics 115:812
3. Appendix A. Rome III diagnostic criteria for functional gastrointestinal disorders. http://www.romecriteria.org/assets/pdf/19-RomeIII-apA-885-898.pdf. Accessed 18 July 2013
4. El-Matary W, Spray C, Sandhu B (2004) Irritable bowel syndrome: the commonest cause of recurrent abdominal pain in children. Eur J Pediatr 163:584
5. Gijsbers CF, Kneepkens CM, Schweizer JJ et al (2011) Recurrent abdominal pain in 200 children: somatic causes and diagnostic criteria. Acta Paediatr 100:e208
6. Headache Classification Committee of the International Headache Society (IHS). (2013) The International Classification of Headache Disorders: 3rd-beta edition. Cephalalgia 33(9):629–808
7. Lee LY, Abbott L, Mahlangu B, Moodie SJ, Anderson S (2012) The management of cyclic vomiting syndrome: a systematic review. Eur J Gastroenterol Hepatol 24:1001–1006
8. Leung AK, Lemay JF (2004) Infantile colic: a review. J R Soc Promot Health 124(4): 162–166
9. Rome Foundation (2006). Guidelines–Rome III diagnostic criteria for functional gastrointestinal disorders. J Gastrointestin Liver Dis 15(3):307–12

Chapter 16
Migraine in the Elderly

Vera V. Osipova, Elena Snopkova, and Guzyal Tabeeva

16.1 Background

It is well known that in the majority of patients migraine completely stops after the age of 50. At the same time in the minority of subjects, migraine attacks or some manifestations could last out. Two cases below illustrate two different ways of migraine evolution in elder age.

16.2 Case Description 1

A 57-year-old woman, married, unemployed since she was 52 (because the institute she worked at closed down), presented with complaints of frequent attacks of pulsating and pressing headache, more frequently on the right side located in the occipito-temporal and supraciliary region, 6–7 points of intensity according to the visual analogue scale, arising two to three times a week (maximum 10–12 days with headache per month) and lasting for 24–72 h. Pain is accompanied by phonophobia, nausea, change in taste preferences (desire of salty and sweet food), face paleness, shiver and feeling of hot flashes to head and shortness of breath, frequent urination, yawning, drowsiness and apathy, as well as tenderness when touching the scalp (allodynia). The allodynia signs are not present between attacks. Among trigger factors there are emotional stress, hunger and alcohol intake. She is postmenopausal. During an attack the patient straps her head with a hot towel and takes two pills of Pentalgin (complex analgesic containing paracetamol, naproxen, caffeine, codeine and pheniramine). In case of pain resumption on the next day, she takes two more doses. The

V.V. Osipova, MD (✉) • E. Snopkova, MD, PhD • G. Tabeeva, MD
Department of Neurology, "Ivan Sechenov" First Moscow Medical University,
Rossolimo, 11, Moscow 119021, Russia
e-mail: osipova_v@mail.ru; kalinka-dr@mail.ru; grtabeeva@gmail.com

A. Siva, C. Lampl (eds.), *Case-Based Diagnosis and Management of Headache Disorders*, Headache, DOI 10.1007/978-3-319-06886-2_16

total number of painkillers for the last quarter ranged between 20 and 30 doses per month.

16.2.1 Case History

Headache attacks, similar to the described above, first appeared at the age of 17, became regular by the age of 20 and occurred four to six times a month. Similar headaches had been detected in her aunt. Attacks were triggered by menstruation, physical exertion, emotional stress, hunger and alcohol intake. In the young age the pain was of very high intensity (9–10 VAS points); however, the attacks were well controlled by combined analgesics and usually eliminated within 24 h. During the examination period in the university, the attacks could occur every day, whereas during vacations pain episodes became considerably less frequent. During both pregnancies in the middle of the 2nd trimester and lactation periods, headache attacks completely stopped and resumed only after the cessation of lactation. After menopause (at the age of 52), headache pattern remained the same with a frequency of three to five attacks per month.

For many years the patient has been managed by a neurologist (who considered the case as "attributed to autonomic dysfunction") and received numerous nonspecific treatments including cardiovascular and nootropics agents, as well as physiotherapeutic treatments with no effect. The patient has never received specific antimigraine prophylaxis (beta-blockers, calcium channel blockers, anticonvulsants, etc.).

The present visit to the neurologist was due to the increased duration and frequency of attacks over the last 2 months (eight to ten times a month) on the background of severe stressful situation (death of a family member) and excessive use of painkillers.

16.2.2 Neurological Examinations

No organic signs revealed during neurological examination (cognitive sphere, cranial nerves, tendon reflexes, sensation, coordination and pelvic functions appear normal). During the examination the patient appeared depressed and anxious.

16.2.3 Comorbid and Concomitant Conditions

Apart from headache episodes the patient complains about depressed mood, increased anxiety, sleep disturbances and mild memory impairment. During the last month in the nighttime, she experienced the episodes of palpitation accompanied by difficulties in breathing, anxiety and fear (similar episodes were observed at the age of 51 during the premenopausal period and stopped spontaneously 6 months later). Throughout the whole life as well as at present, the patient has had low blood pressure and experienced symptoms of hyperventilation (sensation of incomplete breath, laboured breathing) in stuffy rooms and under emotional stress. Over the last 15 years apart from headache attacks described above one to two times a month, the patient has been also experiencing episodes of mild diffuse pressing headache triggered by emotional stress and successfully aborted with ibuprofen.

16.2.4 Additional Examinations

Instrumental examinations that were repeatedly carried out over past 20 years (transcranial and ultrasonic Doppler of brachiocephalic vessels, EEG, X-ray of the skull) revealed no specific changes. Below are the results of the examinations performed within 2010–2011: *Complete blood count:* the parameters are in normal range. *Biochemical blood analysis:* elevated cholesterol (6.6 mmol/l). *ECG:* disorder of intra-atrial conductivity of myocardium. *X-ray of cervical spine:* moderate osteochondrosis and spondylosis. *TCD of BCA:* non-stenosing atherosclerosis and haemodynamically insignificant tortuosity (crimpiness) of the extravertebral parts of vertebral arteries. *Brain MRI:* no pathologic changes revealed in the brain tissue; empty ephippium (sella turcica). *Ophthalmologic investigation*: retinal angiopathy. *Neuropsychological examination:* moderate level of depression (Beck Depression Inventory score – 23), high level of reactive and personal anxiety (57 and 68 points of State-Trait Anxiety Inventory), strong influence of headache on the quality of life (69 points according to HIT-6) and high level of painkiller dependence (22 points according to Leeds Dependence Questionnaire).

16.2.5 Neurological Diagnosis

Migraine without aura, medication overuse (combined analgesics), episodic tension-type headache, anxiety and depression syndrome and panic attacks.

16.2.6 Treatment

Taking into consideration the increasing severity of migraine (increase in the frequency and duration of attacks), medication overuse (20–40 doses of combination analgesics per month) and comorbid emotional disorders, the following recommendations were given to the patient: (1) discontinuation/significant restriction of analgesics (possibly to be replaced by NSAIDS, triptans or ergotamine-containing drugs not more than 6–8 doses per month in total), (2) antidepressant therapy (paroxetine 20 mg/day) for 6–8 months and (3) behavioural therapy. Beta-blockers, calcium channel blockers and sartans were not recommended due to the marked arterial hypotension. To correct mild cognitive (memory) shortage, piracetam was added. In the future in case of insufficient therapeutic effect, anticonvulsants are planned to be recommended.

16.2.7 Follow-Up

After 8 weeks on prescribed therapy and discontinuation of analgesic overuse (now the patient takes not more than 6–8 doses of simple analgesics or triptans per month), the headache attack frequency reduced up to 3 per month, patients' mood improved, anxiety decreased and panic attacks ceased completely. It was recommended to continue taking paroxetine for the next 4 months.

16.3 Case Description 2

A 52-year-old man (married, an engineer, moderate smoker) addressed us because of depressed mood, anxiety and repeated episodes of visual phenomena which appear in one hemivisual field (mostly right sided), 1–2 times per 1–2 month; such episodes appeared after the age of 35 and were not accompanied by headache. He describes his symptoms as "blurred vision and fluorescent and flaring (scintillating) zigzag lines moving from the centre of visual field to the periphery" (Fig. 16.1).

16.3.1 Case History

Since the age of 11 one-two times per year, the patient has been experiencing attacks of intensive bilateral throbbing headache without associated symptoms lasting 8–12 h usually aborted with sleep. At the age of 22 for the first time, he experienced visual symptoms described above with the duration of 20–30 min. Until the age of 35, visual symptoms were followed by headache phase every time. At the age of 35, the headache attacks stopped while visual symptoms have persisted until now. In his 40s the patient noticed that the duration of visual episodes increased to 40–60 min and began to be accompanied by difficulties in speech (dysarthria); after the disappearance of visual symptoms, speech is completely recovered. Among factors provoking these episodes, the patient mentions bright light and intensive visual activity while using PC. A 19-year-old son of the patient since childhood has been suffering from similar headache attacks preceded by visual phenomena.

16.3.2 Neurological Examination

Without any significant findings, the patient is overweight; there is bilateral tenderness of the pericranial and cervical muscles during manual palpation; the patient looked very depressed and expressed anxiety associated with his condition (Fig. 16.1).

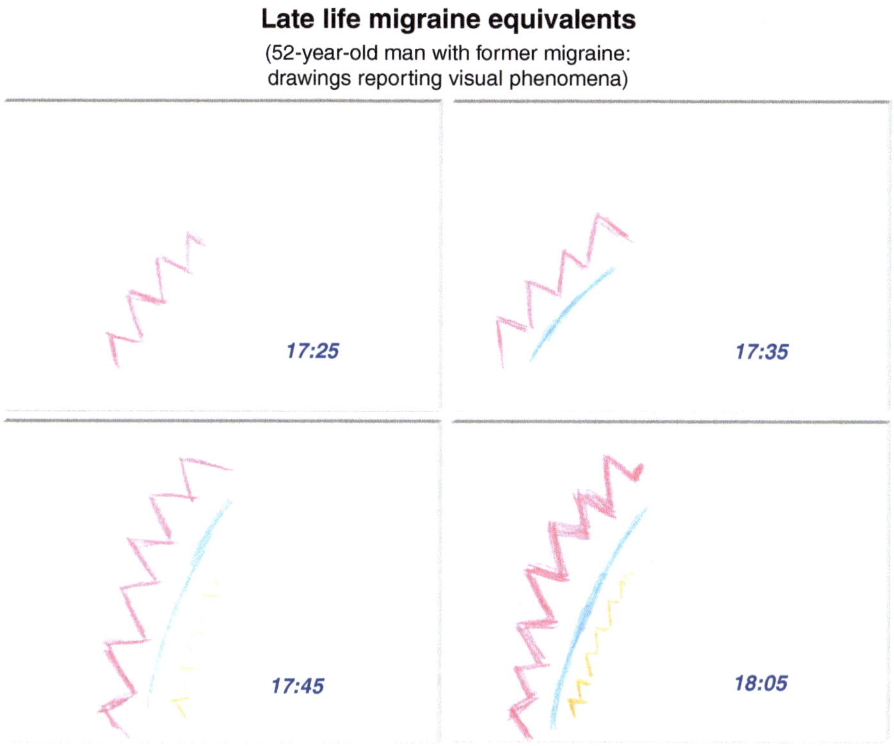

Fig. 16.1 Late Life Migraine Equivalents (52-year-old man with former migraine: drawings reporting visual phenomena)

16.3.3 Comorbid and Concomitant Conditions

Depressed mood, anxiety, episodic back and neck pain, sleep disturbances and arterial hypertension.

16.3.4 Additional Examinations

Complete blood count and biochemical analysis: the parameters are in normal range; cholesterol on the upper range. BP, 135/90; *Brain MRI and MR angiography* did not reveal any organic lesions. *Ophthalmologic investigation*: hypertensive retinal angiopathy.

16.3.5 Neurological Diagnosis

Late-life migrainous equivalent (LLME, Fisher's syndrome), migraine with aura (in the past), anxiety and depression syndrome and pericranial muscles dysfunction.

16.3.6 Treatment

For his arterial hypertension for the last 15 years, the patient received beta-blockers. Taking into account his severe depression and anxiety, the combination of antidepressant and neuroleptic (escitalopram + ticersin) was recommended for 6–8 months.

16.3.7 Follow-Up

When seen repeatedly over 2 years (at the age of 54), the patient demonstrated the same visual and occasionally speech defect symptoms; his mood has significantly improved; no complications or new symptoms were registered. The possibility of adding calcium channel blockers (nimodipine) should be considered in the future.

16.4 Summary of the Cases

Two presented cases illustrate different ways of migraine evolution in elder age. The 1st demonstrates the severe migraine course (*migraine persistence*) in a woman aged 57 and the 2nd, the incomplete migraine cessation (preservation of migraine aura without pain episodes) in a 53-year-old man which could be classified as *late-life migrainous accompaniment* (LLMA).

In the 1st case despite menopause lasting for 5 years, an elderly woman keeps on developing typical migraine attacks with the same accompanying symptoms, pain characteristics and triggers that were present in the young age. It is worth mentioning the following details of this case:

1. For many years the patient was managed by neurologist with the wrong "non-migraine" diagnosis and received erroneous nonspecific "non-migraine" treatment without significant improvement.
2. Although during the lifetime migraine attack occurrence and frequency were closely related to the hormonal state of a patient (onset during menarche, menstrually related migraine in the young age, remission during pregnancy and lactation), the attacks did not stop after menopause.
3. Migraine exacerbation in the relatively late age was triggered by significant emotional stress and subsequent psychiatric disorders (depression and anxiety).
4. On the background of emotional stress, another primary form of headache has developed (TTH).
5. Allodynia occurring during migraine attacks is typical for a patient with long migraine history and high attack frequency and reflects phenomenon of central sensitization.
6. Although the diagnostic criteria for MOH in this patient are not fulfilled, she obviously has medication overuse which occurred for the first time only recently.

Thus main predictors/risk factors of migraine persistence in this patient include:

- Emotional stress and related psychiatric conditions (depression and anxiety)
- Ineffective preceding treatment due to erroneous diagnosis which could facilitate disease progression
- Medication overuse

The 2nd case illustrates age-related transformation of migraine with visual aura into more complicated aura (visual and speech disturbances) without headache ("headless migraine"). Such complex of symptoms was described by C. M. Fisher in 1986 and is also called "late-life migrainous accompaniment". The past history of typical migraine without aura, normal instrumental examinations and benign course of the condition allowed us to exclude the possibility of other causes of aura symptoms. At the same time considering risk factors in our patient (arterial hypertension, mild obesity, elevated cholesterol and smoking), possible preventive therapy with calcium channel blockers could be further recommended.

16.5 Brief General Information

It is well known that migraine is the disease of young age with an onset in childhood or adolescence. Late onset (after 50) is reported only in 1–3 % of cases, and in the majority of patients, migraine completely stops after the age of 50.

At the same time in the minority of subjects, migraine attacks or some manifestations could last out. The exact data on frequency of each outcome is not available due to the absence of epidemiological studies. In the majority of patients (presumably 50–60 %), migraine stops completely; about 7 % continue experiencing more or less typical attacks. The prevalence of LLMA in general population does not exceed 1.4 % (1.33 % in females and 1.08 % in males); manifestation of Fisher's syndrome after the age of 50 is registered in 77 % of cases and in 1/4th in more young age. According to isolated published data in some patients after 45–50 years, old migraine becomes less severe (decrease in attack frequency, duration and intensity, loss of typical associated symptoms); in others migraine severely persists. Migraine outcomes after the age of 50 are summarized in Table 16.1 (according to the recent Russian study, 2011). Clinical predictors of migraine outcomes are listed in Table 16.2.

Elderly patients with migraine have some clinical peculiarities that should be taken into account (Table 16.3). Polymorbidity (conditions comorbid to migraine and concomitant somatic diseases) leads to polypragmasia. Such categories of patients often have more than one headache type as well as pain syndromes of other location (cervical and back pain, arthritis). Medical treatment of these additional pain conditions could significantly increase the medication overuse and possibility of MOH development.

Compared to young migraine subjects in elder patients, differential diagnosis requires more attention. In Table 16.4 the more common causes of headache in patients older than 50 are listed.

Table 16.1 Migraine outcomes in the elder age [5]

Cessation
Incomplete (no pain, preservation of M aura = late-life migrainous accompaniment (LLMA)
Complete (no aura, no pain attacks)
Preservation
Regressing migraine (mild course)
Persistent migraine (severe course)

Table 16.2 Clinical predictors of migraine evolution in the elderly

Mild/regressing M
M with aura
Low attack frequency in the young age
Menopause (=stable hormonal state)
Severe/persistent M
M without aura
Frequent attacks in the young age
Regular menstrual cycle or premenopause (non-stable hormonal state)
Late-life migrainous accompaniment (Fisher's syndrome)
M with aura

Table 16.3 General peculiarities of the elderly migraine patients

Polymorbidity = comorbid and concomitant disorders (sleep disturbances, depression, cognitive, cardiovascular and cerebrovascular disorders, etc.)	Polypragmasia
Combination of several headache types + Other pain syndromes	
Additional analgesics consumption	Increasing medication overuse and risk of MOH

Table 16.4 Differential diagnosis of migraine in the elderly *(ICHD-3 beta, 2013)*

Tension-type headache
Hypnic headache
Trigeminal autonomic cephalalgias (cluster headache, paroxysmal hemicrania, hemicrania continua, etc.)
Headache attributed to giant cell arteritis
Headache attributed to transient ischemic attack
Headache related to intracranial venous dysfunction
Headache attributed to arterial hypertension
Headache attributed to glaucoma
In case the usual clinical course of migraine changes with age, patient should be carefully examined to exclude secondary headache disorder

Key Points and Important Practical Considerations

- Migraine could persist in the late age with more or less typical symptoms. There is a group of elderly subjects with severe migraine course.
- Migraine after the age of 50 is often misdiagnosed and mistreated.
- The loss of reproductive function and age-related hormonal level stabilization cannot be considered as determinant factors for migraine discontinuance.
- Quality of life in the elderly migraineurs is most likely determined not by pain-related characteristics but (to a higher extent) by age-related concomitant somatic and cerebrovascular disorders and conditions comorbid to migraine (depression, anxiety, sleep abnormalities being the most important).
- Revealing concomitant pain syndromes and determining the total amount of painkillers are of great importance in the aged migraineurs: the use of analgesics for other pain syndromes could significantly increase medication overuse and the risk of MOH in migraine patients.
- Key factors leading to migraine persistence in the elderly include:
  1. Emotional stress, personality abnormalities and related psychiatric disorders (depression, anxiety, somatization, etc.).
  2. Inappropriate and ineffective preceding prophylactic and acute treatment due to erroneous "non-migraine" diagnosis.
  3. Medication overuse (including that due to extra-treatment of pain syndromes other from headache).
  4. Other general factors responsible for migraine progression/chronification should be also considered (high attack frequency in the young age, excessive caffeine intake, obesity, sleep apnoea, etc.).
- Elder subjects with late-life migrainous accompaniment do not need any prophylaxis until cardiovascular risk factors (obesity, diabetes, arterial hypertension, cholesterolaemia, smoking, etc.) are revealed. Calcium channel blockers (nimodipine) are the drug of choice in patients with LLMA and risk factors.

Suggested Reading

1. Edmeads JG, Wang SJ (2006) Headache in the elderly. The headaches. pp 1105–1010
2. Fisher CM (1986) Late-lafe migraine accompaniments – further experience. Stroke 17:1033–1042
3. Fisher CM (1999) Late-life (migrainous) scintillating zigzags without headache: one person's 27-year experience. Headache 39:391–397
4. Kelman L (2006) Migraine changes with age: impact on migraine classification. Headache 46:1161–1171

5. Maksyukova E, Sergeev A, Osipova V (2011) Migraine in older age: clinical and psychological analysis. J Neurol 258(Suppl 1):S271
6. Martins KM, Bordini CA, Bigal ME, Speciali JG (2006) Migraine in the elderly: a comparison with migraine in young adults. Headache 46:312–316
7. Mazzotta G, Gallai V, Alberti A, Bileci AM, Coppola F, Sarchielli P (2003) Characteristics of migraine in out-patient population over 60 years of age. Cephalalgia 23:953–960
8. Schwaiger J, Kiechl S, Seppi K, Sawires M, Stockner H, Erlacher T, Mairhofer ML, Niederkofler H, Rungger G, Gasperi A, Poewe W, Willeit J (2008) Prevalence of primary headaches and cranial neuralgias in men and women aged 55–94 years (Bruneck Study). Cephalalgia 29:179–187
9. Snopkova EV, Sergeev AV, Tabeeva GR, Osipova VV (2013) Clinical predictors of migraine evolution in elder age. Cephalalgia 33(Suppl 8):82

Chapter 17
Is It Migraine Aura in the Elderly or Transient Ischaemic Attack?

Koen Paemeleire

17.1 Case Description

A 65-year-old right-handed retired dentist presented to the outpatient neurology clinic after experiencing five episodes of transient focal neurological symptoms in a 1-year period. In fact, he had experienced similar episodes at a lower frequency in the past few years. A single episode was most often characterized by isolated visual symptoms; however, on some occasions these were followed by sensory symptoms and/or language impairment. There were never motor symptoms. The visual disturbance is described as a 'moonshaped grey-brown spot' which is growing over time and evolving into its maximum size over about 20 min on average, followed by a rather fast and complete resolution of the symptoms. He had evaluated his vision with both eyes separately and noticed the symptoms were binocular and present in either the right or left visual hemifield. Sensory symptoms and mild language impairment had on a few occasions followed the visual disturbance and were described as progressive tingling in one arm starting in the hand and moving up the forearm, and word finding difficulties; a detailed description could not be given. These focal neurological symptoms were followed by a mild, generalized, featureless headache which he rated 3–4/10 on a verbal rating scale. These headaches tended to respond well to ibuprofen and disappear within a few hours after onset. These attacks could on occasion be triggered by bright light but most attacks came on spontaneously. His past medical history was remarkable for arterial hypertension, successfully treated with perindopril, and mild reflux esophagitis.

K. Paemeleire, MD, PhD
Department of Neurology, Ghent University Hospital,
De Pintelaan 185, Ghent B-9000, Belgium
e-mail: koen.paemeleire@uzgent.be

A. Siva, C. Lampl (eds.), *Case-Based Diagnosis and Management of Headache Disorders*, Headache, DOI 10.1007/978-3-319-06886-2_17

17.2 Differential Diagnosis

Differential diagnoses to be considered in an elderly patient presenting with recurrent transient visual phenomena with mild headache mainly include transient ischemic attacks (TIAs) and migraine aura, as well as partial seizures.

17.3 Diagnostic Workup of the Case

It turned out this patient had undergone a workup a couple of years earlier in another centre, which included an ophthalmological examination, brain MRI including MR angiography of the circle of Willis, MR angiography of the cervical arteries, echocardiography as well as EEG. All results were normal. A detailed anamnesis revealed a clear history of migraine with aura since the age of 41 years. The exact timing remained unclear, but the patient remembers he was gradually less and less disabled by headache, and associated symptoms faded as the years went by. We instructed him to make a detailed drawing of his visual symptoms, and some time later we received 3 sketches of which one, digitized on the computer by his wife, is shown in Fig. 17.1. Analysis of all three sketches showed that visual symptoms were not monocular and were indeed experienced in either both left or right visual hemifields. Furthermore, his drawing showed that the slowly expanding grey-brown scotoma had a flickering (or 'dancing' as he described it) brighter edge, i.e. a

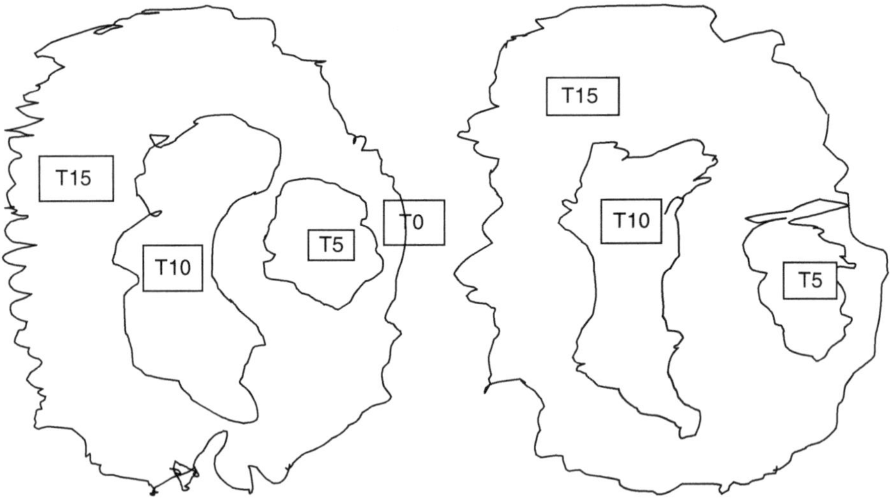

Fig. 17.1 Patient's drawing of a typical episode of transient visual disturbance. At the start ($T=0$ min), the patient noticed an initial change in the centre of his visual fields. At $T=5$ min into the attack he experienced a grey-brown blurred spot on the left of his centre of vision in both eyes. At $T=10$ min into the attack, the spot had enlarged into a moon shape with a flickering edge. At $T=15$ min he indicated the visual disturbance was present in almost the entire visual hemifield of the left and right eye. Finally, at $T=20$ min everything had returned to normal

combination of negative and positive symptoms known as a scintillating scotoma. No further testing was performed.

17.4 Summary of the Case

The patient had a well-established antecedent history of migraine with aura for more than 20 years. He presented with slowly progressing symptoms as illustrated by his drawing, a combination of positive (flickering edge of the scotoma, tingling in case of sensory aura symptoms) and negative symptoms (scotoma, word finding difficulties in case of language aura symptoms), and temporally related mild headache. The diagnosis was made with taking a detailed history and physical examination. Additional testing was not necessary, especially as the patient had undergone a complete workup some years earlier and symptoms were essentially unchanged. The situation would have been very different in an elderly patient lacking an established history of migraine with aura and presenting with aura symptoms for the first time, in which case a full differential diagnostic work-up, especially for TIA, would have been warranted.

17.5 Definition According to the International Classification of Headache Disorder 3rd Edition Beta Version (ICHDIIIbeta)

The ICHDIIIbeta 1.2.1 migraine with typical aura criteria were fulfilled, as the patient experienced multiple rather stereotyped episodes consisting of visual, sensory and/or speech/language symptoms, each fully reversible, but no motor, brainstem or retinal symptoms. Moreover, his visual aura symptoms spread gradually over ≥5 min, and, if present, sensory and language symptoms succeeded the visual symptoms, rather than appearing at the same time. Visual aura symptom duration was within the 5–60 min interval put forward in the criteria. Visual symptoms and, if present, sensory symptoms were always unilateral. A mild headache accompanied the aura, or immediately followed the aura symptoms, which is within the 60 min interval allowed in the criteria. The patient fulfils ICHDIIIbeta 1.2.1.1 subtype criteria for typical aura with headache, as the aura symptoms are accompanied or immediately followed by a headache that lost its migraine features over the years.

17.6 Brief General Information

A typical migraine aura consists of visual and/or sensory and/or speech/language symptoms and is characterized by gradual development, duration of each symptom no longer than 1 h, a mix of positive and negative features and complete reversibility. Visual disturbances are the most common aura symptoms in migraine with aura. Sensory symptoms and speech/language disturbances seldom occur without preceding visual symptoms. Motor, brainstem or retinal symptoms are coded elsewhere in the ICHDIIIbeta under hemiplegic migraine, migraine with brainstem aura and retinal migraine. The average visual aura duration is close to 30 min. Aura symptoms can be differentiated from TIA by their progressive onset, spreading over time and quality, often a combination of both positive and negative symptoms (Table 17.1). The prototype of visual aura is the scintillating scotoma, in which a gradually expanding scotoma is bordered by a flickering edge. A subclassification of migraine with aura is made in the ICHDIIIbeta into typical aura with (1.2.1.1) or without (1.2.1.2) headache. In the former subtype aura is accompanied or followed within 60 min by a headache with or without migraine characteristics.

Late life visual aura symptoms are not rare. Data from the Framingham study suggest visual migraine aura symptoms occur in at least 1 % of the population in mid or late life. These episodes may occur for the first time after age 50 years, in the absence of headache, and a history of recurrent headaches may not be present. They appeared not to be associated with increased risk of stroke in this population. More recent epidemiological studies have shown that certain patients with migraine with aura are at greater risk for stroke, namely, women under the age of 40 years, especially those using an oestrogen-containing contraceptive and smoking.

Cortical spreading depression is a slowly propagating neuronal and glial depolarization that spreads at a characteristic rate of 3–5 mm per minute. It has been studied in mammalian cortices, and closely resembling phenomena have been documented in the human cortex following ischaemic stroke, intracerebral haematoma, subarachnoid haemorrhage and brain trauma, and there is indirect evidence to suggest it is the underlying mechanism of migraine aura. There are however some unresolved questions about the relationship between CSD and aura, and an additional role for astrocytic calcium waves has been suggested.

TIAs are not usually associated with headache, but has been estimated that approximately 20 % of persons with TIAs have accompanying headache, especially with posterior fossa ischaemia. Brief hypoxic-ischaemic episodes could induce CSD which may generate aura and, possibly, migrainous headache. Some cases of aura induced by a focal reduction in cerebral blood flow during cerebral angiography have been reported. Cases of migraine with aura induced by ischaemia, e.g. due

Table 17.1 Differential diagnosis between aura and TIA

	TIA	Migraine aura
Onset	Sudden	Progressive
Progression	None	Slow
Different symptoms	Simultaneous	In succession
Type of visual symptoms	Negative	Negative or positive
Territory	Vascular	Cortical
Duration	Short (10–15 min)	Long (30–60 min)

Adapted from Schoenen and Sándor [14]

to severe internal carotid stenosis/occlusion, have been document-induced. In a mouse model, particulate or air microemboli were able to trigger cortical spreading depression (often without causing microinfarction), suggesting that migraine aura may be provoked by hypoperfusion disorders along with TIAs. In older persons, in whom vascular disease is more prevalent, TIA must therefore be ruled out when migraine aura occurs as a new phenomenon. In the absence of headache with migraine characteristics, a distinction of aura from mimics becomes more difficult. It is suggested in the ICHDIIIbeta that 'when aura occurs for the first time after age 40, when symptoms are exclusively negative (e.g. hemianopia) or when aura is prolonged or very short, other causes, particularly TIAs, should be ruled out'.

Some additional differential diagnoses have to be considered, including occipital seizures, amaurosis fugax, retinal migraine, ocular problems and arteriovenous malformations.

Occipital seizures are characterized by a sudden onset of symptoms with a fast rate of progression, positive and coloured visual symptoms of short duration (minutes). They differ in many respects from visual migraine aura with progressive and slow onset of symptoms, most typically with a combination of negative and positive symptoms and longer duration (up to 60 min). They share the sudden onset of with TIA symptoms, that are however of a negative nature and intermediate duration (10–15 min).

A specific form of TIA within the eye due to compromised ocular arterial circulation is amaurosis fugax. It is defined as a monocular transitory blindness or blurred vision that usually lasts for a few minutes. The most common cause is carotid artery disease with thromboembolism from an atherosclerotic plaque. It may also occur due to distal embolism from heart or aorta, local thrombosis within the optic nerve or retina and thromboembolism from non-atherosclerotic carotid artery disease including dissection. In the elderly giant cell arteritis should be considered. Amaurosis fugax should be considered a medical emergency and requires similar workup as other TIAs.

Structural lesions, such as occipital arteriovenous malformation, can produce similar symptoms to migraine with aura and have to be considered when aura symptoms are attributable to one fixed hemisphere.

Ocular problems, including glaucoma, may present with visual disturbances and headache, but a distinction from aura of TIA should not pose a major problem.

Retinal migraine is defined by the ICHD-IIIbeta as a fully reversible monocular visual disturbance associated with migraine headache and a normal neuro-ophthalmological examination between attacks. Its true incidence is unclear as some have shown that most cases labelled as retinal migraine in fact are not migraine. Retinal migraine most likely represents a heterogeneous group of underlying disorders. Retinal cortical spreading depression is often cited as the mechanism of retinal migraine; however, retinal CSD has not been observed in mammalian/human retina but has mainly been studied in the chick retina after its discovery in the frog retina. Vasospasm of retinal blood vessels has been observed in a small number of cases. Most cases of transient monocular visual loss diagnosed as retinal migraine would be more properly diagnosed as 'presumed retinal vasospasm'.

Key Points

- Aura symptoms can be differentiated from TIA by means of onset, progression and duration of symptoms, quality of the symptoms (most typically a combination of positive and negative symptoms) and, if more than one type of symptoms are present (visual and/or sensory and/or speech/language), by means of succession of symptoms that are not attributable to the same vascular territory.
- Late life visual aura symptoms are not rare.
- Ischaemia may induce cortical spreading depression and aura symptoms.
- The ICHDIIIbeta suggests that 'When aura occurs for the first time after age 40, when symptoms are exclusively negative (e.g. hemianopia) or when aura is prolonged or very short, other causes, particularly TIAs, should be ruled out'.
- Retinal migraine is very rare and most cases of transient monocular visual loss diagnosed as retinal migraine would be more properly diagnosed as 'presumed retinal vasospasm'.

Suggested Reading

1. Beekman R, Nijssen PCG, van Rooij WJ et al (2001) Migraine with aura after intracranial endovascular procedures. Headache 41:410–413
2. Charles A, Baca SM (2013) Cortical spreading depression and migraine. Nat Rev Neurol 9:637–644
3. Dalkara T, Nozari A, Moskowitz MA (2010) Migraine aura pathophysiology: the role of blood vessels and microembolisation. Lancet Neurol 9(3):309–317
4. Dennis M, Warlow C (1992) Migraine aura without headache: transient ischaemic attack or not? J Neurol Neurosurg Psychiatry 55:437–440
5. Evans RW, Tietjen GE (2001) Migrainous aura versus transient ischaemic attack in an elderly migraineur. Headache 41:201–203
6. Hill DL, Daroff RB, Ducros A et al (2007) Most cases labeled as "retinal migraine" are not migraine. J Neuroophthalmol 27:3–8
7. Koudstaal PJ, van Gijn J, Kappelle J (1991) Headache in transient or permanent cerebral ischemia. Stroke 22:754–759
8. Kunkel RS (2005) Migraine aura without headache: benign but a diagnosis of exclusion. Cleve Clin J Med 72:529–534
9. Lauritzen M (1994) Pathophysiology of the migraine aura. The spreading depression theory. Brain 117(Pt 1):199–210
10. Nozari A, Delikoz E, Sukhotinsky I et al (2010) Microemboli may link spreading depression, migraine aura, and patent foramen ovale. Ann Neurol 67:221–229
11. Olesen J, Friberg TS, Olsen TS et al (1993) Ischemia induced (symptomatic) migraine attacks may be more frequent than migraine-induced ischemic insults. Brain 116:187–202
12. Rother J, de Crespigny AJ, D'Arceuil H et al (1996) MR detection of cortical spreading depression immediately after focal ischemia in the rat. J Cereb Blood Flow Metab 16:214–220
13. Saarela M, Sundararajan S, Strbian D (2014) Young patient with headache and amourosis fugax. Stroke 45:e3–e4

14. Schoenen J, Sándor PS (2004) Headache with focal neurological signs or symptoms: a complicated differential diagnosis. Lancet Neurol 3:237–245
15. Headache classification committee of the international headache society. The international classification of headache disorders, 3rd edition beta version (2013) Cephalalgia 33: 629–808
16. Wijman CAC, Wolf PA, Kase CS et al (1998) Migrainous visual accompaniments are not rare in late life. The Framingham Study. Stroke 29:1539–1543

Chapter 18
Migraine Without Aura, with a Discussion of Trigger Factors

Mustafa Ertas and Hayrunnisa Bolay

18.1 Case Description

A 38-year-old Caucasian woman suffering from headache attacks that interfered with activities of daily living visited a headache specialist for the first time. The frequency and severity of her headache attacks had increased over the previous 4 months, and she was suffering one or two attacks every week. Her attacks were throbbing and mostly one-sided, either on the right or the left side of her head. The pain would start from the neck and spread to the forehead in some attacks, but in most it would start from the temple on one side and spread behind the ipsilateral eye. During headache attacks, any movement of her head would increase the intensity of headache, and light and noise would disturb her. Severe attacks were associated with nausea without vomiting. She experienced increased sensitivity to touch on her scalp, predominantly on the headache side and particularly during severe headache attacks. Just before an attack, she would yawn repeatedly. She had never experienced any visual, sensory, or speech problem or any transient neurological dysfunction preceding the headache. In the absence of taking any painkiller such as ibuprofen or another nonsteroidal anti-inflammatory drug, the headaches could last up to 3 days. The intensity of her headache attacks was generally severe. She was a manager in public relations in a large company. If she had a severe headache she was unable to perform any work activities and sometimes had to go home when she could not successfully treat the pain. Five months earlier, her position in the company had changed and she was given additional responsibilities. She was married with two daughters, 13 and 5 years old. Her headache attacks had started nearly 1 year after her first delivery. The frequency of attacks was one or two times a month up to the second pregnancy. For 2 years after the first delivery she was taking oral contraceptive pills (OCPs), but

M. Ertas (✉) • H. Bolay
Department of Neurology, Liv Hospital, Ulus, Istanbul, Turkey
e-mail: mustafaertas@superonline.com

A. Siva, C. Lampl (eds.), *Case-Based Diagnosis and Management of Headache Disorders*, Headache, DOI 10.1007/978-3-319-06886-2_18

had to stop taking them because of a marked increase in the frequency of headache attacks. During the second pregnancy she had almost no headache attacks, but 1 week after the delivery her attacks returned, with pain more severe than before.

The attacks were occurring 1 or 2 days before almost every menstrual period. In addition to the menstrual cycle, other triggering factors were warm windy weather, locally called "Lodos," skipping meals, excessive sleep, loss of sleep, bright lights such as sunlight, excessive effort, and any excessive emotional changes such as anger, sorrow, and even gladness. She noticed that drinking red wine brought on a headache. If she ate dessert such as baklava or chocolate, or had a craving for almost anything sweet, she would have a headache within an hour. She also noticed that strong perfumes might trigger her headaches; therefore, she stopped using perfumes and did not allow her husband to use aftershave. She had used neither prophylactic treatment for her headache attacks nor specific acute-attack medication for migraine, such as triptans and ergots. Her daily routine includes regular consumption of 6 cups of black tea and 2 cups of Turkish coffee; water consumption is limited, she occasionally drinks wine, and she does not smoke. Her sleep pattern has changed; frequent awakenings had occurred during the past few months when her stress level had increased. Physical and neurological examinations did not reveal any abnormalities.

18.2 Differential Diagnosis and How to Work Up This Type of Patient

This patient suffers from primary headache disorder whose diagnosis depends on the history and detailed introspection of the patient for the pain and associated symptoms. One of the major problems with primary headache disorders is the fact that there are no diagnostic biological markers. The differential diagnosis of the presented case includes migraine without aura, episodic tension-type headache, and medication-overuse headache. The patient has never described aura symptoms. The features of pain fulfill the episodic migraine headache criteria, as the frequency of headache days is less than 15 days per month. Neuroimaging studies and blood tests are usually not needed unless the clinical history is not diagnostic and exclusion of secondary causes for headache or accompanying disease is considered. As the neurological history was consistent with a diagnosis of migraine without aura and her examination was within normal limits, no laboratory tests or neuroimaging studies were needed.

18.3 Diagnostic Workup of the Case

The features of this patient's headache fulfill the criteria of *International Classification of Headache Disorders* (2nd edition, 2004 and 3rd beta edition, 2013) for migraine without aura. The patient had more than one type of headache. One starts from the neck and spreads to the forehead, whereas the other radiates from the temple to the back of the eye. Many patients with migraine have more than one type of headache sharing common migrainous features. The attack duration of this patient is between 2 and 3 days. Women with migraine have longer-lasting migraine attacks than men with migraine, on average one and a half days in women and 1 day in men. The intensity of her pain is generally severe. Her headache is mostly lateralized to one side, pulsatile in quality, and aggravated by head movements. Some patients with migraine experience migrainous headache almost always at the same side of the head, while the majority of patients report side-shifting. Fewer patients always have migraine headache bilaterally. Light and noise cause disturbance during the headache attacks (photophobia and phonophobia). The patient has nausea but no vomiting during these episodes. She describes increased sensitivity to touch and mechanical pressure on the scalp during attacks (allodynia). Around 60 % of migraineurs have allodynia on the scalp during the headache phase that may continue even after the headache recedes. Migraineurs may describe the symptom of allodynia as an unpleasant sensation while combing hair or wearing eyeglasses. Yawning and craving for sweets before the onset of pain are common prodromal symptoms of migraine attacks. This patient experiences yawning some minutes before the headache. Although there is no certain starting age for migraine, in general the buildup is around the age of 20–25 years. During pregnancy, the increasing estrogen level without fluctuation is the major protecting factor against migraine attacks. After delivery, the estrogen level goes down. With the termination of breast feeding, estrogen fluctuations return, together with migraine attacks. Sometimes migraine attacks resume immediately after delivery, as in the second delivery of this patient. She had never previously visited a physician about headache. Epidemiological studies have shown that at least one-third of patients with migraine do not go to a physician for their headaches, not necessarily because the headache is not severe enough to demand professional help. The percentage of migrainous patients under prophylactic treatment for migraine is much less than it need be. The reason for this is not only the reluctance of patients to visit physicians but also the underestimation by the physicians of the disability attributable to migraine. Accordingly, this patient has never used a specific medication for migraine attacks and has never received any treatment for the prevention of migraine attacks.

18.4 Brief General Information: Headache Triggers

Triggers are very important, both in the clinical diagnosis of migraine as per the classification criteria and in the management of migraine. Some triggers share the same role in different primary headache disorders such as migraine, tension-type headache, and cluster headache, whereas others are discriminating. This patient reports several triggers for her headache. She experiences migraine attacks 2–3 days before nearly every menstrual period. More than half of women with migraine have a very high chance of experiencing migraine attack in the perimenstrual period (from day −2 to day +3). However, this is not only the case in migraine but also in tension-type headache. Although not to as great an extent as for migraine, one-fourth of women with pure tension-type headache, without accompanying migraine, have a much higher chance of experiencing perimenstrual headache attacks. In the perimenstrual period, migraine attacks may occur mostly 1 or 2 days before menstruation. The chance of having a migraine attack at the end of the menstruation period or on days following menstruation is less. Alterations in the intrinsic or extrinsic milieu triggers migraine headache, and women of reproductive age are continuously prone to waxing and waning effects of female sex hormones. Migraine attacks frequently occur during menstruation when serum levels of estradiol and progesterone steeply decline, and attacks are lower before puberty and after the menopause when the level of ovarian hormones in serum is stable and low. Clinical observations suggest that sex steroids differentially influence attacks in patients with both migraine with aura and migraine without aura. In migraine without aura, attacks are significantly reduced during pregnancy when the level of ovarian hormones in serum are stable and high, but in migraine with aura, new attacks often occur during pregnancy. Menstrual migraine attacks occur almost invariably without aura even in women who experience migraine with aura. OCP use is likely to lead to significant worsening of attacks in patients with migraine with aura (Table 18.1).

This patient's attacks are also triggered by stress, skipping meals, excessive sleep, daytime sleep, and loss of sleep. Such triggers may provoke both migraine and tension-type headache. Mood changes may trigger both migraine and tension-type headache. However, while stress is the most frequent trigger for both migraine and tension-type headache, joyfulness may only trigger migraine, as in this patient. Although skipping meals and sleep disturbances may commonly trigger migraine attacks, occasionally they may also trigger tension-type headaches.

Changes in the weather and warm winds have long been known to affect individuals with migraine, and are correlated with the emergence of headache. Major atmospheric weather variables such as atmospheric pressure, temperature, humidity, and wind or thunderstorm activity are all implicated as potential triggers for headache. It is noteworthy that weather change is usually accompanied by alteration of more than one atmospheric variable. For instance, low atmospheric pressure stimulates movement of air from surrounding areas, and is generally associated with winds, increased temperature, and humidity, facilitating the development of clouds, precipitation, and thunderstorms. Dust-laden weather originating in the African desert has been implicated as a possible trigger by providing molecules and nanoparticles to induce migraine headaches. Outbreaks of Saharan dust are seasonal and very frequent in transitional seasons, and are associated with warm winds and low pressure. Lightning and associated meteorological changes were recently associated with a 28 % increase in the frequency of migraine headaches. Other environmental factors such as high altitude, loud noises, and exposure to glare or flickering lights are also documented as triggers. Atmospheric changes such as windy weather, barometric changes, and bright sunlight are much more frequently reported by migraineurs than by patients with tension-type headaches. Odors such as perfumes, smoke, and strong smells trigger migraine specifically, and are nearly never reported by patients with pure tension-type headache.

Drinking alcoholic beverages is a common trigger for both migraine and cluster headache but not for tension-type headache. However, as this patient reports, red wine and beer are the most common triggering alcoholic beverages for migraine,

Table 18.1 Common triggers in migraine headache

Emotional	Chronic high-level stress
	Abrupt change in the stress level
	Anxiety
	Depression
Sex hormones	Puberty
	Menstruation/ovulation
	Oral contraceptives and hormone replacement therapy
	Pregnancy
	Perimenopausal period
Environmental	Bright lights, sun glare
	Loud sounds
	Smoking
	Scents such as perfume or paint thinner
	Exposure to heat or cold (hot weather, hot baths)
	Traveling
	Jet lag
Atmospheric weather	Change of weather conditions (low barometric pressure, warm winds, high temperature, precipitation, lightning)
	High altitudes (hiking, skiing)
Food	Citrus fruits
	Fermented foods and beverages
	Chocolate, nuts
	Aged cheese, dairy products
	Foods containing nitrates (bacon, hot dogs, salami, cured meats)
	Foods containing monosodium glutamate, aspartame
	Processed, marinated, or pickled foods
Beverages	Alcoholic beverages (i.e., beer, red wine)
	High caffeine consumption (coffee, tea, energy drinks)
	Limited water consumption
Drugs	Abuse of over-the-counter pain medication
	Overuse of painkillers containing caffeine, butalbital, codeine
	Nitroglycerin, nifedipine
	Hormone replacement therapy, OCP
Daily living habits	Changes in wake-sleep pattern, not enough or too much sleep, frequent wake-ups
	Skipping meals, insufficient meal, fasting
	Abnormal head and neck position while working (computer, screen viewing, etc)
Others	Colds, flu, or a sinus infection
	Intense physical exertion, sexual activity
	Head injury

while any kind of alcohol triggers cluster headaches. Foodstuffs may trigger headache in about 10 % of persons with migraine, and may trigger migraine attacks rather than tension-type headaches. However, sometimes a strong desire for certain foods such as chocolate and sweets may be a premonitory symptom of migraine rather than being triggers of attacks. Certain foods may trigger migraine in certain migraineurs, although triggering foods may differ from one migraineur to another. Excessive consumption of caffeine or stopping consumption of regular caffeine may also be a triggering factor for migraine. Caffeine can be found in many products including energy drinks, chocolate, and over-the-counter painkillers. Missing meals or eating insufficient snacks instead of a balanced meal can also induce a migraine attack. Fasting is another trigger, and this also varies depending on fasting habits in different cultures. Migraine headache generally occurs during the first week of the fasting period for Muslims that lasts 30 days (the Ramadan month), whereas headache in Hindu patients, for whom alternating days of fasting occur, are triggered throughout the whole period.

Some additives such as monosodium glutamate, nitrates, and aspartame are other well-known triggers. Inadequate water consumption and mild dehydration can have an impact on persons with migraine. As already mentioned, there is some evidence that wine, and particularly red wine, may trigger a migraine, and many migraineurs avoid drinking red wine. In addition, migraine is related to delayed-type allergy and immunoglobulin G antibodies to various foods.

Tiredness may also trigger both migraine and tension-type headache. While tiredness resulting from hard work may trigger tension-type headache, sportive physical activity, even intensely, may be used by patients with pure tension-type headache as a means to improve their symptoms, and these kinds of activities are nearly never reported as headache triggers by patients with tension-type headache. However, migraineurs mostly avoid intense physical activities, even though such activities, such as playing tennis, swimming, playing soccer or basketball, are pleasant for people other than migraineurs.

Allodynia is described as a painful response to typically nonpainful stimuli. Combing hair, touching the scalp, and wearing eyeglasses are not painful stimuli. However, many migraineurs avoid these actions during a migraine attack. Allodynia is reported to occur during their attack by nearly 60 % of patients with migraine. Headache patients with either migraine or pure tension-type headache and with cutaneous allodynia on their scalp during headache are more responsive to triggers. Figure 18.1a–c shows triggers for migraine and pure tension-type headache and the effect of scalp allodynia during headache from a home-based population headache study in Turkey.

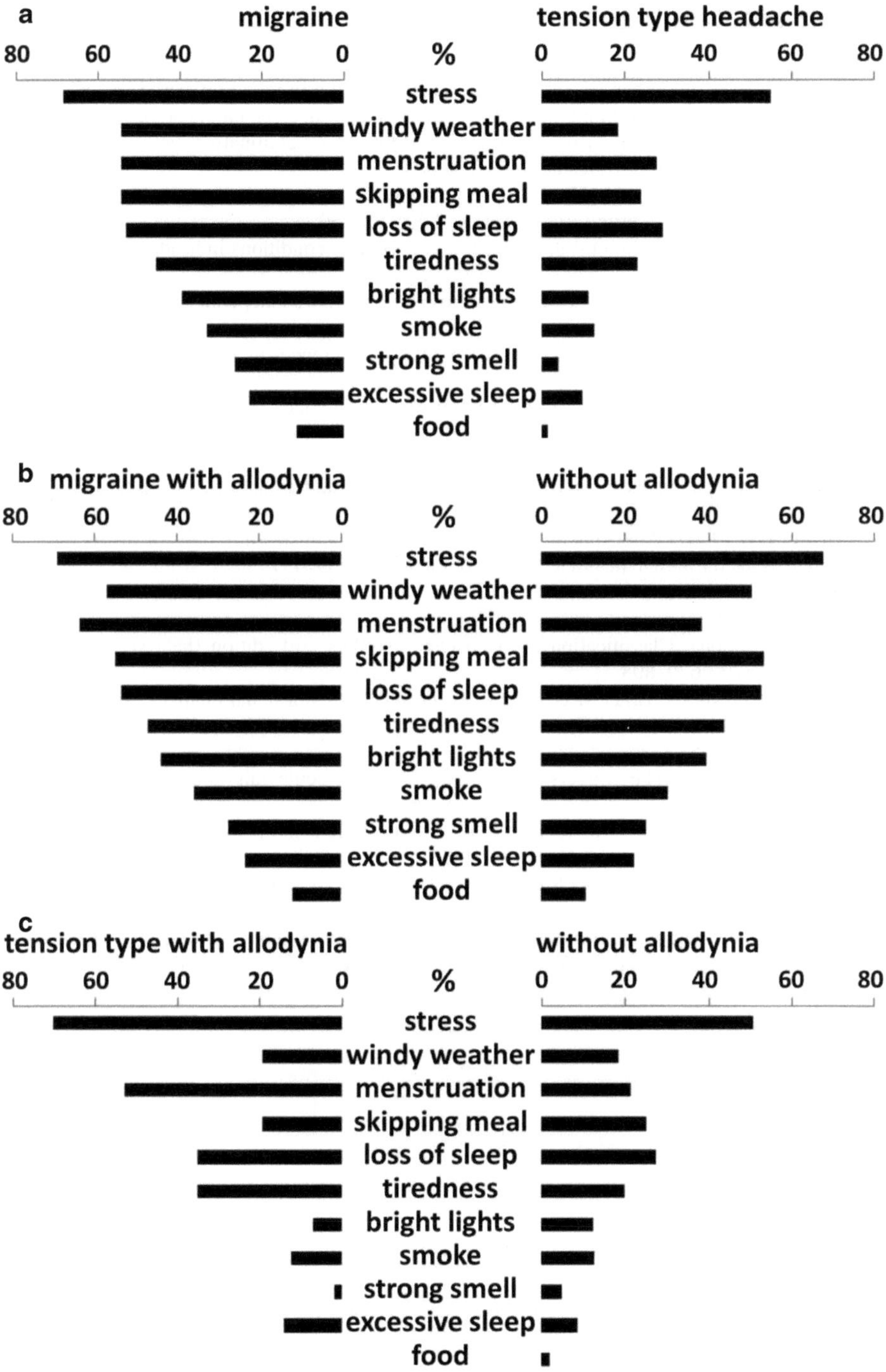

Fig. 18.1 Percentage distribution of headache triggers (**a**) in migraine versus tension-type headache; (**b**) in migraine according to allodynia; (**c**) in tension-type headache according to allodynia (Data from Turkish Headache Prevalence Study, 2008)

Suggested Reading

1. Alpay K, Ertas M, Orhan EK, et al (2010) Diet restriction in migraine, based on IgG against foods. A clinical double-blind, randomised, cross-over trial. Cephalalgia 30:829–837
2. Aydinlar EI, Dikmen PY, Tiftikci A et al (2013) IgG-based elimination diet in migraine plus irritable bowel syndrome. Headache 53:514–525
3. Baldacci F, Vedovello M, Ulivi M et al (2013) Triggers in allodynic and non-allodynic migraineurs. A clinic setting study. Headache 53:152–160
4. Bolay H (2013) En'lightning' the impact of atmospheric conditions in headache. Cephalalgia 33:362–364
5. Bolay H, Rapoport A (2011) Does low atmospheric pressure independently trigger migraine? Headache 51:1426–1430
6. Bolay H, Berman NE, Akcali D (2011) Sex-related differences in animal models of migraine headache. Headache 51(6):891–904
7. Doganay H, Akcali D, Goktas T et al (2009) African dust-laden atmospheric conditions activate the trigeminovascular system. Cephalalgia 29:1059–1068
8. Ertas M, Baykan B, Orhan EK et al (2012) One-year prevalence and the impact of migraine and tension-type headache in Turkey: a nationwide home-based study in adults. J Headache Pain 13:147–157
9. Griffin DW (2007) Atmospheric movement of microorganisms in clouds of desert dust and implications for human health. Clin Microbiol Rev 20:459–477
10. The International Classification of Headache Disorders: 2nd edition (2004). Cephalalgia 24 Suppl 1:9–160
11. The International Classification of Headache Disorders, 3rd edition (beta version) (2013). Cephalalgia 33:629–808
12. Karli N, Baykan B, Ertas M et al (2012) Impact of sex hormonal changes on tension-type headache and migraine: a cross-sectional population-based survey in 2,600 women. J Headache Pain 13:557–565
13. Kelman L (2007) The triggers or precipitants of the acute migraine attack. Cephalalgia 27(5):394–402
14. Levy D, Strassman AM, Burstein R (2009) A critical view on the role of migraine triggers in the genesis of migraine pain. Headache 49:953–957
15. Lipton RB, Bigal ME, Ashina S et al (2008) Cutaneous allodynia in the migraine population. Ann Neurol 63:148–158
16. Wober C, Holzhammer J, Zeitlhofer J, Wessely P, Wober-Bingol C (2006) Trigger factors of migraine and tension-type headache: experience and knowledge of the patients. J Headache Pain 7:188–195

Chapter 19
Migraine Patients with Comorbid Disorders and Their Management

Stefan Evers

19.1 Case Description

Case 1 A 45-year-old female patient was admitted to a headache clinic because she experienced an increase of frequency in her known migraine without aura attacks. Since puberty, she suffered from menstrual migraine attacks with a duration of 3–4 days. The attacks were accompanied by nausea, photophobia, and phonophobia. In the first years, she took paracetamol or acetylsalicylic acid to treat the attacks which was of limited success; often 5–10 tablets were needed during the headache period. After introduction of the triptans, she switched to sumatriptan 100 mg tablets which gave her relief for a whole day; later she took also zolmitriptan 5 mg. She never was put on a short-term prophylaxis or other prophylactic treatment.

The patient had two pregnancies, during which no migraine attacks occurred. However, after the lactation period, migraine recurred and the menstrual migraine continued. In the last years, the menstruation of the patient became irregular, and the frequency of migraine attacks increased up to three or four attacks per month which were of shorter duration (only 1 or 2 days) but with increased pain severity. In addition, the patient developed mild arterial hypertension and was put on ramipril 2.5 mg. In this situation, the patient was referred to a supraregional headache clinic in order to recommend further drug treatment.

In the consultation, the patient was informed about the possibilities of preventive drug treatment of migraine. The indication was given and the patient agreed to prophylactic treatment with a beta blocker. This drug was chosen because it could control both arterial hypertension and migraine. The patient was put on 47.5 mg metoprolol succinate and was asked to keep a headache diary and to return after 3

S. Evers
Department of Neurology, Krankenhaus Lindenbrunn,
Lindenbrunn 1, Coppenbrügge 31863, Germany
e-mail: everss@uni-muenster.de

A. Siva, C. Lampl (eds.), *Case-Based Diagnosis and Management of Headache Disorders*, Headache, DOI 10.1007/978-3-319-06886-2_19

months. Further, the patient was assured that she could take a triptan (zolmitriptan 5 mg) despite her arterial hypertension, since this was controlled by drugs.

At the control visit after 3 months, the patient reported a decrease of migraine attacks to only one per month. This single attack could well be treated by zolmitriptan. However, after starting metoprolol, the patient developed heavy dreams, even sometimes nightmares, which she was not used to. Also, mild somnolence occurred in the morning, but this was tolerated by the patient in opposite to the nightmares which were very frightening for the patient. The arterial hypertension was well controlled under metoprolol.

It was agreed to switch the prophylactic drug to candesartan 16 mg per day. After another 3 months, the patient reported no heavy dreams or nightmares any more. Migraine was still about one attack per month which could be aborted by zolmitriptan. Arterial hypertension was well controlled. It was agreed to continue the intake of candesartan 16 mg for 1 year and then to try and discontinue the prophylactic treatment.

Case 2 A 23-year-old male patient suffered from myoclonic jerks and dialeptic seizures since the age of 14 onwards. The myoclonic jerks happened primarily in the morning every day. Dialeptic seizures occurred under stress and were observed nearly every day. The diagnosis of primary juvenile myoclonus epilepsy (Janz syndrome) was confirmed by generalized epileptiform discharges in the EEG. The patient was treated with levetiracetam 500 mg bid, which controlled the seizures nearly completely. At the age of 21, the patient developed also generalized tonic-clonic seizures about once per week. The dose of levetiracetam was increased, but even in a daily dose of 2,000 mg bid, which was well tolerated without any side effects, generalize tonic-clonic seizures still occurred rarely, whereas myoclonic jerks and dialeptic seizures completely disappeared.

Together with the generalized tonic-clonic epileptic seizures, the patient also developed migraine attacks with half-sided severe headache, which was aggravated by physical activity, with photophobia, nausea, and visual disturbances. These migraine attacks occurred in an irregular frequency of about three times per month. They lasted about 1 day and could sufficiently but not completely be controlled by ibuprofen 800 mg. Triptans were tried but not tolerated by the patient because of pressure feeling in the chest.

When the patient was admitted to the headache clinic, he was dissatisfied with the frequency of migraine attacks and with the incomplete efficacy of ibuprofen. Interestingly, he was not bothered by the rarely occurring generalized tonic-clonic epileptic seizures. The patient was informed about the possibility to treat both migraine and primary epilepsy by valproic acid or by topiramate. Since he was asthenic (BMI under 20), he chose valproic acid and was put on 450 mg bid in a slow-release formulation. After 3 months, he returned to the headache clinic and reported no tonic-clonic seizures anymore and a decrease of migraine attack frequency by about 50 %. The migraine attacks could now be treated by ibuprofen very efficiently; the patient was pain-free within 2 h after drug intake and could continue working without problems.

Case 3 A 55-year-old female patient was admitted in a psychiatric outpatient clinic because of a depressive episode. Such episodes occurred for about 20 years from time to time and were mostly treated by psychotherapy, only rarely an antidepressant drug was necessary in addition. This time, the patient complained about more severe depressive symptoms; however, the sleep was mostly unaffected. It was agreed to initiate a short behavioural psychotherapy for 4 weeks and to start with citalopram 20 mg in the morning as antidepressant.

The patient also suffered from up to five migraine attacks per month since her menopause. In the decades before, only rarely migraine attacks occurred. The treatment was successful with a triptan (rizatriptan 10 mg), but the patient was advised not to take a triptan while also taking citalopram because of a possible serotonergic syndrome.

The patient's depression resolved clearly within 4 weeks but migraine attacks remained. Therefore, the patient was admitted to a headache clinic, where the diagnosis of migraine without aura was confirmed. The patient was advised that citalopram is not efficacious in the prophylaxis of migraine and that a tricyclic antidepressant would be better for her migraine. In agreement with the psychiatrist, the patient was put on amitriptyline 25 mg on the evening which was increased after 2 weeks to 50 mg. Also, the patient had the impression that the migraine attacks were less severe under this medication. However, she became very tired, sometimes even somnolent, and also obstipated. She refused to take amitriptyline any further and asked for alternatives.

The patient was then put on venlafaxine slow release 75 mg bid which was well tolerated except a mild restlessness in the morning. After about 4 weeks, the depression was controlled as it was under citalopram and the migraine attacks decreased in frequency. The patient was advised that there was no contraindication to take a triptan along with venlafaxine and that she should continue venlafaxine for at least months.

19.2 Diagnosis and How to Work Up This Kind of a Patient

The cases illustrate how important it is to consider comorbidity when migraine drug treatment is discussed with the patient. Comorbidity might occur most just by chance (e.g. arterial hypertension in migraine), or comorbidity has been shown to be significant in epidemiological studies such as stroke and migraine with aura or restless legs syndrome and migraine without aura. The latter comorbidities do not necessarily mean that there is a causal link between migraine and the other disorders.

In case no. 1, the female migraine patient developed an increase of severity and frequency of migraine when the menopause started. This is typical for some women with a menstrually related migraine. In this period, she also developed arterial hypertension. Thus, it is obvious to choose a drug treating both conditions. The drug of first choice is a beta blocker which is normally well tolerated in this age. However, this patient developed heavy dreams and nightmares which is a rare but typical side effect of many beta blockers. Therefore, she was switched to candesartan which is not approved for migraine prophylaxis because evidence from the literature suggests that candesartan is effective in migraine prophylaxis. In particular, a very recent study was published showing a similar efficacy of candesartan and propranolol. Candesartan is well tolerated, and in this case the patient showed sufficient benefit from it. Another aspect of this case is that triptans are not contraindicated in patients with comorbid arterial hypertension as long as the hypertension is under control.

Case no. 2 presents a patient with both migraine and primary generalized epilepsy. There is conflicting data in the literature as to whether all types of epilepsy are significantly associated with migraine. An association has only been shown consistently for the benign Rolando's epilepsy. However, epileptic seizures might occur together with migraine attacks (called migralepsy), and very rarely epileptic seizures might have features of migraine attacks. Concomitant epilepsy has to be considered when choosing the best prophylactic treatment of migraine. The only two anticonvulsive drugs with consistently proven efficacy in migraine are valproic acid and topiramate. Both drugs are also efficacious in primary epilepsy (whereas carbamazepine and others should not be used in primary epilepsy). On the other hand, levetiracetam can control primary epilepsy but has not been shown to be efficacious in migraine prophylaxis. The patient in this case was put on valproic acid because this drug could cause weight gain whereas topiramate causes weight loss as a side effect. In addition, valproic acid is the drug of first choice in primary epilepsy, at least in female patients, with respect to efficacy.

In case no. 3, we observe the typical comorbidity of migraine and depression. This comorbidity is bidirectional, meaning that patients with migraine are of increased risk to develop depression and vice versa. If migraine and depression are both relevant, the treatment should be carefully chosen since some interactions might occur. Beta blockers and flunarizine, for example, can increase the severity or even induce a depressive episode. On the other hand, citalopram or other SSRI-type antidepressants would not improve migraine frequency or severity. Furthermore, there is a contraindication to take SSRI and triptans together because of the possible development of a serotonergic syndrome (which, however, has never been reported in the literature). In this case, amitriptyline was given to treat both depression and migraine. This drug was not tolerated which is often the case, at least in migraine patients. Somnolence and obstipation are typical side effects of amitriptyline. As an alternative, venlafaxine can be given although there is not much evidence for efficacy in migraine. Venlafaxine is often better tolerated than amitriptyline, it can be given together with triptans, and there are published studies suggesting an efficacy in migraine.

In summary, the cases illustrate how one can try and treat migraine and comorbid disorders by the same drug and how to consider contraindications or specific labels when prescribing a specific drug in migraine patients.

Key Points

- A comorbidity of migraine with several other disorders has been shown by epidemiological studies (Table 19.1). This comorbidity does not necessarily reflect a causal link. Furthermore, migraine can be comorbid with a disorder just by chance.
- Comorbidity of migraine should be considered when choosing the prophylactic drug treatment. This refers to both types of comorbidity. It is often possible to treat both conditions with one drug (Table 19.2).
- Comorbidity should also be considered in the acute drug treatment of migraine attacks. It might be that the acute drug is contraindicated under specific comorbid circumstances (e.g. triptans in patients with coronary heart disease).

Table 19.1 Disorders comorbid with migraine as shown in at least two population-based epidemiological studies

Category	Disorder
Psychiatry	Depression including bipolar disorders
	Anxiety disorders
	Compulsive-obsessive disorders
Neurology	Epilepsy
	Tourette's syndrome
	Restless legs syndrome
Vascular disorders	Raynaud's phenomenon
	Ischemic stroke, subclinical stroke
	White matter abnormalities
Cardiac	Patent foramen ovale
	Mitral valve prolapse
	Atrial septal aneurysm
	Myocardial infarction
Other	Asthma/allergy
	Systemic lupus erythematosus
	Non-headache pain
	Different types of vertigo
	Temporomandibular disorder

Table 19.2 Recommended drugs when treating migraine with a comorbid disorder

Comorbid disorder	Prophylactic drug
Arterial hypertension	Metoprolol or propranolol
	Candesartan
Epilepsy	Valproic acid
	Topiramate
	Gabapentin
Depression	Amitriptyline
	Venlafaxine
Restless legs syndrome	Gabapentin

Suggested Reading

1. Buse DC, Silberstein SD, Manack AN, Papapetropoulos S, Lipton RB (2013) Psychiatric comorbidities of episodic and chronic migraine. J Neurol 260:1960–1969
2. Cianchetti C, Pruna D, Ledda M (2013) Epileptic seizures and headache/migraine: a review of types of association and terminology. Seizure 22:679–685
3. Evers S, Afra J, Frese A, Goadsby PJ, Linde M, May A, Sandor P (2009) EFNS guideline on the drug treatment of migraine – revised report of an EFNS task force. Eur J Neurol 16:968–981
4. Katsarava Z, Weimar C (2010) Migraine and stroke. J Neurol Sci 299:42–44
5. Linde M, Mulleners WM, Chronicle EP, McCrory DC (2013) Antiepileptics other than gabapentin, pregabalin, topiramate, and valproate for the prophylaxis of episodic migraine in adults. Cochrane Database Syst Rev (6):CD010608
6. Mehle ME (2012) Migraine and allergy: a review and clinical update. Curr Allergy Asthma Rep 12:240–245
7. Nappi RE, Nappi G (2012) Neuroendocrine aspects of migraine in women. Gynecol Endocrinol 28(Suppl 1):37–41
8. Ozyalcin SN, Talu GK, Kiziltan E, Yucel B, Ertas M, Disci R (2005) The efficacy and safety of venlafaxine in the prophylaxis of migraine. Headache 45:144–152
9. Sathe S (2013) Migraine and neurogenetic disorders. Curr Pain Headache Rep 17:360
10. Schwedt TJ (2009) The migraine association with cardiac anomalies, cardiovascular disease, and stroke. Neurol Clin 27:513–523
11. Stovner LJ et al (2013) A comparative study of candesartan versus propranolol for migraine prophylaxis: a randomised, triple-blind, placebo-controlled, double cross-over study. Cephalalgia 34:523–532
12. Tronvik E et al (2003) Prophylactic treatment of migraine with an angiotensin II receptor blocker: a randomized controlled trial. JAMA 289:65–69

Chapter 20
Tension-Type Headache

Lars Bendtsen and Sait Ashina

20.1 Case Description

A 59-year-old woman referred by a neurologist to the Danish Headache Center, a tertiary headache centre, for the treatment of refractory migraine presents for the initial consultation. The patient has suffered from frequent headaches since childhood and in the last couple of years from daily headaches. She told me that she was so tired of the headaches that have ruined her life and of all the various treatments she has received during her life. None of the treatments has had any effect, several have been costly and several had bothersome side effects. She had almost given up hope. The patient did not fill out the 4-week headache diary that has been mailed to her from the headache centre prior to the initial consultation, and it was difficult for her to give a detailed headache history. She reported that her headaches could be unilateral or bilateral, of moderate to severe intensity, throbbing and at times pressing in character and could be aggravated by waking stairs. She also reports frequent nausea and sometimes sensitivity to sounds and light. The headaches are clearly provoked by psychological stress and to a lesser extent by physical activity. Sometimes headaches are preceded by visual disturbances. She had been on sick leave due to the headaches in the past 3 months. She reports being often anxious but she denies depressed mood. She works as

L. Bendtsen (✉)
Department of Neurology, Faculty of Health and Medical Sciences,
Danish Headache Center, Glostrup Hospital, University of Copenhagen,
Nordre Ringvej, Glostrup DK-2600, Denmark
e-mail: bendtsen@dadlnet.dk

S. Ashina
Department of Pain Medicine and Palliative Care, Icahn School of Medicine
at Mount Sinai, Beth Israel Medical Center, New York, NY, USA

Department of Neurology, Headache Program, Icahn School of Medicine
at Mount Sinai, Beth Israel Medical Center, New York, NY, USA

A. Siva, C. Lampl (eds.), *Case-Based Diagnosis and Management of Headache Disorders*, Headache, DOI 10.1007/978-3-319-06886-2_20

a teacher and had some stress at work. Otherwise, she is healthy. Her mother had suffered from life-long migraines. Her paternal uncle had brain aneurysm. At the first consultation, it was obvious that the patient suffered from migraine, tension-type headache (TTH) and anxiety on the most severe headache days. General and neurological examination demonstrates increased pericranial myofascial tenderness. Her blood pressure and pulse are within normal limits. Electrocardiogram and routine blood tests are unremarkable. What to do for this severely incapacitated woman?

20.2 Differential Diagnosis and How to Work Up This Kind of a Patient

The major diagnostic problem in this case is differentiation between episodes of tension-type headache and migraine. In the general population, 94 % of migraineurs also experience TTH and 56 % of migraineurs experience frequent episodic TTH. In contrast, TTH occurs with similar prevalence in those with and without migraine. However, the majority of patients seen by headache specialists will suffer from both disorders. Due to lack of accompanying symptoms and the relatively milder pain intensity in TTH, patients rarely complain of severe incapacitation due to their pain. TTH is the most featureless of the primary headaches and because many secondary headaches may mimic TTH, a diagnosis of TTH should be made only after exclusion of other organic disorders.

A general and neurological examination and prospective follow-up using a headache diary for at least 4 weeks in which all drugs taken are recorded are essential to make the diagnosis. The diary may also reveal triggers of headache and medication overuse, and it will establish the baseline against which to measure the efficacy of treatments. Identification of a high intake of analgesics is important because medication overuse requires specific treatment. There are no reliable imaging or laboratory tests that are reliably useful in the differential diagnosis. Manual palpation of the pericranial muscles and their insertions should be done to demonstrate a possible muscular factor for the patient and to plan the treatment strategy, where physical training and biofeedback/relaxation therapy are important treatment modalities. Paraclinical investigations, in particular brain imaging, are necessary if secondary headache is suspected (e.g. the headache characteristics are atypical), if the course of headache attacks changes or if persistent neurological or psychopathological abnormalities are present.

20.3 Diagnostic Workup and Management of the Case

At the first consultation, the patient was informed about general aspects of headaches such as basic knowledge about pathophysiological mechanisms and common trigger factors, and she was instructed how to fill out a 4-week headache diary. At follow-up after 4 months (shorter would have been optimal but was not possible due to workload in the centre), the diary demonstrated that the most frequent headache was located bilaterally and the character was pressing and intensity moderate with no worsening with physical activities. There occasionally was phonophobia but no accompanying photophobia or nausea. Two days per month, she had unilateral, severe, throbbing headaches with aggravation during physical activity and concomitant nausea and photo- and phonophobia. Approximately two times per year, she experienced scintillating scotomas lasting 30 min which sometimes were followed by headache within 15 min. It was now clear that she suffered from chronic tension-type headache 28 days per month, migraine without aura 2 days per month and infrequent attacks of migraine with visual aura. She was also suffering from anxiety but this was only in relation to her migraine attacks. Both TTH and migraines were provoked by psychological stress. There was no acute medication overuse.

The patient had been treated by her general practitioners since childhood, by a dentist and by three different neurologists for her headaches all without any effect on her headache. Previous non-pharmacological therapies included relaxation therapies, physical therapies, acupuncture, chiropractor and numerous alternative therapies. Among these, only relaxation therapy had had a minor effect. Previous attack medications included aspirin, several NSAIDs, paracetamol and triptans. Previous prophylactic treatments included metoprolol 100 mg daily and others that she did not remember. At the time of referral, she was using ibuprofen 200–600 mg per day approximately 8 days per month and amitriptyline 10 mg daily. At the first consultation in the headache centre, the patient was referred to the psychologists and the physical therapists in the headache centre with the aim of a stress and management course (cognitive-behavioural therapy) and physical therapy with focus on the improvement of posture, individual exercise programmes, relaxation and biofeedback. She was prescribed sumatriptan for migraine attacks and candesartan for migraine prophylaxis.

At the second consultation, after 4 months, she reported that now she could distinguish between TTH and migraine. She had great benefit from both psychological and physical treatments. She experienced a good effect in using sumatriptan for migraine attacks. She had not started candesartan, because she realized by means of her headache diary that she only had 1–2 migraines per month well treated by a triptan and because she would like to avoid daily medications if possible. She was recommended to increase the dose of amitriptyline by 10 mg per week to a daily dose of maximally 70 mg at bedtime and referred to evaluation by a dentist working in the headache centre, because she reported muscle tensions in the jaws.

At the third consultation, 6 months later, she has much improved with only 8 days with TTH per month and 2 days with migraine. The dentist did not have any further suggestions for the treatment. She had not increased the dose of amitriptyline from 10 mg/day as suggested because of the much improved headache and because she would avoid prophylactic medications if possible and fear for side effects. The physician suggested that amitriptyline should be stopped to test whether it had any effect in such a low dose. The patient was still followed with long intervals by the psychologist and physical therapist to make sure that she continued to use the psychological and physical skills that she had learnt.

At the fourth consultation, after another 6 months, she was still doing well. Headache had worsened when she stopped amitriptyline, so she resumed taking the low dose of 10 mg before night-time. She had TTH 8–10 days per month for which she took aspirin 500 mg 4 days per month and migraine without aura 1–2 days per month well controlled by sumatriptan 100 mg. She had not experienced any migraines with aura since admission to hospital. She was very happy with her situation and was discharged from the headache centre and had to follow up with her GP.

20.4 Summary of the Case

The case is a 59-year-old woman who has been suffering from frequent headaches since childhood and by daily headaches during the past couple of years before the referral. She has been treated by her GP, several neurologists, a dentist and numerous other health care professionals without success. She was referred to a tertiary headache centre, where it was evident that she suffered from both TTH and migraines, but the relative importance of these two disorders and the role of provoking factors were obscure. A detailed headache history provided by the patient and the headache diary made it clear that she was suffering from chronic TTH and infrequent migraines and that psychological stress played an important role for both disorders. Physical examination demonstrated increased tenderness of pericranial myofascial structures. She underwent a stress and management course and physical therapy and was prescribed specific treatment for her migraine attacks. She continued on low dose of amitriptyline as preventative therapy for both TTH and migraine. After 16 months of management, she was taken over by her GP. At this time she has been doing well for 1 year with 8 days with TTH and 2 migraine days per month.

The case illustrates the importance of a correct diagnosis and of identification of triggering factors such a psychological stress and musculoskeletal factors.

20.5 Definition According to the International Classification of Headache Disorders

Tension-type headache is classified into three subtypes according to headache frequency: infrequent episodic TTH (<1 day of headache per month), frequent episodic TTH (1–14 days of headache per month) and chronic TTH (≥15 days per month). TTH is characterized by a bilateral, pressing, tightening pain of mild to moderate intensity not aggravated by routine physical activity. The headache is not associated with typical migraine features such as vomiting and severe photophobia or phonophobia. In the chronic form, one symptom of mild nausea and photo- or phonophobia may be present.

20.6 Brief General Information

Non-pharmacological management of TTH is not always as successful as in the presented case. Pharmacological management of individual attacks with acetaminophen, aspirin and nonsteroidal anti-inflammatory drugs has a documented effect in patients with episodic TTH but rarely has an effect in chronic TTH. Prophylactic pharmacotherapy should be considered in patients with frequent episodic or chronic TTH. The tricyclic antidepressant amitriptyline is the first drug of choice. Amitriptyline should be started at low dosages (10–25 mg/day) and titrated by 10–25 mg weekly until the patient has either good therapeutic effect or until side effects are encountered. It is important that patients are informed that this is an antidepressant agent but has an independent action on pain. The maintenance dose is usually 30–75 mg daily administered 1–2 h before bedtime to help to circumvent any sedative adverse effects. A significant effect of amitriptyline may be observed already in the first week on the therapeutic dose. It is therefore advisable to change to other prophylactic therapies, if the patient does not respond after 4 weeks on maintenance dose. The side effects of amitriptyline include dry mouth, drowsiness, dizziness, constipation, palpitations and weight gain. Mirtazapine, of which the major side effects are drowsiness and weight gain, or venlafaxine, of which the major side effects are vomiting, nausea, dizziness and loss of libido, should be considered if amitriptyline is not effective or not tolerated. Discontinuation should be attempted every 6–12 months. The physician should keep in mind that the efficacy of preventive drug therapy in TTH is often modest and that the efficacy should outweigh the side effects.

Key Points

- An accurate diagnosis, in which the individual headache episode is distinguished from migraine and from a secondary headache, especially medication-overuse headache, is essential. The use of a headache diary is helpful for diagnosis and treatment planning. Possible triggers and comorbidity with other disorders, in particular depression and anxiety, should be assessed and addressed.
- Nondrug management should always be considered. Information, reassurance and identification of trigger factors may be rewarding. EMG biofeedback has a documented effect in TTH, while cognitive-behavioural therapy and relaxation training most likely are effective. Physical therapy and acupuncture may be valuable options for patients with frequent TTH.
- Simple analgesics and nonsteroidal anti-inflammatory drugs are recommended for the treatment of episodic TTH. Combination analgesics containing caffeine are the second drugs of choice. It is crucial to avoid frequent and excessive use of analgesics to prevent the development of medication-overuse headache.
- Amitriptyline is the first drug of choice for the prophylactic treatment of chronic TTH. Mirtazapine and venlafaxine are the second drugs of choice.

Suggested Reading

1. Ashina M (2004) Neurobiology of chronic tension-type headache. Cephalalgia 24:161–172
2. Ashina S, Bendtsen L, Ashina M, Magerl W, Jensen R (2006) Generalized hyperalgesia in patients with chronic tension-type headache. Cephalalgia 26:940–948
3. Bendtsen L (2000) Central sensitization in tension-type headache – possible pathophysiological mechanisms. Cephalalgia 20:486–508
4. Bendtsen L, Evers S, Linde M, Mitsikostas DD, Sandrini G, Schoenen J (2010) EFNS guideline on the treatment of tension-type headache – report of an EFNS task force. Eur J Neurol 17:1318–1325
5. Bendtsen L, Jensen R (2011) Treating tension-type headache – an expert opinion. Expert Opin Pharmacother 12(7):1099–1109
6. Cathcart S, Petkov J, Winefield AH, Lushington K, Rolan P (2010) Central mechanisms of stress-induced headache. Cephalalgia 30:285–295
7. Fernandez-de-Las-Penas C, Cuadrado ML, Arendt-Nielsen L, Simons DG, Pareja JA (2007) Myofascial trigger points and sensitization: an updated pain model for tension-type headache. Cephalalgia 27:383–393
8. Holroyd KA, O'Donnell FJ, Stensland M, Lipchik GL, Cordingley GE, Carlson BW (2001) Management of chronic tension-type headache with tricyclic antidepressant medication, stress management therapy, and their combination: a randomized controlled trial. JAMA 285:2208–2215
9. Jensen R, Zeeberg P, Dehlendorff C, Olesen J (2010) Predictors of outcome of the treatment programme in a multidisciplinary headache centre. Cephalalgia 30:1214–1224
10. Leistad R, Sand T, Westgaard R, Nilsen K, Stovner L (2006) Stress-induced pain and muscle activity in patients with migraine and tension-type headache. Cephalalgia 26:64–73
11. Nestoriuc Y, Rief W, Martin A (2008) Meta-analysis of biofeedback for tension-type headache: efficacy, specificity, and treatment moderators. J Consult Clin Psychol 76:379–396
12. Sandrini G, Rossi P, Milanov I, Serrao M, Cecchini AP, Nappi G (2006) Abnormal modulatory influence of diffuse noxious inhibitory controls in migraine and chronic tension-type headache patients. Cephalalgia 26:782–789

Chapter 21
Tension-Type Headache

Rigmor Jensen and Lars Bendtsen

21.1 Case Description

Case 1 A 46-year-old woman was referred for a headache problem for at least 25 years. Started with episodic headaches once or twice a week, became chronic and near daily 5 years ago and can now report 1–2 monthly episodes of additional severe unilateral headaches with aggravation by physical activity especially in relation to menstrual period. These "migraine-like" headaches responded very well to triptans, whereas the "normal" headaches were nonresponsive. She was referred to the headache clinic for a refractory chronic headache. Her physical and neurological examination was completely normal besides severe tenderness in the pericranial muscles, especially in the trapezius and splenius muscles in the neck. Her blood pressure was 140/86 mmHg and the pulse rate was 82 beats/min. A prior Cranial CT-Scan (CTC) was also normal. A diagnostic diary is presented in Fig. 21.1.

Case 2 A 32-year-old man was referred with a chronic, almost constant bilateral, pressing mild to moderate headache for the last 10 years. Started as short episodes (2–8 h) of a similar headache at the age of 15, which responded well to simple analgesics as paracetamol or NSAIDs. Now there is no effect of simple analgesics, opioids nor of triptans. Before the referral to the headache centre, the patient has received multiple treatments at chiropractor, physical therapist, acupuncture and other complimentary strategies without effect. At present the patient took no medication. His physical and neurological examination was completely normal and there was only mild tenderness in the trapezius muscles in the neck. His blood pressure was 126/82 mmHg and the pulse rate was 61 beats/min. A prior cerebral MRI was also normal. His diagnostic diary is presented in Fig. 21.2.

R. Jensen (✉) • L. Bendtsen
Department of Neurology, Danish Headache Center, Glostrup Hospital,
University of Copenhagen, Nordre Ringvej 67, Building 24, Glostrup 2600, Denmark
e-mail: rigmor.jensen@regionh.dk; bendtsen@dadlnet.dk

A. Siva, C. Lampl (eds.), *Case-Based Diagnosis and Management of Headache Disorders*, Headache, DOI 10.1007/978-3-319-06886-2_21

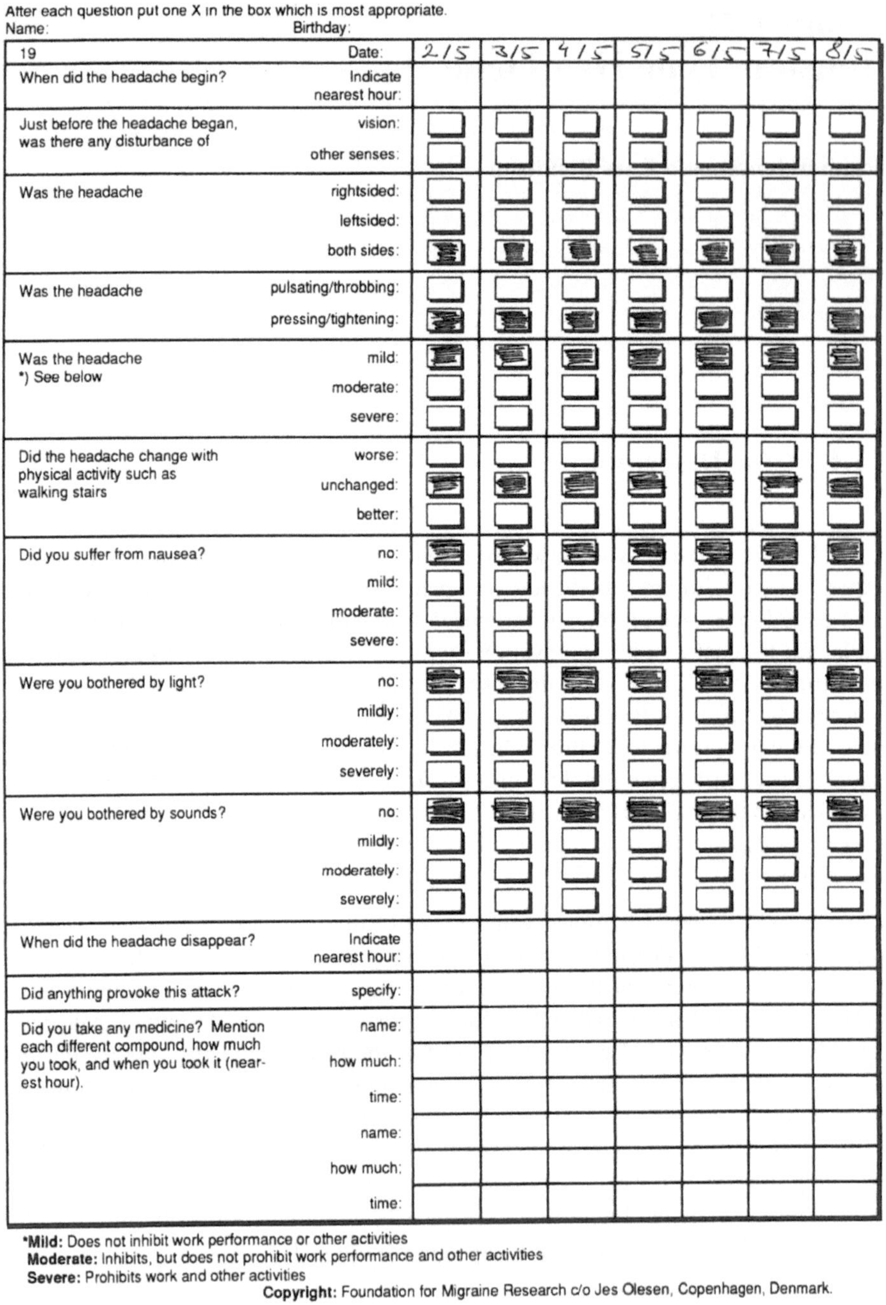

After each question put one X in the box which is most appropriate.
Name: Birthday:

19	Date:	2/5	3/5	4/5	5/5	6/5	7/5	8/5
When did the headache begin?	Indicate nearest hour:							
Just before the headache began, was there any disturbance of	vision:	☐	☐	☐	☐	☐	☐	☐
	other senses:	☐	☐	☐	☐	☐	☐	☐
Was the headache	rightsided:	☐	☐	☐	☐	☐	☐	☐
	leftsided:	☐	☐	☐	☐	☐	☐	☐
	both sides:	■	■	■	■	■	■	■
Was the headache	pulsating/throbbing:	☐	☐	☐	☐	☐	☐	☐
	pressing/tightening:	■	■	■	■	■	■	■
Was the headache *) See below	mild:	■	■	■	■	■	■	■
	moderate:	☐	☐	☐	☐	☐	☐	☐
	severe:	☐	☐	☐	☐	☐	☐	☐
Did the headache change with physical activity such as walking stairs	worse:	☐	☐	☐	☐	☐	☐	☐
	unchanged:	■	■	■	■	■	■	■
	better:	☐	☐	☐	☐	☐	☐	☐
Did you suffer from nausea?	no:	■	■	■	■	■	■	■
	mild:	☐	☐	☐	☐	☐	☐	☐
	moderate:	☐	☐	☐	☐	☐	☐	☐
	severe:	☐	☐	☐	☐	☐	☐	☐
Were you bothered by light?	no:	■	■	■	■	■	■	■
	mildly:	☐	☐	☐	☐	☐	☐	☐
	moderately:	☐	☐	☐	☐	☐	☐	☐
	severely:	☐	☐	☐	☐	☐	☐	☐
Were you bothered by sounds?	no:	■	■	■	■	■	■	■
	mildly:	☐	☐	☐	☐	☐	☐	☐
	moderately:	☐	☐	☐	☐	☐	☐	☐
	severely:	☐	☐	☐	☐	☐	☐	☐
When did the headache disappear?	Indicate nearest hour:							
Did anything provoke this attack?	specify:							
Did you take any medicine? Mention each different compound, how much you took, and when you took it (nearest hour).	name:							
	how much:							
	time:							
	name:							
	how much:							
	time:							

***Mild:** Does not inhibit work performance or other activities
Moderate: Inhibits, but does not prohibit work performance and other activities
Severe: Prohibits work and other activities

Fig. 21.1 Diagnostic diary for case 1, indicating a chronic, daily tension-type headache and 1 day with migraine without aura

After each question put one X in the box which is most appropriate.
Name: Birthday:

19	Date:	3/9	4/9	5/9	6/9	7/9	8/9	9/9
When did the headache begin?	Indicate nearest hour:	7	2	10 30	7	7	7	9
Just before the headache began, was there any disturbance of	vision:							
	other senses:							
Was the headache	rightsided:				X			
	leftsided:							
	both sides:	X	X	X		X	X	X
Was the headache	pulsating/throbbing:		X		X			
	pressing/tightening:	X		X		X	X	X
Was the headache *) See below	mild:	X	X	X		X	X	
	moderate:				X			
	severe:							
Did the headache change with physical activity such as walking stairs	worse:							
	unchanged:	X	X	X	X	X	X	X
	better:							
Did you suffer from nausea?	no:	X	X	X	X	X	X	X
	mild:							
	moderate:							
	severe:							
Were you bothered by light?	no:	X	X			X	X	X
	mildly:			X	X			
	moderately:							
	severely:							
Were you bothered by sounds?	no:	X	X	X	X	X	X	
	mildly:							X
	moderately:							
	severely:							
When did the headache disappear?	Indicate nearest hour:							
Did anything provoke this attack?	specify:							
Did you take any medicine? Mention each different compound, how much you took, and when you took it (nearest hour).	name:							
	how much:							
	time:							
	name:							
	how much:							
	time:							

***Mild:** Does not inhibit work performance or other activities
Moderate: Inhibits, but does not prohibit work performance and other activities
Severe: Prohibits work and other activities

Fig. 21.2 Diagnostic diary for case 2, indicating a chronic tension-type headache, with a very constant and identical presentation on a daily basis

21.2 Diagnosis and Differential Diagnosis

Tension-type headache (TTH) is characterized by a bilateral, pressing tightening pain of mild to moderate intensity, occurring either in short episodes of variable duration, infrequent TTH ≤1 days/month or as frequent episodic TTH occurring between 1 and 14 days/month or continuously in the chronic form ≥15 days/month. The headache is pressing in quality, often bilateral and not aggravated by physical activity as in migraine. Furthermore, TTH is not associated with the typical migraine features as vomiting, severe nausea, photophobia and/or phonophobia. Only one of the migraine accompanying symptoms is allowed, so either photophobia, phonophobia or nausea is accepted. Due to lack of accompanying symptoms and the relatively mild pain intensity, patients are rarely severely incapacitated by their pain to the same degree as to migraine and cluster headache. In the clinic, TTH patients often call these headaches "normal" or their "background" headache. Likewise, migraine or medication-overuse headache (MOH) patients tend to underestimate these headaches in the direct interview, and a diagnostic diary where all headaches are registered is therefore a very useful instrument. As TTH also is the most featureless of the primary headaches and because many secondary headaches may mimic TTH, a diagnosis of TTH requires exclusion of other organic disorders.

A general and neurological examination and a prospective follow-up using diagnostic headache diaries with registration of all consumed drugs are therefore of utmost importance to reach the diagnosis. There are no reliable specific paraclinical tests that are useful in the differential diagnosis. Manual palpation of the pericranial muscles and their insertions should always be done to demonstrate a possible muscular factor for the patient and to plan the treatment strategy, where physical training and relaxation therapy are important components.

The differential diagnosis is most frequently migraine and MOH, as they most frequently coexist with TTH. A migraine attack may start as a TTH-like headache, high-frequency TTH may trigger a latent migraine and a long-lasting severe migraine attack may also be accompanied by a TTH in the postictal phase. Based on the medical history, the diagnostic diary and the phenotype, secondary headaches as MOH, posttraumatic headaches and idiopathic intracranial hypertension should also be ruled out. MOH can be identified by a detailed interview and a prospective diary if all pain medications are indicated. Posttraumatic headache is required to have occurred in close relation (within 8 days) to a head trauma and, despite the headaches, is most often accompanied by a variety of cognitive complaints, fatigue, isolation, alcohol intolerance and sleep problems. IIH can present in variable forms but most often manifest as a severe more migraine-like constant headache, along with pulsating tinnitus, and transitory visual obscurations in obese, young individuals. In all cases of chronic headache, a detailed funduscopy in the search for papilledema is required.

In case 1, there is a very typical coexisting migraine once or twice a month but this headache is fully responsive to triptans, whereas the "normal" featureless background headache, the chronic tension-type headache, is unresponsive to triptans or simple analgesics, which is the most significant problem for the patient.

In case 2, the patient is suffering from a "pure" chronic TTH without any other primary or secondary headaches, and the headaches are completely constant without day to variation.

21.3 Treatment

A correct diagnosis should be assured by means of a headache diary recorded over at least 4 weeks (Figs. 21.1 and 21.2). The diagnostic problem most often encountered is to discriminate between TTH and mild migraines. The diary may also reveal triggers and medication overuse, and it will establish the baseline against which to measure the efficacy of treatments. Identification of a high intake of analgesics is essential as other treatments are largely ineffective in the presence of medication overuse. Significant co-morbidities, e.g. anxiety or depression, should be identified during the consultation and treated concomitantly.

Information about the nature of the disease is important. It can be explained that muscle pain can lead to a disturbance of the brain's pain-modulating mechanisms, so that normally innocuous stimuli are perceived as painful, with secondary perpetuation of muscle pain and risk of anxiety and depression. The very fact that the physician takes the problem seriously may have a therapeutic effect, particularly if the patient is concerned about serious disease, e.g. brain tumour, and can be reassured by thorough muscle and neurological examination. The most frequently reported triggers for TTH are stress (mental or physical), irregular or inappropriate meals, high intake of coffee and other caffeine-containing drinks, dehydration, sleep disorders, too much or too little sleep, reduced or inappropriate physical exercise, psychological problems as well as variations during the female menstrual cycle and hormonal substitution. It should be explained to the patient that frequent TTH only seldom can be cured, but that a meaningful improvement can be obtained with the combination of non-pharmacological and pharmacological treatments. These treatments are described separately in the following but should go hand in hand.

Non-pharmacological management should be considered for all patients with TTH and is widely used. However, the scientific evidence for efficacy of most treatment modalities is sparse. Physical therapy is the most used non-pharmacological treatment of TTH and includes the improvement of posture, relaxation and exercise programmes. Active treatment strategies are generally recommended (here to case 1). It has been reported that adding craniocervical training to classical physiotherapy was better than physiotherapy alone and a recent study indicated the effect of manual therapy. There are conflicting results regarding the efficacy of acupuncture for the treatment of TTH.

Psychological treatment strategies have reasonable scientific support for effectiveness. Relaxation training is a self-regulation strategy that provides patients with the ability to consciously reduce muscle tension and autonomic arousal that can precipitate and result from headaches. Electromyographic (EMG) biofeedback has been demonstrated to be effective. During EMG biofeedback, patients are presented

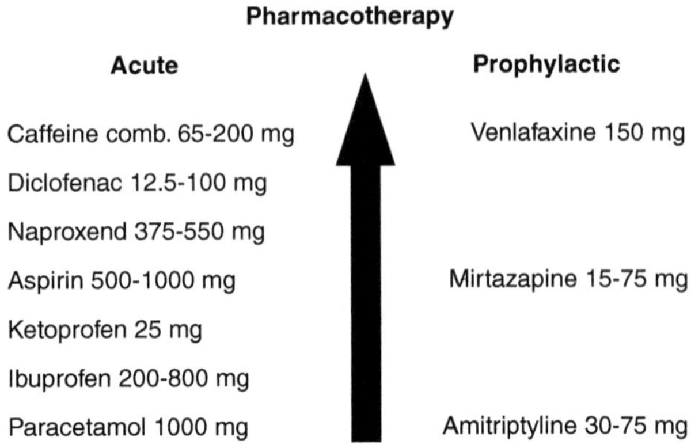

Fig. 21.3 Pharmacological treatment paradigm for tension-type headache

with an auditory or visual display of electrical activity of the muscles in the face, neck or shoulders. This feedback helps the patients to develop control over pericranial muscle tension. It is most likely that cognitive changes (i.e. self-efficacy) rather than reductions in muscle tension account for the improvement in TTH with EMG biofeedback. Cognitive-behavioural therapy (stress management) aims to teach the patient to identify thoughts and beliefs that generate stress and aggravate headaches (here to case 1). The exact degree of effect of psychological treatment strategies is difficult to estimate, but cognitive-behavioural therapy has been found to be comparable with treatment with tricyclic antidepressants, while a combination of the two treatments seemed to be more effective than either treatment alone.

Acute pharmacological therapy refers to the treatment of individual attacks of headache in patients with episodic and chronic TTH. Most headaches in patients with episodic TTH are mild to moderate, and the patients often can self-manage by using simple analgesics. The efficacy of the simple analgesics tends to decrease with increasing frequency of the headaches. In patients with chronic TTH, the headaches are often associated with stress, anxiety and depression, and simple analgesics are usually ineffective and should be used with caution because of the risk of MOH at a regular intake of simple analgesics above 14 days a month or triptans or combination analgesics above 9 days a month. Other interventions such as nondrug treatments and prophylactic pharmacotherapy should be considered.

Simple analgesics and nonsteroidal anti-inflammatory drugs (NSAIDs) including ibuprofen, ketoprofen, aspirin, naproxen, diclofenac and paracetamol have been demonstrated effective (Fig. 21.3). Combination analgesics containing caffeine are also effective, but are recommended as the second drugs of choice, because of a possible higher risk of inducing medication-overuse headache.

The combination of analgesics with codeine, sedatives or tranquilizers is frequently used. However, combination analgesics should generally be avoided because of the risk of dependency, abuse and chronification of the headache. Triptans do not have a clinically relevant effect, and muscle relaxants have not been demonstrated effective in TTH.

To summarize, simple analgesics and NSAIDs are the mainstays in the acute therapy of the episodic forms of TTH (Fig. 21.3). Paracetamol is probably less effective than the NSAIDs but has a better gastric side effect profile and is therefore considered the first drug of choice by some experts. If acetaminophen is not effective, ibuprofen 400 mg may be recommended because of a favourable gastrointestinal side effect profile compared with other NSAIDs. Physicians should be aware of the risk of developing MOH as a result of frequent and excessive use of analgesics in acute therapy. Triptans, muscle relaxants and opioids do not have a role in the treatment of TTH.

Prophylactic pharmacotherapy should be considered in patients with chronic TTH who do not respond to non-pharmacological treatment (here to case 2). The tricyclic antidepressant amitriptyline is the only drug that has proven to be effective in several controlled trials in TTH. The two most recent studies reported that amitriptyline 75 mg/day reduced headache index (duration x intensity) with 30 % compared with placebo. The effect is long-lasting (at least 6 months) and not related to the presence of depression. It is important that patients are informed that this is an antidepressant agent but has an independent action on pain. Amitriptyline should be started at low dosages (10 mg/day) and titrated by 10 mg weekly until the patient has either good therapeutic effect or until side effects are encountered. The maintenance dose is usually 30–75 mg daily administered 1–2 h before bedtime to help to circumvent any sedative adverse effects. A significant effect of amitriptyline may be observed already in the first week on the therapeutic dose. It is therefore advisable to change to other prophylactic therapy, if the patient does not respond after 4 weeks on maintenance dose. The side effects of amitriptyline include dry mouth, drowsiness, dizziness, constipation and weight gain.

The tricyclic antidepressant clomipramine and the tetracyclic antidepressants maprotiline and mianserin have been reported more effective than placebo, while the selective serotonin reuptake inhibitors (SSRIs) have not been found effective. Interestingly, antidepressants with action on both serotonin and noradrenalin seem to be as effective as amitriptyline with the advantage that they are tolerated in doses needed for the treatment of a concomitant depression. Thus, the noradrenergic and specific serotonergic antidepressant mirtazapine 30 mg/day reduced headache index by 34 % more than placebo in difficult-to-treat patients including patients who had not responded to amitriptyline. The serotonin and noradrenalin reuptake inhibitor venlafaxine 150 mg/day reduced headache days from 15 to 12 per month. Tizanidine, botulinum toxin, propranolol or valproic acid is not recommended for the prophylactic treatment of TTH.

To summarize, the initial approach to prophylactic pharmacotherapy of chronic TTH is through the use of amitriptyline (Fig. 21.3). Concomitant use of daily analgesics should be avoided. If the patient does not respond to amitriptyline, mirtazapine or venlafaxine could be attempted. SSRIs could be considered in patients with concomitant depression, if tricyclics, mirtazapine or venlafaxine is not tolerated. The physician should keep in mind that the efficacy of preventive drug therapy in TTH is often modest and that the efficacy should outweigh the side effects. Discontinuation should be attempted every 6–12 months.

As neither non-pharmacological nor pharmacological management is highly efficient, it is usually recommended to combine multiple strategies although proper evidence is lacking. It is therefore reassuring that the first study that has evaluated the efficacy of a multidisciplinary headache clinic reports positive results. Treatment results for all patients discharged within 1 year were evaluated. Patients with episodic TTH demonstrated a 50 % reduction in frequency, 75 % reduction in intensity and 33 % in absence rate, whereas chronic TTH patients responded with 32, 30 and 40 % reductions, respectively.

21.4 Brief of General Information

The substantial societal and individual burdens associated with tension-type headache constitute a major public health issue. Episodic infrequent TTH affects almost all adults and is more a nuisance than a disease, but for those suffering from the frequent subforms, especially those 3–5 % with chronic TTH, the total burden is significant. Pericranial myofascial nociception is probably important for the pathophysiology of TTH, while sensitization of central nociceptive pathways seems to be responsible for the conversion of episodic to chronic TTH. The headache-related disability can usually be reduced by identification of trigger factors combined with non-pharmacological and pharmacological treatments, but specific effective treatment modalities are lacking. In the individual patient, there is especially a great need for identification and treatment of medication overuse and other coexisting headaches. Overall, there is an unmet need for pathophysiological studies and experimental models.

Suggested Reading

1. Ashina M (2004) Neurobiology of chronic tension-type headache. Cephalalgia 24:161–172
2. Ashina S, Bendtsen L, Ashina M, Magerl W, Jensen R (2006) Generalized hyperalgesia in patients with chronic tension-type headache. Cephalalgia 26:940–948
3. Bendtsen L (2000) Central sensitization in tension-type headache – possible pathophysiological mechanisms. Cephalalgia 20:486–508
4. Bendtsen L, Evers S, Linde M, Mitsikostas DD, Sandrini G, Schoenen J (2010) EFNS guideline on the treatment of tension-type headache – report of an EFNS task force. Eur J Neurol 17:1318–1325
5. Bendtsen L, Jensen R (2006) Tension-type headache: the most common, but also the most neglected, headache disorder. Curr Opin Neurol 19:305–309
6. Bezov D, Ashina S, Jensen R, Bendtsen L (2011) Pain perception studies in tension-type headache. Headache 51:262–271
7. Buchgreitz L, Lyngberg AC, Bendtsen L, Jensen R (2008) Increased pain sensitivity is not a risk factor but a consequence of frequent headache: a population-based follow-up study. Pain 137:623–630
8. Castien RF, van der Windt DA, Grooten A, Dekker J (2011) Effectiveness of manual therapy for chronic tension-type headache: a pragmatic, randomised, clinical trial. Cephalalgia 31:133–143
9. Cathcart S, Petkov J, Winefield AH, Lushington K, Rolan P (2010) Central mechanisms of stress-induced headache. Cephalalgia 30:285–295

10. Fernandez-de-Las-Penas C, Schoenen J (2009) Chronic tension-type headache: what is new? Curr Opin Neurol 22:254–261
11. Jensen R (1999) Pathophysiological mechanisms of tension-type headache: a review of epidemiological and experimental studies. Cephalalgia 19:602–621
12. Lyngberg AC, Rasmussen BK, Jorgensen T, Jensen R (2005) Has the prevalence of migraine and tension-type headache changed over a 12-year period? A Danish population survey. Eur J Epidemiol 20:243–249
13. Nestoriuc Y, Rief W, Martin A (2008) Meta-analysis of biofeedback for tension-type headache: efficacy, specificity, and treatment moderators. J Consult Clin Psychol 76:379–396
14. Stovner LJ, Hagen K, Jensen R et al (2007) The global burden of headache: a documentation of headache prevalence and disability worldwide. Cephalalgia 27:193–210
15. Stovner LJ, Zwart JA, Hagen K, Terwindt GM, Pascual J (2006) Epidemiology of headache in Europe. Eur J Neurol 13:333–345

Chapter 22
Chronic Tension-Type Headache

Necdet Karli and Mehmet Zarifoğlu

22.1 Case Description

A 42-year-old woman was admitted to the emergency room (ER) for the worsening of a continuous headache. She reported of having very frequent headaches for the last couple of years. Last year she had had headaches every day. Headache severity was mild to moderate, bilateral, starting from back of her head, and spreading to the vertex and forehead. She said she took NSAIDs when the pain is moderate. The pain responds moderately to the NSAIDs. Her blood pressure (BP) was found to be 150/90 mmHg; otherwise, the physical examination was normal. She received a diagnosis of headache secondary to hypertension and was treated accordingly. Her BP returned to normal in an hour and then she was referred to the cardiology hypertension outpatient clinic. There, she was diagnosed with essential hypertension and was given an ACE inhibitor. Five months after the first evaluation, despite that her BP remained normal, her headaches did not improve and she went back to her cardiologist who then referred her to the neurology headache outpatient clinic.

She described her headaches that started when she was in her early twenties. In the first few years, her headaches were infrequent and mild and would last about 3–4 h. Once in a while, she took an over-the-counter NSAID, which brought pain relief. Headache frequency increased in her mid-thirties. It was bilateral, continuous, and mild to moderate and sometimes became severe particularly during menstruation with similar characteristics. She described a tightening headache, with no photophobia or phonophobia associated. Menstruation, emotional stress, and sleep deprivation were the trigger factors, while sleeping and resting would relieve her headaches. Within the last year, her headache worsened in severity and frequency, becoming daily. In previous years, she was seen by a number of different physicians

N. Karli (✉) • M. Zarifoğlu
Department of Neurology, University of Uludağ, School of Medicine, Bursa, Turkey
e-mail: nkarli@yahoo.com

A. Siva, C. Lampl (eds.), *Case-Based Diagnosis and Management of Headache Disorders*, Headache, DOI 10.1007/978-3-319-06886-2_22

including neurologists, ENT specialists, neurosurgeons, and internists who all make different diagnoses. Migraine, sinusitis, neck problems, psychogenic headache, and tension-type headache were among those diagnoses. She was given different medications including NSAIDs, muscle relaxants, antibiotics, and antidepressant agents (i.e., fluoxetine, sertraline) without any result.

Her past medical and neurological histories were insignificant. Her sister was also suffering from headaches and had a diagnosis of migraine. Both her parents were alive and had hypertension.

22.2 Differential Diagnosis and How to Work Up This Kind of Patient

Among physicians there is a tendency to consider organic disease whether intracranial or not in patients with a long headache history and high headache frequency. On the contrary, longer headache history means less possibility of organic diseases, particularly intracranial disorders. Such a slow progression of headache with no accompanying neurological or physical abnormality suggests chronic forms of primary headaches, particularly migraine and tension-type headache (TTH). No neurological abnormality or symptoms, absence of nausea or vomiting, and just increasing frequency or severity of headache strongly support primary headache diagnosis.

In this case, the presence of high blood pressure at the time of ER admittance led the ER physicians to a wrong pathway, thinking that headache was secondary due to high BP. This is another misbelief among physicians that arterial hypertension causes headache most of the time. In ICHD-3 beta version, headache due to arterial hypertension is defined as, usually bilateral and pulsating, caused by a paroxysmal rise of arterial hypertension (systolic – 180 mmHg and/or diastolic – 120 mmHg). It remits after normalization of blood pressure. Long-term hypertension periods do not cause headache due to adaptive mechanisms. On the other hand, paroxysmal and sudden and significant increases in blood pressure might cause headache, which most of the time is relieved by antihypertensive medication and with the normalization of the blood pressure. In our case, even 5 months after normalization of the blood pressure, patient's headache did not improve. So, in our case, headache could not be secondary to hypertension according to ICHD-3 beta.

Tension-type headache is the most frequent primary headache type. According to ICHD-3 beta, tension-type headache is a bilateral, mild to moderate, tightening headache not aggravated by routine physical activity. No nausea or vomiting accompanies the episodic TTH, but either photophobia or phonophobia may be seen during the headache. Patient's description allowed us to classify her headache as TTH. Severe headaches of the patient during the menstruation period might suggest migraine or menstrual headache. However, the patient described her headache during menstruation similar to her regular headaches other than severity. Therefore, menstruation can be accepted as a worsening factor for her TTH. If someone suffers from TTH 15 days or more per month on average for more than 3 months, then it is

Table 22.1 Recommended drugs and dose for prophylactic therapy of C-TTH

Substance	Daily dose (mg)
First choice	
Amitriptyline	30–75
Second choice	
Mirtazapine	30
Venlafaxine	150
Third choice	
Clomipramine	75–150
Maprotiline	75
Mianserine	30–60

Adapted from: Bendtsen et al. [4]

classified as chronic TTH (C-TTH) (Table 22.1). According to the criteria, our patient was suffering from C-TTH as her headache occurred almost every day during the previous year. There are two main differences between episodic and chronic TTH in the classification: the frequency of headache and the presence of mild, not moderate, or severe nausea. Differential diagnosis between chronic migraine (CM) and C-TTH might be difficult in some patients. Although that some features of headaches in some days may not be typical of migraine in individuals with CM, at least 8 days of the 15 or more days of headaches should have the characteristics of migraine according to the ICHD-3 beta. In CM, the presence of migraine attacks consistent with the IHS criteria before chronification and to a certain extent the response to triptans further help to differentiate it from C-TTH.

No tests are needed for the diagnostic work-up of C-TTH, unless there is suspicion of secondary headaches.

22.3 Diagnostic Workup of the Case

According to her headache history and characteristics, C-TTH was the diagnosis. Her neurological exam was normal. She was started 25 mg amitriptyline daily and increased to 50 mg 10 days after. Three months later, her headache days decreased to 6–7 days a month. Her amitriptyline dosage increased to 75 mg/day. At the fifth month of her treatment, she had only 2–3 headache days per month.

22.4 Definition of Chronic Tension-Type Headache

According to the ICHD-3 beta, the definition of C-TTH headache is headaches occurring on ≥15 days per month on an average of >3 months (≥180 days per year), lasting hours or may be continuous; has at least two of the following characteristics: bilateral location, pressing/tightening (non-pulsating) quality, mild or moderate intensity, and not aggravated by routine physical activity such as walking or climbing stairs; and both of the following associating symptoms: no more than one of photophobia, phonophobia, or mild nausea and neither moderate or severe nausea nor vomiting.

22.5 Summary of the Case

A 42-year-old woman was admitted to the ER for the worsening of her continuous headache. This headache was daily, bilateral, tightening, and moderate, starting from the neck radiating to the vertex without any associating symptoms. Her BP was 150/90 mmHg, treated with antihypertensive agents and referred to the cardiology hypertension outpatient clinic. She was put on antihypertensive medication for essential hypertension. Her BP stayed normal for 5 months but her headache did not change. She was then referred to the neurology outpatient clinic and was diagnosed with C-TTH. She was given 50 mg amitriptyline daily, and 3 months later, her headache frequency dropped to 6–7 days a month. Her dosage increased to 75 mg daily and her headache days decreased to 2–3 days a month.

22.6 Brief General Information

TTH is the most frequent headache type among adults. Reported prevalence rates differ between 25 and 55 % worldwide. It is mostly bilateral, tightening, and mild to moderate, may last from 30 min to 7 days, is not aggravated by routine physical activity, is not associated by nausea or vomiting, but may be accompanied by either photophobia or phonophobia. C-TTH may be associated with mild nausea and its frequency should be at least 15 days per month for 3 months according to ICHD-3 beta. The prevalence of C-TTH is up to 2–3 % in the general population. The high prevalence rates and high frequency of C-TTH are also a cause of significant burden. Chronification of TTH may take years. Medication overuse may also accompany C-TTH but is seen less when compared with CM. Its management includes preventive medications, acute medications mainly NSAIDs (if not associated with medication overuse), close follow-up, interdisciplinary handling of the case, and alternative treatment approaches for medically resistant cases. For preventive treatment, antidepressant agents, TCAs (amitriptyline, nortriptyline), are the first choice, while mirtazapine and venlafaxine can be used as the second choice.

Suggested Reading

1. Ailani J (2009) Chronic tension-type headache. Curr Pain Headache Rep 13(6):479–483
2. Ashina M (2004) Neurobiology of chronic tension-type headache. Cephalalgia 24:161–172

3. Bendtsen L, Jensen R (2011) Treating tension-type headache – an expert opinion. Expert Opin Pharmacother 12(7):1099–1109
4. Bendtsen L et al (2010) EFNS guideline on the treatment of tension-type headache – report of an EFNS task force. Eur J Neurol 17(11):1318–1325
5. Fernández-de-las-Peñas C, Schoenen J (2009) Chronic tension-type headache: what is new? Curr Opin Neurol 22(3):254–261
6. Garza I, Schwedt TJ (2010) Diagnosis and management of chronic daily headache. Semin Neurol 30(2):154–166
7. Gipponi S et al (2010) Hypertension is a factor associated with chronic daily headache. Neurol Sci 31(Suppl 1):171–173
8. Headache Classification Committee of the International Headache Society (IHS) (2013) The International Classification of Headache Disorders, 3rd edition (beta version). http://www.ihs-headache.org
9. Kruszewski P et al (2000) Headache in patients with mild to moderate hypertension is generally not associated with simultaneous blood pressure elevation. J Hypertens 18:437–444
10. Monteith TS, Oshinsky ML (2009) Tension-type headache with medication overuse: pathophysiology and clinical implications. Curr Pain Headache Rep 13(6):463–469
11. Sahler K (2012) Epidemiology and cultural differences in tension-type headache. Curr Pain Headache Rep 16(6):525–532

Chapter 23
Treatment-Resistant Chronic Cluster Headache

Nu Cindy Chai and Alan M. Rapoport

23.1 Case Description

A 40-year-old man with a history of episodic cluster headache (CH) was referred to the headache clinic for intractable headache that has been persistent for the past year without remission. His initial diagnosis of CH (obtained 2 years previously) was based on a 3-week episode of daily, severe, unilateral headache attacks in and above the right eye twice per day for 45 min associated with conjunctival injection, tearing, and rhinorrhea. This was successfully treated with subcutaneous sumatriptan (6 mg) and 100 % oxygen at 15 l/min via rebreathing mask for acute episodes and verapamil preventively (titrated up to 360 mg daily). All medicines were discontinued 5 weeks after the cluster period started.

He was pain-free for 1 year and subsequently began to experience severe unilateral head pain again. On this occasion, his head pain occurred three to four times a day and lasted up to 90 min per episode. The pain was always right sided, periorbital, knifelike, and excruciating with an intensity of 10/10 and consistently associated with ipsilateral conjunctival injection, tearing, miosis, ptosis, and rhinorrhea. He was again treated with subcutaneous sumatriptan and high flow oxygen therapy, which provided symptomatic benefit only 25 % of the time. He was started on verapamil (titrated up to 480 mg daily) for preventive treatment. However, he continued to have recurrent pain daily even after 2 months of treatment. High-dose corticosteroids were added with a 2-week taper but without efficacy. Due to lack of response,

N.C. Chai, MD (✉)
Department of Neurology, Johns Hopkins School of Medicine,
1800 Orleans Street, Baltimore, MD 21287, USA
e-mail: nchai1@jhmi.edu

A.M. Rapoport, MD
Department of Neurology, The David Geffen School of Medicine at UCLA,
239 South Orange Drive, Lost Angeles, CA 90036, USA
e-mail: alanrapoport@gmail.com

A. Siva, C. Lampl (eds.), *Case-Based Diagnosis and Management of Headache Disorders*, Headache, DOI 10.1007/978-3-319-06886-2_23

lithium (900 mg daily) and topiramate (up to 300 mg/day) were tried, each for 6 weeks, without efficacy. He was switched to intranasal zolmitriptan with some efficacy but continued to experience three attacks of head pain daily. He was hospitalized for 1 week both for severe pain and suicidal ideation.

He was otherwise healthy with no significant past history. He did not take any other prescription medications and reported no allergies to medication. He was smoking one pack of cigarettes per day for 15 years. He stopped drinking alcohol 2 years previously after receiving a diagnosis of cluster headache. His mother suffered from migraine. He had no family history of cluster headache.

At the time of the neurological exam, he was pain-free, and his exam was normal with the exception of slight ptosis on the right.

23.2 Differential Diagnosis and How to Evaluate This Kind of Patient

This patient has a history of CH. While it is possible for episodic CH to transform into chronic cluster headache (CCH), any significant change in headache characteristic and duration warrants further investigation. Differential diagnosis for CCH must include other primary headache disorders with autonomic features, such as chronic migraine and other trigeminal autonomic cephalalgias (TACs). In addition, secondary headache conditions can occasionally mimic symptoms of chronic CH, especially lesions in the parasellar area or dissection of a carotid artery.

CCH can be differentiated from chronic migraine by the unilateral and ipsilateral nature of its accompanying autonomic symptoms and especially by its timing (short duration and frequent episodes daily). In comparison, migraine patients are much more likely to describe bilateral lacrimation, conjunctival injection, periorbital edema, ptosis, and rhinorrhea, although unilateral symptoms can occur. Migraineurs also have much longer duration of attacks with more associated symptoms such as nausea, photo- and phonophobia, and worsening with exertion. While other TACs can also cause head pain with ipsilateral autonomic symptoms, they can be distinguished from CH most readily based on their duration and frequency. CH can be distinguished from hemicrania continua by its short, more intense painful attacks with predictable interictal pain-free periods and its circadian or circannual periodicity.

Vascular abnormalities such as carotid dissection, aneurysms, venous sinus thrombosis, and cavernous sinus dural arterial-venous (AV) fistulas as well as structural disease of the sellar and parasellar structures have all been reported to mimic treatment-resistant CH. There have also been rare reports of multiple sclerosis lesions in the pontomedullary trigeminal nuclei presenting as unrelenting cluster-like head pain. Therefore, when a patient, even one with a prior history of CH, presents with intractable severe headache different from the prior CH episode, a thorough updated history as well as a general and neurological examination must be performed. Consideration should also be given to a repeat MRI, as a new lesion may not be detectable by history and neurological exam alone. On exam, visual field deficits may be suggestive of a sellar mass such as a prolactinoma. Cranial nerve palsies with severe unilateral retro-orbital pain may be suggestive of Tolosa-Hunt syndrome or other structural abnormalities in the cavernous sinus. Focal weakness, numbness, or vision changes, especially interictally, may suggest structural lesions, vascular abnormalities, or multiple sclerosis.

Finally, secondary headaches from infections or other local diseases of ophthalmological, nasal, dental, or sinus origins can cause headache pain together with symptoms of lacrimation, conjunctival injection, or rhinorrhea. Patients suffering from these secondary headaches tend to have more associated symptoms, such as fever, chills, and cough. In addition, they tend to suffer from continued pain instead of the episodic pain and interictal pain-free periods characterizing CH.

Screening laboratory studies including white blood cell count (WBC), erythrocyte sedimentation rate (ESR), and C-reactive protein (CRP) can help to identify an infectious or inflammatory etiology that may be causing or contributing to the head pain. In addition, serum melatonin levels can be obtained, as decreased nocturnal melatonin secretion with low melatonin levels has been linked with CH, and may provide a source of therapy when abnormality is identified. To definitively rule out secondary causes of severe, unilateral cluster-like headache, imaging studies must be performed. Magnetic resonance imaging (MRI) of the brain with and without contrast and magnetic resonance studies focusing on the arteries and veins in the brain and the neck (MRA and MRV) are the preferred initial imaging studies. A head CT may be able to identify certain mass lesions and vascular lesions but is much less sensitive than MRI. If the suspicion is high clinically for chronic sinusitis as the etiology or as a contributing factor for the headache (i.e., background pain outside of cluster attacks, pain upon palpation of the maxillary sinuses, bad smelling or tasting post nasal drip, etc.), a CT scan of the paranasal sinuses is the best study. If vascular malformation or aneurysm is suspected or suggested by MRA or MRV, further vessel imaging with contrasted CT scan, CT angiography, or even more invasive (and more sensitive) cerebral angiography may be necessary.

23.3 Diagnostic Workup and Management of This Case

This patient's neurological exam revealed right-sided ptosis. While it is possible for CH sufferers to have persistent ipsilateral ptosis and/or pupil changes even interictally, given the change in the treatment responsiveness of his headache, an MRI of the brain with and without contrast was performed. This was found to be normal. In addition, MRA of his head and neck and MRV of his head were performed with contrast, and they were also normal. His basic laboratory studies were unremarkable. With these normal results, secondary causes of his headache were effectively ruled out.

By the time he presented to the headache clinic, he had already tried and failed several pharmacologic options for CH at appropriate doses. He had also been hospitalized once for suicidal ideation, which further attested to the devastating impact CH had on this patient. Occipital nerve block was performed ipsilaterally, without significant benefit. After confirming a normal EKG and no history of coronary artery disease or arrhythmias, he was started on methylergonovine maleate (0.2 mg three times a day) for prevention over the next 3 months. He was concurrently referred for greater occipital nerve stimulation (ONS). He received ipsilateral placement of an occipital nerve stimulator and was set on continuous stimulation. He continued to use high flow oxygen for acute pain. At 3-month follow up, his headache frequency had decreased by 75 %, and his headache intensity decreased by 50 %. Methylergonovine maleate was stopped after 3 months of use to decrease the risk of fibrosis, and he was able to maintain the decreased frequency and intensity of the headache on ONS.

23.4 Summary of the Case

Our patient had an initial diagnosis of episodic CH and transformed into CCH. While his symptoms (unilateral severe pain with associated ipsilateral autonomic dysfunction occurring with predictable periodicity) fulfilled the diagnostic criteria for CH, the change in the treatment responsiveness of his head pain and the shift to chronic cluster with its unrelenting pain were red flags that something else might have been going on. This led to further brain and vessel imaging to rule out secondary causes of cluster-like headache pain.

Interventional treatment options are available for those with CCH in which pharmacologic therapies have been found ineffective or insufficient. Further, a high prevalence of depression and self-inflicted injuries have been reported in the population of active and CCH sufferers, and clinicians must take great care to identify those at risk. (The patient in this case was hospitalized for suicidal ideation.)

23.5 Definition of Chronic Cluster Headache

CH is a devastating headache disorder characterized by its unilateral severe nature and its associated ipsilateral cranial autonomic symptoms, and it is defined in particular by its short duration and its circadian and circannual periodicity. CH is considered chronic when there have been no pain-free periods over the course of 1 year, or if a pain-free period lasts less than 1 month.

23.6 Brief General Information

CH is one of the more common TACs, but is still relatively rare compared to migraine or tension-type headache. The lifetime prevalence of cluster headache is about 124/100,000. There is a 5–18-fold increased risk of developing CH for first-degree relatives of patients with CH. About one in six CH patients suffers from the chronic form. Men are three to four times more likely than women to suffer from CH and are more likely to have chronic CH.

There remains significant diagnostic delay for CH patients – with only 21 % receiving the correct diagnosis at initial presentation. About 10 % cluster patients are refractory to treatment. Suicidality is a major and serious comorbidity of CH, with more than 50 % sufferers having reported suicidal ideation.

23.6.1 Acute Care Therapy

First-line abortive therapy for CH consists of 12–15 L/min oxygen via a rebreathing mask in the sitting position and triptan medications (e.g., sumatriptan 6 mg subcutaneous injection approved in the USA and zolmitriptan 5 or 10 mg nasal spray approved in the EU). (See Chapter on "Episodic cluster headache.") Older age and female gender have both been linked to less responsiveness to triptans; nausea/vomiting, photophobia/phonophobia, and restlessness have all been linked to poor responsiveness to oxygen. Women CH sufferers have been reported to be more responsive to intranasal lidocaine. Other acute therapies such as ergotamine tartrate by tablet and suppository and dihydroergotamine intranasally and by injection, intranasal capsaicin, intravenous somatostatin, subcutaneous octreotide, and sodium oxybate by mouth at night have all been reported to have some efficacy in CH and can be tried in those with refractory cases.

23.6.2 Preventive Therapy

Preventive therapy is especially critical for those with CCH, as it aims to decrease the frequency and severity of the attacks. Verapamil is the drug of choice and lithium is also the first-line treatment but may have more significant adverse effects (see Chapter on "Episodic cluster headache"). Other pharmacologic treatments including topiramate, valproic acid, a brief burst of steroids, methysergide (not available in the USA), and methylergonovine maleate have all been shown to be probably efficacious, though definitive positive results from randomized controlled trials are not yet available. Case reports and observational studies attesting to the efficacy of pizotifen, candesartan, indomethacin, melatonin, baclofen, gabapentin, clonidine, clomiphene citrate, testosterone supplement, leuprolide, rotigotine, mycophenolate mofetil, and botulinum toxin are also available for CCH, though randomized trials have either been negative (e.g., candesartan) or not available. Civamide nasal solution, a TRPV-1 receptor modulator, has been studied as a preventive treatment for cluster headache, but a larger phase III trial is needed. Finally, while both psilocybin (lysergic acid diethylamide/LSD) and cannabis have been used by CH patients with anecdotal benefit, they cannot be recommended given the lack of definitive evidence of efficacy and the uncontrolled nature of the substances.

23.6.3 Invasive Procedures

CH patients can usually be managed conservatively with pharmacologic agents. Hospitalization may be necessary for IV DHE, steroids, and other treatments. Rarely, however, more invasive strategies need to be used in those with resistant pain. Historically, primarily destructive surgical procedures aiming at the trigeminal system and the parasympathetic pathways were the mainstay (and last resort) for those with recalcitrant cluster headache. However, more recently, techniques such as greater occipital nerve block (ONB) or stimulation (ONS), sphenopalatine ganglion (SPG, also known as the pterygopalatine ganglion, PPG) stimulation, as well as deep brain stimulation (DBS) in the hypothalamic region have replaced the previous destructive surgeries.

ONB with lidocaine and a steroid (triamcinolone, betamethasone, or methylprednisolone) injected ipsilaterally has been investigated in a few clinic-based studies yielding positive results and have been in use for many years. ONB is generally well tolerated and can demonstrate benefit within a few days, with lasting benefit reported for up to 4 weeks. Response rate varies between 60 and 80 %, and complete remission from cluster period has been reported.

ONS has been reported to decrease attack intensity, frequency, and duration in approximately 80 % of patients, though its effect may not be evident until 2 months after implantation. In addition, patients rarely become completely headache-free after ONS, and many continue to require some pharmacologic therapy. Hardware-related complications (infection, lead dislocation and breakage, etc.) are not uncommon and reported to be approximately 50 % in one clinic-based prospective observational study. Predictive factors for responsiveness to ONS have not been established based on current literature. Therefore, it is reasonable to conduct a trial phase with lead electrodes to select for responders before implantation of the stimulator.

SPG stimulation has also been reported to decrease both mean attack frequency and intensity of CH for up to 18 months, and this effect may be more robust in those with episodic CH compared to those with CCH. The main adverse effect of SPG stimulation includes postoperative epistaxis and numbness in the second division of the trigeminal nerve, rare unintentional complete destruction of SPG (resulting in dry eyes, hyperesthesia of the hard palate), and partial lesion of the nervus maxillaris (resulting in paresthesia in the upper jaw or soft palate).

Finally, hypothalamic DBS is an emerging therapeutic option for those with refractory CCH, reported to be effective in much greater than 50 % of patients implanted for treatment-refractory cluster headache. The rationale for this therapeutic option lies in the observation of activation of the ipsilateral posterior hypothalamus during nitroglycerine-induced and spontaneous cluster attacks. DBS for cluster headache involves inserting a lead containing stimulation electrodes in the posterior ipsilateral hypothalamic gray matter. Benefit can be seen in about 1–2 months after implantation. While there are risks of infection, seizure, intracranial hemorrhage, as well as interruptions of hypothalamic function (sleep, mood, appetite, etc.), hypothalamic DBS actually has been generally well tolerated based on available reports.

However, similar to SPG stimulation, there continues to be a lack of information regarding which patients will respond to this particular therapeutic option. It tends to be the last option, although an often effective one.

23.6.4 Other Therapies

Patients with treatment-resistant CH need to be managed with a multidisciplinary approach. In addition to pharmacologic and procedural therapies, behavioral therapy and psychological support are often needed. In addition, sleep studies may be beneficial for obese CH patients, as obstructive sleep apnea is comorbid with CH and is treatable. Although not completely effective on their own in cluster, these therapies often help to improve the condition of patients with CCH.

23.7 Key Epidemiological Data Regarding Treatment-Resistant Cluster Headache

- About 1 in 1,000 people suffers from cluster headache.
- Only 21 % cluster headache patients receive the correct diagnosis at initial presentation.
- About one in six cluster headache patients suffers from the chronic form.
- Men are three to four times more likely than women to suffer from cluster headache and are more likely to have chronic cluster headache.
- About 10 % cluster patients are refractory to treatment.
- More than 50 % cluster headache sufferers have reported suicidal ideation.

Key Points Regarding the Diagnostic Workup for Patients with Treatment-Resistant Cluster Headache

- Even clinically typical cluster headaches can be caused by structural lesions.
- Even secondary cluster-like headaches can show some improvement symptomatically with cluster headache treatment.
- Any significant change in cluster headache characteristics (location, severity, duration, treatment responsiveness, continuous background pain while not during a cluster headache attack) deserves further diagnostic workup, even in a patient with a previous history of cluster headache.
  - Laboratory studies recommended include CBC, ESR, CRP, TSH, and melatonin level.
  - Imaging studies recommended include MRI of the brain with and without contrast, MRA of the head and neck with contrast, and MRV of the head.

Key Points Regarding Management of Treatment-Resistant Chronic Cluster HA

- Both acute abortive and preventive treatments should be used.
- For preventive treatments, monotherapy is preferred, though occasionally polytherapy will be needed.
- Occipital nerve block is the least invasive procedure for cluster headache and should be tried prior to committing patients to more invasive procedures.
- A multidisciplinary approach is necessary for the management of patients with treatment-resistant chronic cluster headache.

Suggested Reading

1. Ashkenazi A, Schwedt T (2011) Cluster headache–acute and prophylactic therapy. Headache 51(2):272–286
2. Favier I, van Vliet JA, Roon KI, Witteveen RJ, Verschuuren JJ, Ferrari MD, Haan J (2007) Trigeminal autonomic cephalgias due to structural lesions: a review of 31 cases. Arch Neurol 64(1):25–31
3. Fischera M, Marziniak M, Gralow I, Evers S (2008) The incidence and prevalence of cluster headache: a meta-analysis of population-based studies. Cephalalgia 28(6):614–618
4. Gaul C, Christmann N, Schroder D, Weber R, Shanib H, Diener HC, Holle D (2012) Differences in clinical characteristics and frequency of accompanying migraine features in episodic and chronic cluster headache. Cephalalgia 32(7):571–577
5. Goadsby PJ, May A (1999) PET demonstration of hypothalamic activation in cluster headache. Neurology 52(7):1522
6. Kudrow L (1979) Cluster headache: diagnosis and management. Headache 19(3):142–150
7. Kudrow L, Kudrow DB (1994) Inheritance of cluster headache and its possible link to migraine. Headache 34(7):400–407
8. Kudrow L, McGinty DJ, Phillips ER, Stevenson M (1984) Sleep apnea in cluster headache. Cephalalgia 4(1):33–38
9. Leone M, Franzini A, Proietti Cecchini A, Bussone G (2013) Success, failure, and putative mechanisms in hypothalamic stimulation for drug-resistant chronic cluster headache. Pain 154(1):89–94
10. Luerding R, Henkel K, Gaul C, Dresler T, Lindwurm A, Paelecke-Habermann Y, Leinisch E, Jurgens TP (2012) Aggressiveness in different presentations of cluster headache: results from a controlled multicentric study. Cephalalgia 32(7):528–536
11. Magis D, Gerardy PY, Remacle JM, Schoenen J (2011) Sustained effectiveness of occipital nerve stimulation in drug-resistant chronic cluster headache. Headache 51(8):1191–1201
12. Magis D, Schoenen J (2012) Advances and challenges in neurostimulation for headaches. Lancet Neurol 11(8):708–719
13. Mainardi F, Trucco M, Maggioni F, Palestini C, Dainese F, Zanchin G (2010) Cluster-like headache. A comprehensive reappraisal. Cephalalgia 30(4):399–412
14. May A, Leone M, Afra J, Linde M, Sandor PS, Evers S, Goadsby PJ, EFNS Task Force (2006) EFNS guidelines on the treatment of cluster headache and other trigeminal-autonomic cephalalgias. Eur J Neurol 13(10):1066–1077
15. McGeeney BE (2013) Cannabinoids and hallucinogens for headache. Headache 53(3):447–458

16. Messina G, Rizzi M, Cordella R, Caraceni A, Zecca E, Bussone G, Franzini A, Leone M (2013) Secondary chronic cluster headache treated by posterior hypothalamic deep brain stimulation: first reported case. Cephalalgia 33(2):136–138
17. Mueller O, Diener HC, Dammann P, Rabe K, Hagel V, Sure U, Gaul C (2013) Occipital nerve stimulation for intractable chronic cluster headache or migraine: a critical analysis of direct treatment costs and complications. Cephalalgia 33(16):1283–1291
18. Pedersen JL, Barloese M, Jensen RH (2013) Neurostimulation in cluster headache: a review of current progress. Cephalalgia 33(14):1179–1193
19. Peterlin BL, Purdy RA, Rapoport AM, Gantenbein AR, Sturzenegger M, Riederer F et al (2011) Comment on acute and preventive pharmacologic treatment of cluster headache. Neurology 30(9):921–922
20. Piacentino M, D'Andrea G, Perini F, Volpin L (2014) Drug-resistant cluster headache: long-term evaluation of pain control by posterior hypothalamic deep-brain stimulation. World Neurosurg 81(2):442.e11–5
21. Robbins MS (2013) The psychiatric comorbidities of cluster headache. Curr Pain Headache Rep 17(2):313, 012-0313-8
22. Rozen TD, Fishman RS (2012) Cluster headache in the united states of america: demographics, clinical characteristics, triggers, suicidality, and personal burden. Headache 52(1):99–113
23. Rozen TD, Fishman RS (2012) Female cluster headache in the united states of america: what are the gender differences? Results from the united states cluster headache survey. J Neurol Sci 317(1–2):17–28
24. Russell MB (1997) Genetic epidemiology of migraine and cluster headache. Cephalalgia 17(6):683–701
25. Tfelt-Hansen PC, Jensen RH (2012) Management of cluster headache. CNS Drugs 26(7):571–580
26. Tronvik E, Wienecke T, Monstad I, Dahlof C, Boe MG, Tjensvoll AB, Salvesen R, Zwart JA, Jansson SO, Stovner LJ (2013) Randomised trial on episodic cluster headache with an angiotensin II receptor blocker. Cephalalgia 33(12):1026–1034
27. Wilbrink LA, Ferrari MD, Kruit MC, Haan J (2009) Neuroimaging in trigeminal autonomic cephalgias: when, how, and of what? Curr Opin Neurol 22(3):247–253

Chapter 24
Headache Resembling Hemicrania Continua Caused by Pituitary Adenoma

Christian Wöber

24.1 Case Presentation

This patient presented for the first time in May 2008 to the emergency department of our hospital with a 2-year history of almost daily headaches and migraine with aura occurring several times a year. The daily headache was of moderate intensity and localised bilaterally, radiating from the neck and occipital region to the forehead. It was non-pulsating and not aggravated by routine physical activity, and the patient did not report any associated symptoms, but frequent use of diclofenac. She was treated with 500 mg metamizole and 5 mg diazepam orally and discharged after headache had improved.

In November 2008, she presented again because headache had changed significantly. At that time headache was right sided, strictly unilateral and continuously present with periods of more severe pain lasting for a few hours. During these exacerbations, the patient noticed right-sided reddening and tearing of the eye and dropping of the lid. The headache was radiating from the neck to the forehead with its maximum intensity felt in the frontal and orbital regions. Analgesics and nonsteroidal anti-inflammatory drugs (NSAIDs) were ineffective. The patient was referred to the headache outpatient clinic. Hemicrania continua was suspected. The patient was referred for cranial magnetic resonance imaging (MRI) and she was started on indomethacin 75 mg twice daily. At follow-up 2 weeks later, she reported only a 40 % improvement in headache severity and she presented the MRI showing a pituitary macro-adenoma (17 × 19 × 26 mm) encircling the internal carotid artery at the level of the cavernous sinus on the right side (Fig. 24.1).

C. Wöber, MD
Headache Unit, Department of Neurology, Medical University of Vienna,
Währinger Gürtel 18-20, Vienna 1090, Austria
e-mail: christian.woeber@meduniwien.ac.at

A. Siva, C. Lampl (eds.), *Case-Based Diagnosis and Management of Headache Disorders*, Headache, DOI 10.1007/978-3-319-06886-2_24

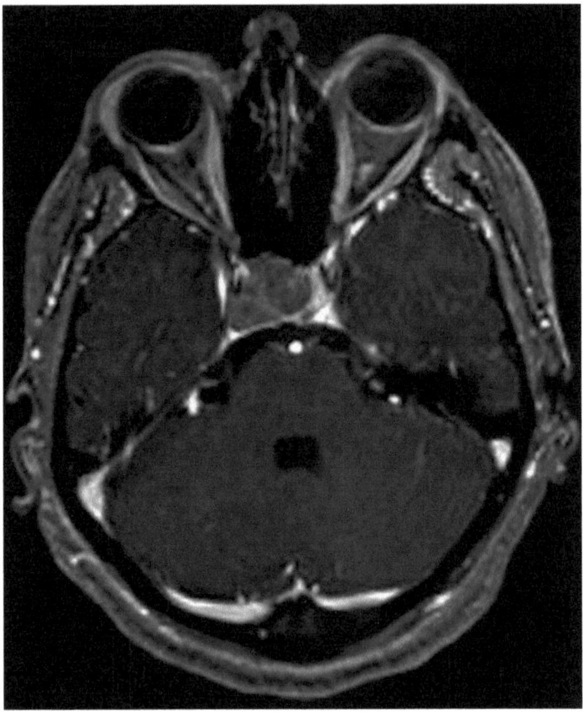

Fig. 24.1 Magnetic resonance imaging showing pituitary macroadenoma

Pituitary hormone tests revealed elevated growth hormone levels. Asking the patients about signs of acromegaly she confirmed recent changes in her face and hands. The ophthalmological examination was normal apart from a minimal visual field defect consistent with a chiasmal lesion.

Surgery was scheduled on February 26, 2009, but the patient said that she would not be able to stand the headache up to this date. Considering that analgesics and NSAIDs had failed, occipital and supraorbital nerve block with a long-acting steroid was performed resulting in complete resolution of the headache for 4 weeks. After transsphenoidal resection of the pituitary adenoma, a residual tumour encircling the right carotid artery had remained. Therefore, the patient underwent gamma knife treatment on June 30, 2009.

The patient was not seen in the headache outpatient clinic up to November 2009, when she presented again, because of persisting continuous right-sided headache associated with conjunctival injection and ptosis during periods of pain exacerbations. Again, an occipital nerve block was performed with significant improvement of headache. At follow-up 4 weeks later, a rounder and fuller face was noticed, and therefore, occipital nerve block was not repeated. Instead, topiramate was described. When the patient presented again in April 2010, she reported about side-shifting headaches with fullness of the ear and subjective hearing impairment. She had stopped topiramate because of side effects. During further follow-up, she continued to have chronic headache, but the side locked strictly to the right side with cranial autonomic symptoms changed to a bilateral headache being most severe on the right frontal and orbital regions and not accompanied with cranial autonomic symptoms anymore. MRI showed complete resolution of the residual tumour and pituitary hormone tests had become normal. She failed several prophylactic treatments and underwent inpatient treatment for medication overuse headache. At the last follow-up visit in April 2014, she reported almost daily headaches of varying intensity and bilateral localisation with a maximum in the right frontal and orbital regions, frequent use (but not overuse) of dexibuprofen and some benefit of amitriptyline 25 mg taken 2 h before bedtime.

In conclusion, this is the complex history of a patient with pre-existing migraine with aura who developed first daily headaches, headache resembling tension-type headache and later a continuous, strictly unilateral side-locked headache with exacerbations and ipsilateral cranial autonomic symptoms leading to the detection of a pituitary macroadenoma. After surgery and gamma knife treatment, headache evolved first to a unilateral headache with side shift and later to a bilateral headache with its intensity being most prominent on the right fronto-orbital region without cranial autonomic symptoms complicated by medication overuse requiring inpatient treatment. Obviously, the resolution of the hemicrania continua like headache has paralleled with the resolution of the pituitary macroadenoma, thus suggesting a causal relation.

24.2 Diagnosis of Hemicrania Continua

Hemicrania continua was first described by Sjaastad and Spierings in 1984. Since then case reports, small cases series and the largest case series up till now published by Cittadini and Goadsby in 2009 broadened the spectrum of hemicrania continua, but caused also discussions on how to define true hemicrania continua.

With respect to the International Classification of Headache Disorders (ICHD), hemicrania continua was not included in the first edition published in 1988; it was listed among other primary headaches (ICHD-2 4.7) in the 2004 edition, and finally it has been classified as trigeminal autonomic cephalalgia (ICHD-3 beta, 3.4) in 2013 [5]. According to ICHD-3 beta, the diagnosis of hemicrania continua requires a unilateral headache, present for more than 3 months showing pain exacerbations and accompanied by one or more of the following symptoms or signs on the side of the pain: conjunctival injection and/or tearing, nasal congestion and/or rhinorrhoea, eyelid oedema, sweating/flushing in the forehead and face, sensation of fullness in the ear and miosis and/or ptosis. Additionally or alternatively to these symptoms, and signs headache may be accompanied by a sense of restlessness or agitation, or movement may worsen the pain. Furthermore, an absolute response to therapeutic doses of indomethacin is mandatory, and the headache may not better be accounted for by another ICHD-3 diagnosis.

Compared to the initial two patients described by Sjaastad and Spierings [13], other patients diagnosed with hemicrania continua showed intermittent, not continuous pain, side shifting or even bilateral localisation of the headache, and a broader spectrum of cranial autonomic symptoms [2,7,10,11]. Furthermore, there are reports about headaches exactly resembling the phenomenology of hemicrania continua, but showing no or no absolute response to indomethacin [7,11]. All these observations have been included in the ICHD-3 criteria. Definite hemicrania continua still requires an absolute response to indomethacin, but lack of an (absolute) response allows to diagnose probable hemicrania continua, provided that all other ICHD-3 beta criteria of hemicrania continua are fulfilled.

Currently the revisions of the diagnostic criteria of hemicrania continua in ICHD-3 beta are under discussion. Antonaci and Sjaastad [1] argue that headache must be side locked and inclusion of the movement criteria is the consequence of misunderstanding hemicrania continua. They also argue that a response to 50 mg indomethacin intramuscularly is mandatory and a dose of 100–200 mg as given in ICHD- 3 beta is not only too high, but also harmful. Furthermore, Antonaci and Sjaastad do not agree with the inclusion of autonomic features beyond those reported in the initial patients. Goadsby [4] advocates the ICHD-3 beta criteria entitling his reply "Hemicrania continua – building on experience and clinical science".

24.3 Differential Diagnosis of Hemicrania Continua

Hemicrania continua must be differentiated from (1) (chronic) migraine, (2) half-sided tension-type headache, (3) cluster headache and paroxysmal hemicrania and (4) secondary headaches. In a series of 528 patients of a headache clinic, Ramón et al. [9] identified 100 patients with unilateral, side-locked headaches. According to ICHD-II, 8 patients had hemicrania continua, 64 had other primary headaches and the remaining patients had secondary headaches. The most common diagnosis was cluster headache in 38 patients; other trigeminal autonomic cephalalgias were diagnosed in 7 patients, episodic and chronic migraine in 6 and 5 subjects, respectively, and other primary headaches in 8 patients. Secondary headaches comprised 12 different diagnoses, with cervicogenic headache being most common ($n = 10$). In a series of 63 patients with unilateral headaches beyond migraine and cluster headache presenting to a general neurological outpatient clinic, 38 % were classified as having a primary headache, 13 % as a secondary headache and the remaining 49 % could not be classified according to ICHD-II [10]. In the Vågå study, Sjaastad and Bakketeig [12] found one possible case of hemicrania continua among 1838 parishioners in the age group 18–65 years. Further epidemiological data on hemicrania continua are not available.

Considering the low prevalence of hemicrania continua, lack of knowledge about this condition and restrictive previous diagnostic criteria, there is a considerable risk of misdiagnoses and mistreatment. Viana et al. [14] reviewed seven case series and case reports on diagnostic and therapeutic errors in hemicrania continua comprising a total of 56 patients. The diagnostic delay ranged between 3 months and 22 years. Hemicrania continua was most commonly misdiagnosed as migraine and cluster headache. Other misdiagnoses included atypical facial pain, dental pain, temporomandibular disorder, sinus headache and cervicogenic headache.

On the other hand, it is essential to recognise secondary headaches resembling hemicrania continua as shown in the case report above. Hemicrania continua like headaches may be the consequence of intracranial and extracranial disorders. Prakash et al. [8] reported three patients with secondary hemicrania continua and reviewed another 26 cases from the literature. A considerable number of these cases, i.e. 9 of 29, were related to head injury; among various other reasons, one case was related to a sphenoidal tumour and another to sphenoidal sinusitis. Wilbrink et al. [15] reviewed 56 cases of secondary trigeminal autonomic cephalalgias, not covering hemicrania continua, as this disorder was not classified as a trigeminal autonomic cephalalgia up till 2013. Interestingly, pituitary adenomas and other pituitary tumours were the second most common disorder following orbital pseudotumour and accounted for 14 of the 56 cases. The series of Seidel et al. [10] including 63 patients with unilateral headaches beyond migraine and cluster headache demonstrated the diagnostic difficulties with almost half of the patients not classifiable according to ICHD-2 and follow-up findings did not show statistically significant differences between patients with primary, secondary and unclassifiable unilateral headaches.

As there are no warning signs or symptoms indicating secondary hemicrania continua, imaging should be considered in all patients with hemicrania continua, particularly in those with atypical presentation.

24.4 Treatment of Hemicrania Continua

Absolute response to indomethacin is mandatory in definite hemicrania continua according to ICHD-3 beta. According to a recommendation of the EFNS [3], indomethacin should be started at a dose of 25 mg t.i.d. and increased up to 225 mg daily, if necessary. Additional administration of a proton pump inhibitor may be considered.

Indomethacin may be contraindicated or not tolerated. In addition, indomethacin may itself cause headache ([6], Jürgens et al. 2013). Furthermore, probable hemicrania continua may or may not sufficiently respond to indomethacin. For these patients, evidence-based treatment is not available. There are single case reports on the efficacy of verapamil, steroids, naproxen, lamotrigine, gabapentin, methysergide, topiramate, melatonin and caffeine [3].

Key Points in the Management of Hemicrania Continua

- Establish diagnosis according to ICHD-3 beta.
- Consider imaging in all patients, particularly in those with atypical presentation.
- Start indomethacin with 25 mg t.i.d. and increase the daily dose to 225 mg, if necessary.
- Monitor treatment with indomethacin with respect to side effects including headache.

References

1. Antonaci F, Sjaastad O (2014) Hemicrania continua: towards a new classification? J Headache Pain 15:18
2. Cittadini E, Goadsby PJ (2009) Hemicrania continua and unilateral chronic migraine indomethacin negative: a clinical comparison study. Cephalalgia 29(Suppl 1):108–109
3. Evers S, Goadsby P, Jensen R et al (2011) Treatment of miscellaneous idiopathic headache disorders (Group 4 of the HIS classification)–report of an EFNS task force. Eur J Neurol 18:803–812
4. Goadsby PJ (2014) Hemicrania continua – building on experience and clinical science. J Headache Pain 15:9
5. Headache Classification Committee of the International Headache Society (2013) The International Classification of Headache Disorders, 3rd edition (beta version). Cephalalgia 33:629–808
6. Hollingworth M, Young TM (2014) Melatonin responsive hemicrania continua in which indomethacin was associated with contralateral headache. Headache 54(5):916–919
7. Prakash S, Golwala P (2012) A proposal for revision of hemicrania continua diagnostic criteria based on critical analysis of 62 patients. Cephalalgia 32:860–868
8. Prakash S, Shah ND, Soni RK (2009) Secondary hemicrania continua: case reports and a literature review. J Neurol Sci 280:29–34
9. Ramón C, Mauri G, Vega J, Rico M, Para M, Pascual J (2013) Diagnostic distribution of 100 unilateral, side-locked headaches consulting a specialized clinic. Eur Neurol 69:289–291
10. Seidel S, Lieba-Samal D, Vigl M, Wöber C (2011) Clinical features of unilateral headaches beyond migraine and cluster headache and their response to indomethacin. Wien Klin Wochenschr 123:536–541
11. Seidel S, Wöber C (2012) Are the ICHD-II criteria for hemicrania continua too restrictive? Headache 52:827
12. Sjaastad O, Bakketeig LS (2007) The rare, unilateral headaches. VAGA study of headache epidemiology. J Headache Pain 8:19–27
13. Sjaastad O, Spierings EL (1984) Hemicrania continua: another headache absolutely responsive to indomethacin. Cephalalgia 4:65–70
14. Viana M, Tassorelli C, Allena M et al (2013) Diagnostic and therapeutic errors in trigeminal autonomic cephalalgias and hemicrania continua: a systematic review. J Headache Pain 14:14
15. Wilbrink LA, Ferrari MD, Kruit MC, Haan J (2009) Neuroimaging in trigeminal autonomic cephalgias: when, how, and of what? Curr Opin Neurol 22:247–253

Further Reading

Jürgens TP, Schulte LH, May A (2013) Indomethacin-induced de novo headache in hemicrania continua–fighting fire with fire? Cephalalgia 33:1203–1205

May A (2013) Diagnosis and clinical features of trigemino-autonomic headaches. Headache 53:1470–1478

Pareja JA, Cuadrado ML, Fernández-de-las-Peñas C et al (2012) Primary continuous unilateral headaches: a nosologic model for hemicrania continua. Cephalalgia 32:413–418

Chapter 25
Primary Cough Headache

Peter J. Goadsby

25.1 Case Description

The patient, a 51-year-old male, presented with a 10-month history of a new headache, without any previous history of headache and in particular no history of headache with alcohol consumption.

The headaches began in January and he was seen in November. They had commenced one morning at work with a bout of coughing. They felt as a pressure wave that would radiate from the back of the head to the front on both sides. There was a severe, tight sensation for two to three minutes followed by a less severe pain for about an hour.

There was no nausea, photophobia, phonophobia, or osmophobia with these headaches. There was no visual disturbance, including blurring and no migrainous aura. He could walk afterward without discomfort although he was inclined not to do so.

There were no cranial autonomic symptoms, no dizziness, vertigo, or premonitory symptoms.

The headache could also be triggered by sneezing, lifting, and stooping. There was no effect of sexual excitement or of orgasm.

He was on no medications when he was seen.

He took no treatment for headache. He was taking a statin for hypercholesterolemia.

He had been treated with ibuprofen 800 mg and naproxen 440 mg and neither was helpful. He had tried sumatriptan 100 mg, rizatriptan 10 mg, and eletriptan 40 mg each without useful effect. He had an 8-week course of amitriptyline 50 mg nightly that was not helpful and made him drowsy with a dry mouth. He had been

P.J. Goadsby
NIHR-Wellcome Trust Clinical Research Facility, Wellcome Foundation Building, King's College Hospital, London SE5 9PJ, UK
e-mail: peter.goadsby@kcl.ac.uk

A. Siva, C. Lampl (eds.), *Case-Based Diagnosis and Management of Headache Disorders*, Headache, DOI 10.1007/978-3-319-06886-2_25

treated with topiramate 50 mg daily that was not useful and produced marked cognitive side effects that he could not tolerate. He had seen a chiropractor and osteopath and had acupuncture, none of which helped. He had a course of cognitive behavioral therapy that was not useful.

His past history was otherwise unremarkable.

There was no family history of headache, although he had not specifically asked his parents who were both dead.

He was a nonsmoker who took alcohol perhaps twice a week without headache and cannabis weekly. The cannabis did not prevent the headache onset.

On examination he was well, in no distress and weighed 76 Kg. Neck movements were full and the neck was painless to palpation, including the region around the greater occipital nerves. In the cranial nerves, the fields were full and the fundi normal. Color visual was normal as was opticokinetic nystagmus. The eye movements were full with normal full pursuits and normal saccadic movements. There was no trigeminal or cervical sensory change. There was no facial asymmetry. Palate elevation and tongue movements were normal. There was no wasting or abnormal movements. Tone and power were equal and normal, and the reflexes symmetrical and normal with down-going toes. Gait and coordination were normal.

He was attended to in an emergency room once with the problem and had a brain CT that was normal. He declined a lumbar puncture on that visit.

25.2 Differential Diagnosis and Investigation

The patient presents with Valsalva-maneuver or cough headache. He has a typical history and normal examination. We elected to image his brain with MRI particularly to look for a Chiari malformation, given the association of that with cough headache, and our planned management. He had no other tests.

25.3 Diagnostic Workup for the Case

The patient had an MRI brain with and without contrast; this was normal. He had a lumbar puncture. The opening pressure was 12 cm CSF with normal constituents. He had 20 ml of fluid taken off. He had no headache from that day until follow-up 6 months later.

25.4 Summary of the Case

A 51-year-old male with primary cough headache treated with lumbar puncture.

25.5 ICHD-III Beta Definition [2]

4.1 Primary cough headache

Previously used terms: benign cough headache, Valsalva-maneuver headache

Description: headache precipitated by coughing or other Valsalva (straining) maneuvers, but not by prolonged physical exercise, in the absence of any intracranial disorder

Diagnostic criteria:

A. At least two headache episodes fulfilling criteria B–D
B. Brought on by and occurring only in association with coughing, straining, and/or other Valsalva maneuvers
C. Sudden onset
D. Lasting between 1 s and 2 h
E. Not better accounted for by another ICHD-3 diagnosis

25.6 General Information

Primary cough headache is a generalized headache that begins suddenly; lasts for several minutes, sometimes up to a few hours; and is precipitated by coughing; it is preventable by avoiding coughing or other precipitating events, which can include sneezing, straining, laughing, or stooping. The syndrome was first described by Symonds [5] as patients with the "liability to brief, severe pain in the headache precipitated by… especially coughing."

In all patients with this syndrome, serious etiologies must be excluded before a diagnosis of primary cough headache can be established. Pascual and colleagues [3] reported a large series of cough, exercise, and sex headache. They noted that symptomatic cough headache tended to last for days, occurred in younger patients, and was usually associated with posterior fossa signs.

A Chiari malformation or any lesion causing obstruction of CSF pathways or displacing cerebral structures can be the cause of the head pain. Other conditions that can present with cough or exertional headache as the initial symptom include cerebral aneurysm, carotid stenosis, and vertebrobasilar disease. Benign cough headache can resemble primary exercise headache, and the essential clinical differentiation is that cough headache is precipitated by sudden Valsalva actions and exercise headache by prolonged strenuous activity.

From a treatment perspective, Symonds [5] had certainly noted that lumbar puncture could resolve the problem. Raskin [4] noted that six of fourteen cases of primary cough headache responded to lumbar puncture and that ten of sixteen responded to indomethacin. These data formed the basis of the author's practice in primary cough headache which is to offer a lumbar puncture first, as there is a reasonable change for cure with a simple single procedure. As Raskin found, indomethacin, 25 mg three to four times daily, remains the best oral therapeutic option, and when it was available, methysergide can also be useful [1].

Key Points

- Cough headache has both primary and second forms.
- In patients with long attacks, lasting many hours, and in those with abnormal neurological examinations, brain MRI is important to consider a Chiari malformation.
- Lumbar puncture can be curative and, without any contraindication, should be considered.
- Indomethacin is the optimal oral therapy when required.

Suggested Reading

1. Bahra A, Goadsby PJ (1998) Cough headache responsive to methysergide. Cephalalgia 18:495–496
2. Headache Classification Committee of the International Headache Society (2013) The International classification of headache disorders, 3rd edition (beta version). Cephalalgia 33:629–808
3. Pascual P, Iglesias F, Oterino A, Vazquez-Barquero A, Berciano J (1996) Cough, exertional, and sexual headache. Neurology 46:1520–1524
4. Raskin NH (1995) The cough headache syndrome: treatment. Neurology 45:1784
5. Symonds C (1956) Cough headache. Brain 79:557–568

Chapter 26
Emergency Room Headache: A Case with Primary Thunderclap Headache Including Differential Diagnosis from Secondary Ones

Dominique Valade

26.1 Case Description

A 41-year-old man was admitted to the general emergency room (ER) because of an extremely severe headache of instantaneous onset (1 min at most), probably the worst ever in his life. He had described of having two previous similar episodes within a few days all during sexual intercourse, including the final one that brought him to the ER.

His neurological and general examinations were totally normal, and the patient had no more pain for 12 h. No other triggers such as exposure to vasoactive drugs or any other circumstances related to these severe headache episodes other than sexual activity could be demonstrated. However, the absence of any associated symptoms and strictly normal physical and neurological examinations do not exclude a serious underlying life-threatening cause and an urgent diagnostic workup is needed in such cases.

The patient was referred to the emergency headache centre (EHC) for appropriate investigations. His cranial computerized tomography (CT) scan was normal. The initial neuroimaging study then was followed by a spinal tap, which showed a normal opening pressure, no cells and normal biochemistry. Later in the afternoon he was further investigated with MRI, MRA and MRV, with none of them revealing any abnormality. Despite that all these studies were normal, it was decided to carry out a conventional angiography to rule out definitely a reversible cerebral vasoconstriction syndrome (RCVS). This study also disclosed no abnormality, and therefore, as all exams were normal, it was concluded that his diagnosis was "primary headache associated with sexual activity".

D. Valade
Emergency Headache Centre, Lariboisiere Hospital, Paris, France
e-mail: dominique.valade@lrb.aphp.fr

A. Siva, C. Lampl (eds.), *Case-Based Diagnosis and Management of Headache Disorders*, Headache, DOI 10.1007/978-3-319-06886-2_26

26.2 What Is Thunderclap Headache?

It is a severe high-intensity headache of abrupt onset; we must investigate with a detailed questionnaire:

- How long the headache took to peak: less than 1 min.
- What the maximum severity was: more than 7 on a scale 0–10.
- Lasting for more than 5 min, but from minutes to several days.
- It may be single or recur over a few days more often with the same cause.
- It may start spontaneously or during emotional stress, sexual activity, cough, exertion, etc.
- There is no specificity of the type or the location of the pain.

The patient must be urgently referred to an emergency department and if possible to a hospital with neurological department.

26.3 Epidemiology

The prevalence of sexual headache is unknown. In the only population-based epidemiological study, the lifetime prevalence was 1 % with a broad confidence interval and similar to that of primary cough and exertional headaches. The prevalence of this headache may be underestimated, since patients often feel embarrassed about reporting it. In terms of consultation in headache clinics, it accounts for 0.2–1.3 % of all headache patients.

The age of onset of patients consulting due to this headache is 35–39 years (range 20–50 years). Similar to exertional headache, the male-to-female ratio is 3–4/1. The dull type occurs in less than one-quarter of patients. Two-thirds of patients have their headache in a bout: at least two attacks occurring in over 50 % of sexual activities and then none for more than 2 weeks.

26.4 Diagnostic and ICHD-3 Beta Criteria

The number of attacks per bout ranges from 2 to 50, and the mean duration of the symptomatic period is 3 months, though a minority of patients suffer from sexual headache for several years without apparent remission. Most of these patients experience infrequent (<20 % of sexual activities) attacks.

Pain characteristics are also similar to those described for primary exertional headache. The duration of pain is heterogeneous, ranging from 1 min to 24 h. Most patients have severe pain for between 1 and 3 h followed by mild pain for about 4 h. Pain is bilateral in two-thirds of patients, usually occipital or diffuse, and of a dull (47 %), throbbing (47 %) or stabbing (45 %) quality.

Patients with sexual headache are usually healthy people, with no vascular disease. Two-thirds, however, suffer from other headache disorders such as episodic tension-type headache (35 %), migraine (25 %) and chronic tension-type headache (10 %). Comorbid migraine and exertional headache are more frequent in orgasmic headache.

Subarachnoid haemorrhage occurs during sexual activity in 4–12 % of cases.

Decreased levels of consciousness, vomiting, meningeal signs, focal symptoms and severe pain lasting more than 24 h should be interpreted as "red flags" requiring immediate diagnostic workup. A minority of patients experiencing cough headache due to Chiari type I malformation or some other posterior fossa abnormality also notice head pain during orgasm. This is logical if we consider that sexual intercourse is a mixture of prolonged physical exercise and Valsalva manoeuvres.

A. At least two episodes of pain in the head and/or neck fulfilling criteria B–D
B. Brought on by and occurring only during sexual activity
C. Either or both of the following:
   1. Increasing in intensity with increasing sexual excitement
   2. Abrupt explosive intensity just before or with orgasm
D. Lasting from 1 min to 24 h with severe intensity and/or up to 72 h with mild intensity
E. Not better accounted for by another International Classification of Headache Disorders (ICHD-3) diagnosis

26.5 Differential Diagnosis of Primary Thunderclap Headache

1. Vascular causes:
   - Subarachnoid haemorrhage (95 % during the 24 h after bleeding)
   - Intracerebral haemorrhage
   - Intraventricular haemorrhage
   - Acute subdural haemorrhage
   - Dissection of cervical arteries (extracranial, intracranial, carotid or vertebral)
   - Symptomatic aneurysm with mass effect (painful third nerve palsy)
   - Reversible cerebral vasoconstriction syndrome
   - Cerebral venous thrombosis (opening pressure may be high)
   - Brain infarct in patients in whom CT was performed within 3 h of onset
   - Temporal arteritis
   - Myocardial ischaemia
   - Aortic dissection

2. Other causes:
   - Meningitis (bacterial or viral)
   - Brain infarct (after 3 h)
   - Tumour (third ventricle colloid cyst, posterior fossa tumour)
   - Hydrocephalus (aqueductal stenosis, Chiari type 1 malformation)
   - Acute sinusitis (exclusion diagnosis)
   - Posterior reversible encephalopathy syndrome
   - Pituitary apoplexy
   - Intracranial hypotension (opening pressure is low)

26.6 Management

To advise that the course of the condition is limited in time, explain that the headaches recur during several sexual encounters over a period of time and never return again, but also inform that the course may be unpredictable; some patients experience them from time to time throughout their lifetime.

It has been reported that when patients resume sexual activity within days after an attack, the headache may recur, so advising the patients to refrain from sex for a week after an attack might be prudent.

26.7 Pharmacotherapy

Indomethacin 50–100 mg taken 30–60 min before sexual activity or naratriptan 2.5 mg taken 2 h before may be useful as short-term prophylaxis. The acute treatment for an attack that has already begun is, in general, worthless but can be tried with triptans or NSAIDs. For patients with longer lasting bouts or with frequent attacks, propranolol in doses from 40 to 240 mg/day is reported to be effective.

26.8 Does Primary Thunderclap Headache Exist?

It is always dangerous to diagnose primary headache when onset is abrupt or because it is related to sexual activity but also cough or exertion. To conclude to the diagnosis of primary thunderclap headache requires the exclusion of a secondary cause. Nevertheless there is a real doubt about the existence of a primary entity, and in my opinion, all thunderclap headaches are secondary that is only because the diagnosis has been missed by too early or too late investigations or more simply a lack of sensitivity of these investigations. We must have a strict follow-up of these patients with MRA 3 or 4 weeks after the onset of the last attack, and sometimes we need to have an invasive conventional angiography; that is the reason why in the EHC we do not speak of "primary thunderclap headache" but of "thunderclap headache of undefined origin".

Suggested Reading

1. Al-Shahi R, White PM, Davenport RJ, Lindsay KW (2006) Subarachnoid haemorrhage. BMJ 333:235–40
2. Broner S, Lay C, Newman L, Swerdlow M (2007) Thunderclap headache as the presenting symptom of myocardial infarction. Headache 47:724–5
3. Cough JR (2001) Orgasm headache. Headache 41:512–514
4. Cough J, Bearss C (1990) Relief of migraine with sexual intercourse. Headache 30:302
5. Cumurciuc R, Crassard I, Sarov M, Valade D, Bousser MG (2005) Headache as the only neurological sign of cerebral venous thrombosis: a series of 17 cases. J Neurol Neurosurg Psychiatry 76:1084–7
6. Davenport R (2002) Acute headache in the emergency department. J Neurol Neurosurg Psychiatry 72:ii33–ii7
7. Day JW, Raskin NH (1986) Thunderclap headache: symptom of enraptured cerebral aneurysm. Lancet 2:1247–8
8. De Bruijn SF, Stam J, Kappelle LJ, CVST Study Group (1996) Thunderclap headache as first symptom of cerebral venous sinus thrombosis. Lancet 348:1623–5
9. Dodick DW (2002) Thunderclap headache. J Neurol Neurosurg Psychiatry 72:6–11
10. Dodick DW, Wijdicks EF (1998) Pituitary apoplexy presenting as a thunderclap headache. Neurology 50:1510–1
11. Ducros A (2012) Reversible cerebral vasoconstriction syndrome. Lancet Neurol 11:906–17
12. Ducros A, Boukobza M, Porcher R, Sarov M, Valade D, Bousser MG (2007) The clinical and radiological spectrum of reversible cerebral vasoconstriction syndrome. A prospective series of 67 patients. Brain 130:3091–101
13. Ducros A, Fiedler U, Porcher R, Boukobza M, Stapf C, Bousser MG (2010) Hemorrhagic manifestations of reversible cerebral vasoconstriction syndrome. Frequency, features, and risks factors. Stroke 41:2505–11
14. Evans RW, Pascual J (2000) Orgasmic headache: clinical diagnosis and treatment. Headache 40:491–494
15. Evers S, Lance JW (2006) In primary headache attributed to sexual activity. In: Olesen J, Goabsy PJ, Ramadan NM et al (eds) The headaches, 3rd edn. Lippincott William & Wilkins, Philadelphia, pp 841–846
16. Frese A, Eikermann A, Frese K et al (2003) Headache associated with sexual activity. Demography, clinical features and comorbidity. Neurology 61:796–800
17. Frese A, Frese K, Ringelstein EB, Husstedt I-W, Evers S (2003) Cognitive processing in headache associated with sexual activity. Cephalalgia 23:545–551
18. Fugate JE, Ameriso SF, Ortiz G, Schottlaender LV, Wijdicks EF, Flemming KD et al (2012) Variable presentations of postpartum angiopathy. Stroke 43:670–6
19. Headache Classification Committee of the international Headache Society (2013) The international classification of headache disorders. (ICHD-3beta). Cephalalgia 33(9):628–808
20. Landtblom AM, Fridriksson S, Boivie J, Johansson G, Johansson I (2002) Sudden onset headache: a prospective study of features, incidence and causes. Cephalalgia 22:354–60
21. Lasoasa DS (2003) Not so benign sexual headache. Cephalalgia 34:808
22. Linn FH, Rinkel GJ, Algra A, van Gijn J (1998) Headache characteristics in subarachnoid haemorrhage ad benign thunderclap headache. J Neurol Neurosurg Psychiatry 65:791–3

23. Linn FH, Wijdicks EF, van der Graaf Y, Weedesteyn-van Vliet FA, Bartelds A, van Gijn J (1994) Prospective study of sentinel headache in aneurismal subarachnoid haemorrhage. Lancet 344:590–3
24. Lopes Azevedo L, Breder R, de Freitas GR, de A Santos DP (2011) Ischemic stroke presenting as thunderclap headache: report of two cases and review of the literature. Eur Neurol 66:133–5
25. MgGeeney BE, Barest G, Grillone G (2006) Thunderclap headache from complicated sinusitis. Headache 46:517–20
26. Mistry N, Mathew L, Parry A (2009) Thunderclap headache. Pract Neurol 9:294–7
27. Moussouttas M, Mayer SA (2008) Thunderclap headache with normal CT and lumbar puncture: further investigations are unnecessary: against. Stroke 39:1394–5
28. O'Neill J, McLaggan S, Gibson R (2005) Acute headache and subarachnoid haemorrhage: a retrospective review of CT and lumbar puncture findings. Scott Med J 50:151–3
29. Pascual J, Iglesias F, Oterino A et al (1996) Exertional and sexual headaches: an analysis of 72 benign and symptomatic cases. Neurology 46:1520–1524
30. Savitz SI, Edlow J (2008) Thunderclap headache with normal CT and lumbar puncture: further investigations are unnecessary: for. Stroke 39:1392–3
31. Schievink WI, Thompson RC, Loh CT, Maya MM (2001) Spontaneous retroclival hematoma presenting as a thunderclap headache. Case report. J Neurosurg 95:522–4
32. Schievink WI, Wijdicks EF, Meyer FB, Sonntag VK (2001) Spontaneous intracranial hypotension mimicking aneurismal subarachnoid haemorrhage. Neurosurgery 48:513–6, discussion 6-7
33. Schwedt TJ, Matharu MS, Dodick DW (2006) Thunderclap headache. Lancet Neurol 5: 621–31
34. Silbert PL, Edis HR, Stewart-Wynn EGG, Gubbay SS (1991) Benign vascular sexual headache and exertional headache: inter-relationships and long term prognosis. J Neurol Neurosurg Psychiatr 54:417–421
35. Singhal AB, Hajj-Ali RA, Topcuoglu MA, Fok J, Bena J, Yang D et al (2011) Reversible cerebral vasoconstriction syndromes :analysis of 139 cases. Arch Neurol 68:1005–12
36. Timoteo A, Inacio N, Machado S, Pinto AA, Parreira E (2012) Headache as the sole presentation of cerebral venous thrombosis: a prospective study. J Headache Pain 13:487–90
37. Yeh YC, Fuh JL, Chen SP, Wang SJ (2010) Clinical features, imaging findings and outcomes of headache associated with sexual activity. Cephalalgia 30:1329–35

Chapter 27
Hypnic Headache

Christian Lampl

27.1 Case Description

A 61-year-old woman was admitted to our headache outpatient center with a 6-month history of headache attacks occurring every night. She had no history of other types of headache or any other neurological diseases. There was no family history of headache. The attacks always occurred between 1 and 3 o'clock, and the duration was no longer than 120 min. She experienced one attack per night. The pain quality was described as tightness and pressure, always right sided with mild to moderate intensity (3–6/10 on a visual analogue scale). There was no nausea or vomiting, no photophobia, or no phonophobia. After waking up, she has the habit to walk around; however, headache did not worsen by that physical activity. Trigemino-autonomic symptoms, such as ptosis, miosis, conjunctival injection, tearing, and rhinorrhea, were absent. General, as well as neurological, examination was normal. The trapezius muscles were mildly pain sensitive to finger pressure. Blood pressure was normal. Routine blood tests only showed moderately high levels of cholesterol (total cholesterol 277 mg/dL, LDL cholesterol 162 mg/dL), as well as slightly elevated liver enzymes (alanine transaminase (ALT) 47, aspartate transaminase (AST) 41). Numerous treatments, such as aspirin, paracetamol, diclofenac, and several mixed analgesics, failed to improve their headache attacks. She suffered from extreme psychological strain, because of severe sleep disturbances. Lorazepam, used as a sleep-inducing drug, did not abort the headache attacks.

C. Lampl
Headache Medical Center Seilerstaette Linz, Hospital Sisters of Charity, Linz, Austria
e-mail: christian.lampl@bhs.at

A. Siva, C. Lampl (eds.), *Case-Based Diagnosis and Management of Headache Disorders*, Headache, DOI 10.1007/978-3-319-06886-2_27

27.2 Differential Diagnosis and How to Work Up This Kind of a Patient

In individuals who develop such a recurring, moderate headache, exclusively during sleep, without any pathological signs in physical and/or neurological examinations, the probability of a craniocervical pathology is extremely rare. If this kind of headache occurs for the first time, of course, the consulting physician needs to rule out any pathological intracerebral/intracranial events, such as subarachnoid hemorrhage, cervico-cephalic arterial dissection, cerebral venous thrombosis, reversible cerebral vasoconstriction syndrome, colloid cyst of the third ventricle, or spontaneous intracranial hypotension.

Other possible causes of headache developing during and causing wakening from sleep should be ruled out, with additional particular attention given to sleep apnea, nocturnal hypertension, hypoglycemia, and medication overuse. Trigemino-autonomic features must be asked for to rule out any trigemino-autonomic headaches like cluster headache or hemicrania continua. Hypnic headache (HH) usually begins after the age of 50 years but may occur in younger people.

27.3 Diagnostic Workup of the Case

Cervical and transcranial Doppler ultrasonography was normal. A CT scan followed by a digital subtraction arteriography (DSA) shows one small asymptomatic aneurysm at the bifurcation of the right middle cerebral artery. The CT scan was necessary because of the first headache period that patient ever had. DSA was performed because of a reasonable suspicion of an AV malformation. Due to the fact of vessel pathology, she was advised for a reexamination of the CT scan of the brain in 6 months. Psychiatric evaluation showed signs of moderate depression; the Hamilton Depression Scale (HAM-D17) gave 21 points. A follow-up polysomnography detected a poor sleep quality (2 arousals/h) and a mildly decreased oxygen saturation (mean 94 %, 4 min under 86 %). One nocturnal headache attack was captured during the first REM stage of sleep, 3.20 h after falling asleep, and was not associated with oxygen desaturation. Polysomnography showed several episodes of mildly decreased oxygen saturation at the beginning of sleep, which was due to nocturnal hypoventilation secondary to the patient's obesity. The clinical description, the exclusive relationship with sleep, notably always during the same time of the night, and the occurrence in a female patient older than 60 years, without any neurological deficiency and missing trigemino-autonomic features, lead us to the diagnosis of hypnic headache (HH).

27.4 Summary of the Case

A 61-year-old female with recurrent nocturnal headache was admitted to our headache outpatient center. Primary headache disorders which also often occur during nocturnal sleep or upon awakening, such as migraine, cluster headache, and chronic

Table 27.1 Definition of hypnic headache according to "The International Classification of Headache Disorders, 3rd edition (beta version)." Cephalalgia 2013; 33(9) 678–679

4.9. Hypnic headache
Description:
Frequently recurring headache attacks developing only during sleep, causing wakening and lasting for up to 4 h, without characteristic associated symptoms and not attributed to other pathologies
Diagnostic criteria:
A. Recurrent headache attacks fulfilling criteria B–E
B. Developing only during sleep and causing wakening
C. Occurring on ≥ 10 days per month for >3 months
D. Lasting ≥ 15 min and for up to 4 h after waking
E. No cranial autonomic symptoms or restlessness
F. Not better accounted for by another ICHD-3 diagnosis

paroxysmal hemicrania, can readily be diagnosed through clinical evaluation. The clinical presentation of headache attacks in our patient excludes a diagnosis of migraine and paroxysmal hemicrania. HH must also be differentiated from cluster headache, notably by the absence of autonomic signs. Her neurological and physical examinations were normal and there was no neck stiffness. Based on her headache history, the clinical features of a current mild to moderate nocturnal headache, without any trigemino-autonomic signs, HH was diagnosed. Therapy with lithium carbonate, 450 mg at bedtime, improved the headache intensity (2–4/10 on the visual analogue scale) within 3 weeks and decreased the frequency of attacks (2–3 per week instead of every night) (Table 27.1)

27.5 Brief General Information

HH was first described in 1988. It is a benign, recurrent headache disorder occurring exclusively during sleep, often starting during the same time of the night. The recurrence and the time-dependent manner are truly pathognomonic for this kind of headache. Commonly the headache is bilateral, mainly frontotemporal, or holocranial diffuse, with mild to moderate intensity. Concomitant symptoms are unusual. Patients usually suffer from 1 to 2 attacks per night lasting from 30 min to 3 h. Mean age of onset is 63 years with a female/male ratio of 2:1. Case series show an incidence of 0.1 % in outpatient headache centers. There is no known comorbidity with other idiopathic headaches or psychiatric diseases. Polysomnography studies show that attacks occurred during the initial REM sleep stage. Sleep quality is commonly normal, except decreased sleep efficiency and mildly decreased oxygen saturation down to 70 % in some patients. The exclusive relationship of HH with sleep, notably always during the same time of the night, and its tendency to occur in subjects older than 60 years imply a possible association with the changes of sleep physiology occurring in the elderly and the involvement of brain structures responsible for the endogenous circadian rhythm.

Therapeutic options are caffeine (cup of strong cafe) before sleep and lithium carbonate (150–600 mg/day) with control of the thyroid gland and renal function. Other therapeutic options might be indomethacin (100–150 mg/dL) and flunarizine (10 mg). In the acute management, sumatriptan and oxygen inhalation, the first-choice treatment for cluster headache, are not effective. Antidepressant drugs and beta-blockers likewise are not useful.

Suggested Reading

1. Dodick DW (2000) Polysomnography in hypnic headache syndrome. Headache 40:748–752
2. Dodick DW, Mosek AC, Campbell JK (1998) The hypnic ("alarm clock") headache syndrome. Cephalalgia 18:152–156
3. Dodick DW, Eross EJ, Parish JM (2003) Clinical, anatomical, and physiologic relationship between sleep and headache. Headache 43:282–292
4. Evers S, Goadsby PJ (2003) Hypnic headache. Clinical features, pathophysiology, and treatment. Neurology 60:905–910
5. Evers S, Rahmann A, Schwaag S, Lüdemann P, Husstedt IW (2003) Hypnic headache – the first German cases including polysomnography. Cephalalgia 23:20–23
6. Pinessi L, Rainero I, Cicolin A, Zibetti M, Gentile S, Mutani R (2003) Hypnic headache syndrome: association of the attacks with REM sleep. Cephalalgia 23:150–154
7. Raskin NH (1988) The hypnic headache syndrome. Headache 28:534–536

Chapter 28
Headache Attributed to Paracranial Inflammatory Disorders

Morris Levin

28.1 Case Description

A 32-year-old woman was referred to a headache center for intractable headaches occurring almost every day. The pain is generally right temporal but can also occur frontally, either unilaterally or bilaterally. Head pain can radiate to the occiput or even become generalized. There has been no eye pain, but she occasionally describes right ear pain. Head pain can last between 30 min and several days. She denies accompanying nausea, photosensitivity, or visual symptoms. She does notice phonosensitivity with some headaches. Headaches have led her to take modest doses of ibuprofen and acetaminophen almost daily.

She emphasizes the fact that she works in a very stressful setting at a business where she answers the phones and does clerical work on the computer. She says that she notices tight neck muscles and teeth clenching "all the time," "because of my job." She describes that she sits at a computer screen and keyboard all day long. The pain is so bad sometimes that her eyes tear. She relates a long history of "sinus allergies" and has seen otolaryngologists who "have not found anything."

She states that she has seen a number of physicians who have alternately diagnosed migraine, cluster headaches, tension-type headaches, sinus headaches, anxiety, fibromyalgia, and depression. Her dentist thought that she has temporomandibular dysfunction (TMD) and suggested a "bite plate" that was "really expensive." She tried it at night for several days but there was no benefit and was uncomfortable. She does not usually awaken with headache. Her jaw has not "locked."

M. Levin, MD
DHMC Department of Neurology, Geisel School of Medicine at Dartmouth,
1 Medical Center Drive, Lebanon, NH 03756, USA
e-mail: morris.levin@hitchcock.org

A. Siva, C. Lampl (eds.), *Case-Based Diagnosis and Management of Headache Disorders*, Headache, DOI 10.1007/978-3-319-06886-2_28

During her teens she had infrequent moderately severe headaches during menses, sometimes accompanied by nausea, but these resolved during her first pregnancy at age 19 and have not recurred. She does not recall the location of these headaches. She is currently on a low-dose oral contraceptive.

There was some tenderness of the right temporomandibular joint when compressed during jaw excursion. With protrusion or lateral jaw movement, pain seemed to intensify. There was no palpable clicking around the temporomandibular joint during excursion. Forceful palpation of either the right or left masseter muscles was very uncomfortable. Temporalis muscle palpation was not unpleasant, and in fact if it was gentle, it seemed to relieve her pain to some extent. Her range of movement of the jaw was slightly diminished, and there was some discomfort when she attempted to open more fully. Facial morphology was normal. Otoscopic and mastoid examination was normal. There was some conjunctival injection bilaterally, but pupils were normal and funduscopic exam was normal. Paranasal sinuses were nontender and bending forward did not induce head pain. Neck range of motion was reduced, and the Spurling test was positive with head turning to the right. It did not seem to induce headache. Neurological exam was normal, including mental status, cranial nerves, motor and sensory function, reflexes, coordination, and gait.

She brought magnetic resonance imaging (MRI) images of her head which had been read as normal. They revealed bilateral mucous cysts in her maxillary sinuses and a small left nasal septal spur, but no bony erosion or other facial bone or sinus abnormalities. There were no brain abnormalities and there was no meningeal enhancement after gadolinium.

28.2 Summary of the Case

This is a case of a young, relatively healthy woman with daily headaches occasionally accompanied by ear pain and phonosensitivity. History suggests possible stress or sinus causation. Examination points more toward temporomandibular or cervical pathology.

28.3 Discussion

As is true for many people with chronic headaches, there are a number of pain and other symptoms noted by this patient. Also typical is the list of different diagnoses she carries. There are features of migraine, and it seems very likely she had menstrual migraines in her teens. There are also features of tension-type headache (cervical tightness, exacerbated by uncomfortable positions) and even a couple of features of cluster headache (tearing, unilateral pain). But she does not actually meet diagnostic criteria for any of the primary headaches except perhaps chronic tension-type headache (Table 28.1). The positive Spurling test (elicitation of radicular neck or arm pain with downward pressure on the head when the sitting patient

Table 28.1 Diagnostic criteria for chronic tension-type headache (International Classification of Headache Disorders (3rd edition – beta version))

A. Headache occurring on ≥15 days/month on average for >3 months (≥180 day/year), fulfilling criteria B–D
B. Lasting hours to days or unremitting
C. ≥2 of the following four characteristics:
1. Bilateral location
2. Pressing/tightening (non-pulsating) quality
3. Mild or moderate intensity
4. Not aggravated by routine physical activity
D. Both of the following:
1. Not >1 of photophobia, phonophobia, or mild nausea
2. Neither moderate or severe nausea nor vomiting
E. Not better accounted for by another ICHD-3 diagnosis

extends and rotates the head) suggests cervical foraminal stenosis, but typical headache was not elicited so this is probably not the key etiology of her headaches. Sinus mucoceles are common and do not cause headache. The nasal septal spur is interesting since some authors believe this can be the source of head or facial pain (the so-called "contact point headache"), but it is on the wrong side to make that a viable diagnosis in this case.

28.3.1 Clues from History and Physical Examination

The provocative tests of temporomandibular function are very compelling here. In particular, the decreased range of motion of her jaw, pain with movements of the jaw, and right temporomandibular tenderness suggest right TMD. Many causes of TMD are not associated with "clicking," which, even if present, may be intermittent and/or difficult to appreciate even with a stethoscope, so this is not contrary to the diagnosis. Otalgia in the absence of ear or mastoid pathology is also quite suggestive as ear pain is a common referral pain site in TMD.

The International Classification of Headache Disorders (ICHD) has tackled the problem of specifying diagnostic criteria for headache due to TMD in the latest edition (Table 28.2). An alternative set of criteria for diagnosing headache related to TMD has been published by Schiffman et al. and is supported by some compelling validation data (Table 28.3). By either set of criteria, this patient would seem to have a fairly clear case of TMD.

It has become clear that there are a number of distinct causes of painful TMD. These include arthralgia, myalgia, myofascial pain, disc displacement (several varieties), degenerative joint disease, and subluxation. Virtually all can induce head pain and some forms may produce primarily headache. This patient seems to have an arthralgic form, or perhaps both arthralgic and myalgic, since

Table 28.2 Diagnostic criteria for headache due to temporomandibular dysfunction (International Classification of Headache Disorders (3rd edition – beta version))

A. Any headache fulfilling criterion C
B. Clinical and/or imaging evidence of TMD
C. Evidence of causation demonstrated by ≥2 of the following: 1. Headache has developed in temporal relation to onset of TMD 2. Either or both of: (a) HA has significantly worsened in parallel with progression of TMD (b) HA has significantly improved or resolved in parallel with improvement/resolution of TMD 3. Headache produced or exacerbated by active jaw movements, passive movements through range of motion of the jaw, and/or provocative maneuvers such as pressure on TMJ and surrounding muscles of mastication 4. Headache, when unilateral, is ipsilateral to TMD
D. Not better accounted for by another ICHD-3 diagnosis

Table 28.3 Diagnostic criteria for headache due to temporomandibular disorders

A. Any headache fulfilling criterion C
B. Painful TMD demonstrated by clinically based diagnostic criteria
C. Evidence of causation shown by both of the following: 1. History – headache in the temple(s) that is changed with jaw movement, function, and/or parafunction (jaw clenching history) 2. Examination – report of typical headache in the temporal area with: (a) Palpation of the temporalis muscle(s), or (b) Range of motion of the jaw
D. The headache is not better accounted for by another headache diagnosis

After Schiffman et al. [5]

there is clear induction of pain with joint manipulation. There is pain with masseter palpation, but a case can be made that this is actually arthralgic as well since it occurred with forceful palpation, which almost certainly exerted traction on joint tissues.

28.3.2 Diagnostic Testing

Imaging of her temporomandibular joint (TMJ) was not recommended. MRI is generally only indicated if there is locking of the jaw or significantly limited opening, in order to make sure there is no serious disc displacement. Computed tomography (CT) can be done when degenerative arthritis is suspected and might be a good corroborative test here. Of note, however, is that many individuals may have arthritic changes or disc displacement on imaging with virtually no symptoms. This is analogous to the difficulty in diagnosing cervicogenic headache with commonly seen abnormal imaging.

This patient and some of her clinicians have ascribed her pain to the stresses in her life, and, certainly, this can be an exacerbating factor. It is also possible that cervical pain stemming from foraminal stenosis in the setting of poor posture and ergonomics is a contributing factor. But the positive provocative tests of TMD seem most telling. Interestingly, when this patient was presented with this hypothesis, she stated, "Maybe I should tell you something; my boyfriend gets rough with me sometimes…." Upon further questioning, she admitted that he had struck her across her jaw and face on several occasions. This was surely a source of extreme stress but also an apparent cause of permanent TM injury. Of note, Ballegaard et al. found a high incidence of moderate to severe depression in TMD patients as well as a very high comorbidity of primary headaches and TMD.

28.3.3 Management

A number of treatment strategies were entertained here. She was referred to a dentist specializing in TMD who arranged a comfortable nighttime appliance and physical therapy for jaw and neck relaxation and exercises. Nortriptyline was started for treatment of possible tension-type headaches. She was urged to limit analgesics to two days per week in order to alleviate the possibility of medication-overuse headache. She was also told to avoid chewy food and when pain flared to revert to a soft food diet. An appointment was arranged quickly for her to meet with a representative of a confidential support organization for abused individuals.

Physical measures are the mainstay of TMD management. Efforts are made to gently reduce muscular tension, improve mechanical function, and evenly distribute pressure. It seems that a significant fraction of the population has some degree of TMD, and a recent study by Piekartz and Kerstin suggested that successful treatment of TMD can lead to improvement in cervicogenic headache as well. One wonders if this can help other pain disorders in the head and neck as well.

Even when diagnosed properly, treatment of TMD can be very disappointing for a number of reasons. Often patients are not compliant with dietary instructions. Physical therapy resources can be lacking in the patient's community. The joint or muscular pathology can progress. There may be multiple sources of head pain that all must be addressed, such as concomitant migraine or cervicogenic headache. But with careful diagnosis of all factors and combining pharmacological, mechanical, and lifestyle strategies, very gratifying results can be obtained.

Suggested Reading

1. Ballegaard V, Thede-Schmidt-Hansen P, Svensson P, Jensen R (2008) Are headache and temporomandibular disorders related? A blinded study. Cephalalgia 28:832–841
2. Classification Committee, International Headache Society (2013) The international classification of headache disorders, 3rd edition, beta version (ICHD III beta). Cephalalgia 33:629–808

3. McNeely ML, Armijo Olivo S, Magee DJ (2006) A systematic review of the effectiveness of physical therapy interventions for temporomandibular disorders. Phys Ther 86:710–725
4. Piekartz H, Kerstin L (2011) Effect of treatment of temporomandibular disorders in patients with cervicogenic headache: a single-blind randomized controlled study. Cranio 29:43–56
5. Schiffman ES, Ohrbach R, List T, Anderson G, Jensen R, John MT, Nixdorf D, Goulet JP, Kang W, Truelove E, Clavel A, Fricton J, Look J (2012) Diagnostic criteria for headache attributed to temporomandibular disorders. Cephalalgia 32(9):683–692
6. Schiffman E, Ohrbach R, Truelove E et al (2014) Diagnostic criteria for temporomandibular disorders (DC/TMD) for clinical and research applications: Recommendations of the International RDC/TMD Consortium Network and Orofacial Pain Special Interest Group. J Oral Facial Pain Headache 28:6–27

Chapter 29
Headache Attributed to Paracranial Inflammatory Disorders

Joerg R. Weber

29.1 Case Description

A 62-year-old patient reported a common cold several days ago. He has no significant diseases and suffers only from well-treated migraine with aura.

Within the last 24 h, the patient has developed a diffuse headache clearly different from his migraine with a previously never experienced intensity. Additionally the man has 38.8 C fever and malaise. The headache is frontally pronounced and extends down to the neck. His wife is worried because over the last few hours the man has been confused and sensitive to noises and avoided direct light.

29.1.1 Clinical Examination

Moderate neck stiffness is found, whereas Kernig, Brudzinski and Lasègue tests are negative. The patient has neither focal neurological signs nor an involvement of the cranial nerves. He is orientated but has problems to concentrate and to follow even simple instructions. Besides the fever the heart rate is 110 per minute. The patient is a runner in good physical condition with his heart frequency down to 55. The clinical exam reveals no further alterations and a careful inspection of the integument was normal. No infections, etc., in his professional or private environment are reported.

J.R. Weber, MD, PhD
Department of Neurology, Klinikum Klagenfurt,
Feschnigstr. 11, 9020 Klagenfurt, Austria
e-mail: joerg.weber@kabeg.at

A. Siva, C. Lampl (eds.), *Case-Based Diagnosis and Management of Headache Disorders*, Headache, DOI 10.1007/978-3-319-06886-2_29

29.1.2 Laboratory Tests

At admission, leucocytes were 3,500/μl (3.9–10.2) and neutrophils 75 %. CRP was 4.1 mg/dl (≤5). Other parameters of the blood count, coagulation tests, liver and renal parameters, electrolytes, blood glucose and urine tests were within the normal range.

29.2 Differential Diagnosis and How to Work Up This Kind of Patient

The patient developed the key clinical features of bacterial meningitis as headache, malaise, fever and, later on, neck stiffness and photophobia as signs of meningeal irritation. Headache and neck stiffness (meningismus) indicate inflammatory activation of the trigeminal sensory nerve fibres in the meninges.

Neck stiffness may be absent in the disease, in deeply comatose patients, in children and in immunocompromised patients such as in liver cirrhosis. It is important to consider that the classical triad of fever, neck stiffness and altered mental state is present in less than 50 % of adults with proven bacterial meningitis. The above patient finally developed the classical triad.

Approximately 30 % of patients develop focal neurological signs, such as epileptic seizures or paresis of a limb, and up to 69 % present with impaired consciousness or 14 % with coma.

Inspection of the integument may reveal petechiae suggestive of meningococcal infection or Osler's nodes indicative of bacterial endocarditis. Meningococcal disease may present as a fulminant Gram-negative sepsis with prominent cardiovascular insufficiency and disseminated intravascular coagulation, threatening ischaemic tissue damage. A petechial skin rash is not unique to meningococcal disease but may also be present in septicaemia caused by, amongst others, streptococci or *S. aureus*. In our patient, no skin manifestation was observed.

29.2.1 Laboratory Tests

The proof to the diagnosis of bacterial meningitis is the proof of bacteria in the cerebrospinal fluid (CSF) by Gram staining or a positive bacterial culture (Fig. 29.1). Detection rates in the CSF are as high as 90 %, while up to 70 % positive results are observed in blood cultures. Polymerase chain reaction (PCR) is not yet a routine test although it has an important role in strain identification mostly in meningococcal disease.

Latex agglutination-based rapid tests are available for major meningitis pathogens, but imperfect sensitivity and specificity argue against routine clinical use.

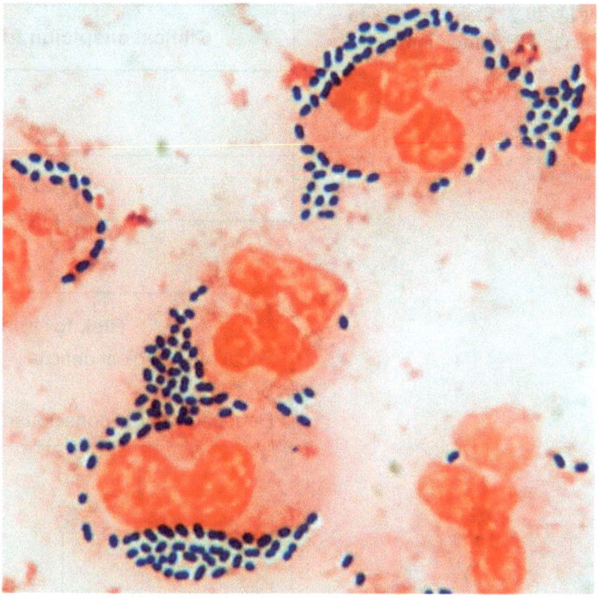

Fig. 29.1 Masses of Gram-positive extracellular diplococci (*Streptococcus pneumoniae*) surrounded by activated leucocytes in the CSF

The CSF in bacterial meningitis is characterized by a strongly elevated white blood cell count (>500 cells/µl) with predominant neutrophils and a strongly elevated protein (>1 g/l), indicating severe blood-CSF barrier disruption. Increased lactate (>0.3 g/l) and decreased glucose CSF/blood ratio (<0.4) support the diagnosis of acute bacterial meningitis.

Lower cell counts and a mixed pleocytosis are observed with *L. monocytogenes, M. tuberculosis* and fungi; also, they may be found in partially or insufficiently treated meningitis. Peripheral white blood cells, serum C-reactive protein and procalcitonin are usually elevated in bacterial meningitis but are of limited diagnostic value in the emergency situation. The later parameters in normal ranges together with lower cell counts predominantly lymphocytotic in the CSF are suggestive for viral or fungal meningitis.

29.2.2 Computer Tomography of the Head (CCT)

A cranial CT provides information concerning intracranial complications such as brain oedema, hydrocephalus and infarcts. Moreover, bone window imaging identifies parameningeal foci such as sinusitis, mastoiditis or odontogenic abscess. Those patients who present with focal neurological deficits or seizures and those who have a disturbed consciousness should have a cranial CT before lumbar puncture. Of those patients without focal signs or seizures and with a normal level of consciousness, CT abnormalities are found in less than 3 % and CSF can be drawn without prior CT scanning. Under no circumstances the CCT should delay antibiotic treatment in

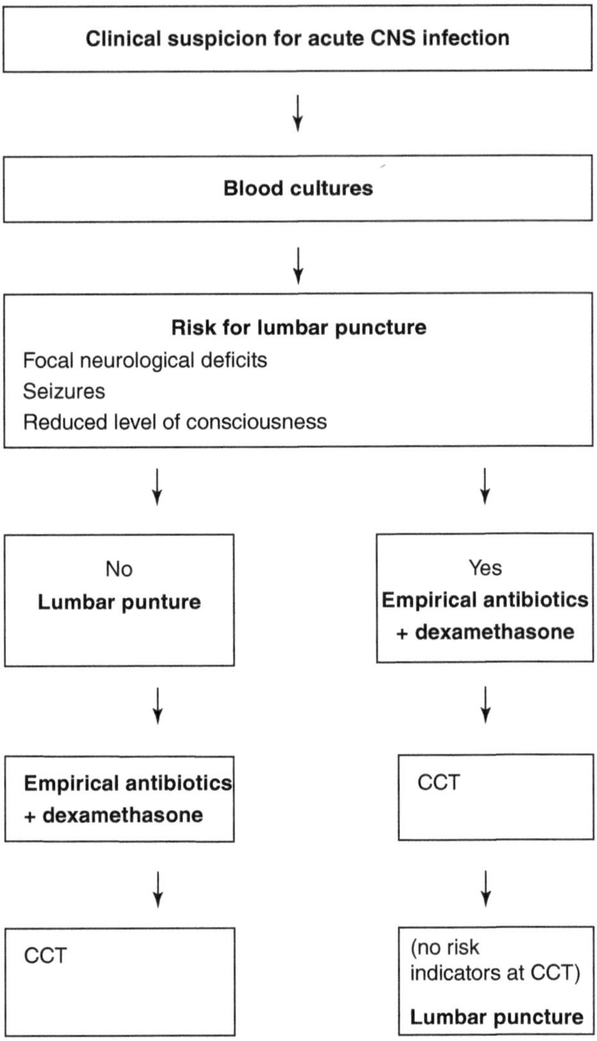

Fig. 29.2 Decision tree in acute CNS infection

highly suspicious cases. MRI scans in the acute setting are not recommended since no further information is gained (Fig. 29.2). In our patient, due to fluctuating qualitative impairment of his consciousness, a CCT scan revealed no pathologies and was performed only because the procedure did not delay treatment (<15 min).

29.2.3 CSF Tests

The CSF was withdrawn and proved the diagnosis of pneumococcal meningitis (12×10^3 leucocytes/ml, 99 % neutrophils, CSF protein 1.3 g/l, lactate 0.8 g/l glucose CSF/blood ratio 0.2). In the CSF extracellular Gram-positive cocci were seen and qualified as pneumococci (Fig. 29.1). The CSF culture confirmed *Streptococcus pneumoniae* as suggested by Gram staining, 36 h later, as well as the blood culture results (Fig. 29.1). The MIC (minimal inhibitory concentration) was <0.1 μg/ml for penicillin. Together with systemically lowered leucocytes, fever of 38.8 C and a heart rate of 110 sepsis criteria are fulfilled.

29.3 Final Diagnosis

Pneumococcal meningitis with sepsis

29.4 Definition of Bacterial Meningitis

Bacterial meningitis is an inflammation of the meninges, in particular the arachnoid and the pia mater, associated with the invasion of bacteria into the subarachnoidal space. A hallmark of bacterial meningitis is the recruitment of highly activated leucocytes into the CSF. Besides bacteria, viruses, fungi and noninfectious causes as in systemic and neoplastic disease as well as certain drugs can induce meningeal inflammation.

Streptococcus pneumoniae and *Neisseria meningitidis* are the most common and most aggressive pathogens of meningitis. Symptomatic headache results from the activation of trigeminal C fibres in the meninges and is categorized as headache attributed to bacterial meningitis and meningoencephalitis (9.1.1, HIS 3rd edition, 2013).

Bacterial meningitis is a medical emergency requiring immediate diagnosis and immediate treatment.

29.5 Management and Treatment Options

Antibiotic treatment (cefotaxime 3×4 g i.v. and ampicillin 6×2 g i.v., Table 29.1) followed the administration of dexamethasone 10 mg i.v. (every 6 h/4 days) and the patient was transferred to our neurocritical care unit for one night. Once pneumococci were confirmed in the CSF culture, only cefotaxime was continued for 10 days.

29.5.1 Antibiotics

Immediate antibiotic therapy must not be postponed by diagnostic delays, e.g. waiting for a CT scan. Prior to treatment, a blood culture should be obtained.

Table 29.1 Empiric antibiotic therapy in adults in bacterial meningitis

	Probable pathogens	Empirical therapy
Infants and children	*N. meningitides* *S. pneumoniae* *S. agalactiae* *E. coli (H. influenzae*[a]*)*	Cephalosporin[b] (+vancomycin or rifampicin[c])
Adults	*S. pneumoniae* *N. meningitidis* *L. monocytogenes*[d] Aerobic streptococci (*H. influenzae*)	Cephalosporin[b]+ampicillin (+vancomycin or rifampicin[c])
Chemoprophylaxis of close contacts	*N. meningitidis*	Adult doses[e]: Rifampicin (600 mg b.i.d., 2 days) Ciprofloxacin (500 mg single dose) Ceftriaxone (250 mg single dose)

[a]*H. influenzae* is unlikely if the child has been vaccinated
[b]Cephalosporins group 3a (e.g. ceftriaxone or cefotaxime) or group 4 (e.g. cefepime) are recommended
[c]Cephalosporin- and penicillin-resistant pneumococci are increasingly frequent, e.g. in areas of the USA, Australia, South Africa and Spain. In these regions, vancomycin or rifampicin (when dexamethasone is given)
[d]*Listeria* causes meningitis in immunocompetent patients in 5–7 %. Addition of ampicillin should be considered especially in patients with atypical CSF findings (mixed pleocytosis)
[e]Rifampicin and ciprofloxacin are not recommended in pregnancy. Recommended dose of rifampicin is 5 mg/kg for neonates and 10 mg/kg for children older than 1 month; alternatively, 125 mg ceftriaxone can be used. Ciprofloxacin should not be given below age 18 (recommendations and approvals differ between countries)

Since microbiological identification of the pathogen is not immediately available, the initial choice of antibiotics is usually empirical (Table 29.1). Factors to consider include regional antibiotic resistance rates, patient age, predisposing conditions and resources. Antibiotic therapy should be adjusted according to the cultural results in order to provide highly active yet narrowly targeted coverage. Treatment durations of 10–14 days are adequate for most pathogens. 3–4 weeks of treatment are recommended for *L. monocytogenes* and Enterobacteriaceae. Suspected meningococcal meningitis requires patient isolation during the first 24 h of treatment; chemoprophylaxis is recommended for close contacts according to local guidelines.

29.5.2 Corticosteroids

In adults, a prospective double-blind study in central Europe reported reduced mortality and lower frequency of hearing loss and neuropsychological sequelae. Subgroup analysis suggests that protective effects of dexamethasone are limited to pneumococcal meningitis. Expert opinion and several societal guidelines recommend routine treatment with dexamethasone for community-acquired meningitis of children (0.15 mg/kg every 6 h for 2–4 days) and adults (10 mg every 6 h for 4 days). Discontinuation of this therapy is advisable if *H. influenzae* (children) and *S. pneumoniae* (adults and children) can be ruled out as the underlying pathogen.

Current data do not support the routine use of corticosteroids in countries with limited resources.

29.5.3 Other Symptomatic Therapies

Severe headache requires sufficient analgesia. Antiepileptic treatment is indicated if seizures occur; prophylactic treatment is not recommended.

Mortality from bacterial meningitis is up to 34 % and is highest with *S. pneumoniae.* Up to 50 % of survivors suffer from neurologic sequelae. Complications are most likely to occur during the first few days of therapy. Severe intracranial complications are brain oedema, vascular alterations and hydrocephalus, all contributing to increased intracranial pressure and parenchymal damage. CT imaging should be performed if patients fail to improve within 48 h of antibiotic treatment and/or new focal signs develop. Hydrocephalus develops in up to 15 % of patients, usually in the form of malresorption due to increased outflow resistance of the CSF, and they may require external ventricular drainage. In particular early hydrocephalus needs special attention. Vascular complications include vasculitis, vasospasm and septic thrombosis of dural sinuses and cortical veins, often leading to the infarction of large cerebral territories. Approximately 30 % of the patients need treatment in a neurocritical care unit.

29.6 Summary

The patient history of a previously healthy 62-year-old man is typical for the differential diagnosis of a newly occurring severe headache and fever. The clinical presentation and the CSF test following Fig. 29.2 prove or exclude intracranial infection. Bacterial meningitis is still a life-threatening medical emergency requiring immediate diagnosis and immediate treatment.

Suggested Reading

1. Bohr V, Paulson OB, Rasmussen N (1984) Pneumococcal meningitis. Late neurologic sequelae and features of prognostic impact. Arch Neurol 41:1045–1049
2. Buchholz G, Ormanns S, Pfister HW et al (2014) Neuroinfectious diseases at a European neurological tertiary care center: one-third of patients require treatment in the neurological intensive care unit. Eur J Neurol. [Epub ahead of print]

3. Cabellos C, Viladrich PF, Ariza J et al (2008) Community-acquired bacterial meningitis in cirrhotic patients. Clin Microbiol Infect 14:35–40
4. de Gans J, van de Beek D (2002) Dexamethasone in adults with bacterial meningitis. N Engl J Med 347:1549–1556
5. Fernandes D, Gonçalves-Pereira J, Janeiro S et al (2014) Acute bacterial meningitis in the intensive care unit and risk factors for adverse clinical outcomes: Retrospective study. J Crit Care 29:347–50
6. Hasbun R, Abrahams J, Jekel J et al (2001) Computed tomography of the head before lumbar puncture in adults with suspected meningitis. N Engl J Med 345:1727–1733
7. Kasanmoentalib ES, Brouwer MC, van der Ende A et al (2010) Hydrocephalus in adults with community-acquired bacterial meningitis. Neurology 75:918–923
8. Kastenbauer S, Pfister HW (2003) Pneumococcal meningitis in adults: spectrum of complications and prognostic factors in a series of 87 cases. Brain 126:1015–1025
9. Klein M, Koedel U, Pfefferkorn T et al (2011) Arterial cerebrovascular complications in 94 adults with acute bacterial meningitis. Crit Care 15:R281
10. Nguyen DP, Nguyen HP, To SD et al (2007) Dexamethasone in Vietnamese adolescents and adults with bacterial meningitis. N Engl J Med 357:2431–2440
11. Scarborough M, Thwaites GE (2008) The diagnosis and management of acute bacterial meningitis in resource-poor settings. Lancet Neurol 7:637–648
12. Sudarsanam T, Rupali P, Tharyan P et al (2013) Pre-admission antibiotics for suspected cases of meningococcal disease. Cochrane Database Syst Rev (8):CD005437
13. Thigpen MC, Whitney CG, Messonnier NE et al (2011) Bacterial meningitis in the United States, 1998-2007. N Engl J Med 364:2016–2025
14. van de Beek D, de Gans J, Spanjaard L et al (2004) Clinical features and prognostic factors in adults with bacterial meningitis. N Engl J Med 351:1849–1859
15. van de Beek D, de Gans J, Tunkel AR et al (2006) Community-acquired bacterial meningitis in adults. N Engl J Med 354:44–53
16. Weber JR, Angstwurm K, Bove GM et al (1996) The trigeminal nerve and augmentation of regional cerebral blood flow during experimental bacterial meningitis. J Cereb Blood Flow Metab 6:1319–1324
17. Weisfelt M, van de Beek D, Spanjaard L et al (2008) A risk score for unfavorable outcome in adults with bacterial meningitis. Ann Neurol 63:90–97

Chapter 30
Tumor-Related Headache

Christian Lampl

30.1 Case Description

A 53-year-old male was admitted to our headache outpatient center with a 3-month history of repeated visual disturbances, in which a central scotoma was bordered by a crescent of scintillating zigzag patterns, which slowly advances to the edge of the visual field. Usually this visual phenomena march slowly across the visual field over a period of 20–30 min, with a frequency of one to two attacks a week. Initially, no headache followed this visual sensation. In the last 2 weeks prior to admission, similar attacks occurred more frequently, up to 5–7 times a day, with accompanying unilateral sensory disturbances, described as pins-and-needles sensations, traveling from the left face to the left hand. Similar to the visual symptoms, paresthesias spread from one side of the left face to the left hand and march slowly down the left arm and limb. Numbness occurs following the paresthesia as well as moderate, throbbing headache with nausea. The duration of these attacks including visual and sensory disturbances and headache lasts approximately 3 h, so nearly the whole day was filled out with these phenomena. Headache symptoms were sufficiently treated with acetylsalicylic acid, however, with no influence on the visual and sensory disturbances.

C. Lampl
Headache Medical Center Seilerstaette Linz, Hospital Sisters of Charity, Linz, Austria
e-mail: christian.lampl@bhs.at

A. Siva, C. Lampl (eds.), *Case-Based Diagnosis and Management of Headache Disorders*, Headache, DOI 10.1007/978-3-319-06886-2_30

In the neurological examination, a mild hemihypesthesia in the left face side, as well as the left forearm, was found. Blood pressure and routine blood tests were normal.

30.2 Differential Diagnosis and How to Work Up This Kind of a Patient

In individuals who develop such a recurring, mixture of moderate headache and visual/sensory disturbances with any pathological signs in the physical and/or neurological examinations, the probability of an intracerebral pathology is extremely high. If this kind of visual and sensory disturbances occurs for the first time, with or without any pathological signs, of course, the consulting physician needs to rule out any pathological intracerebral event. In that particular case, we do have a period of nearly 3 months with singular signs of visual disturbances that can be diagnosed as visual auras. However, this slow march helps to distinguish these aura symptom from conditions in which aura-like symptoms build more rapidly or are maximal from onset, such as seizures and TIAs. Even at that time when headache got a part of that symptom complexity, diagnosis of a migraine attack with aura (or prolonged aura) might be valid. One should be aware of that an aura may also precede a temporal lobe seizure. In that case the aura is actually a small seizure itself, one that has not spread into an observable seizure that impairs consciousness and ability to respond. People who have temporal lobe seizures can remain partially conscious during a seizure, but they also may lose awareness of their surroundings and often do not remember what happened. In our case, no characteristic signs and symptoms of temporal lobe seizures, like loss of awareness of surroundings, staring, lip smacking, or repeated swallowing or chewing, were found.

The International Headache Society (IHS) diagnostic criteria recognize the importance of sequence and duration of symptoms in distinguishing migraine with aura from more serious conditions. The migraine aura is a phenomenon in which one or more visual or sensory disturbances develop over a few minutes and disappear within 1 h. A typical migraine headache usually follows within 1 h, but may occur before or during the aura or may be entirely absent. The IHS diagnostic criteria also describe less common subtypes of migraine with aura, in which the aura may be more prolonged and/or include some degree of hemiparesis. These cases obviously require more careful workup to rule out underlying conditions such as transient ischemic attacks (TIAs) or intracerebral abnormalities. Therefore, a good history will go a long way in differentiating the less common subtypes of migraine with aura from emergent conditions (Table 30.1).

Table 30.1 Definition headache attributed to intracranial neoplasia according to "The International Classification of Headache Disorders, 3rd edition (beta version)." Cephalalgia 2013; 33(9) 719–721

7.4. Headache attributed to intracranial neoplasia Description: Headache caused by intracranial neoplasia Diagnostic criteria: A. Any headache fulfilling criterion C B. Intracranial neoplasia has been diagnosed C. Evidence of causation demonstrated by at least one of the following: 1. Headache has developed in temporal relation to the intracranial neoplasia or led to its discovery 2. Headache has significantly worsened in parallel with worsening of the intracranial neoplasia 3. Headache has significantly improved in temporal relation to successful treatment of the intracranial neoplasia D. Not better accounted for by another ICHD-3
7.4.1 Headache attributed to intracranial neoplasm Description: Headache, usually progressive, worse in the morning and aggravated by Valsalva-like maneuvers, caused by one or more space-occupying intracranial tumors Diagnostic criteria: A. Headache fulfilling criterion C B. A space-occupying intracranial neoplasm has been demonstrated C. Evidence of causation demonstrated by at least two of the following: 1. Headache has developed in temporal relation to the development of the neoplasm or led to its discovery 2. Either or both of the following: (a) Headache has significantly worsened in parallel with worsening of the neoplasm (b) Headache has significantly improved in temporal relation to successful treatment of the neoplasm 3. Headache has at least one of the following three characteristics: (a) Progressive (b) Worse in the morning or after daytime napping (c) Aggravated by Valsalva-like maneuvers D. Not better accounted for by another ICHD-3 diagnosis
7.4.1.1 Headache attributed to colloid cyst of the third ventricle Description: Headache caused by colloid cyst of the third ventricle, presenting very characteristically as recurrent attacks with thunderclap onset and reduced level or loss of consciousness Diagnostic criteria: A. Headache fulfilling criterion C B. A colloid cyst of the third ventricle has been demonstrated

(continued)

Table 30.1 (continued)

C. Evidence of causation demonstrated by both of the following:
  1. Headache has developed in temporal relation to the development of the colloid cyst or led to its discovery
  2. Either or both of the following:
     (a) Headache is recurrent, with thunderclap onset and accompanied by reduced level or loss of consciousness
     (b) Headache has significantly improved or resolved in temporal relation to successful treatment of the colloid cyst

D. Not better accounted for by another ICHD-3 diagnosis

30.3 Diagnostic Workup of the Case

Since the patient's symptom complex was not further investigated so far, an MR scan of the brain was performed. It showed a 5.6 cm in maximal diameter, partially necrotic, contrast-enhancing temporo-occipital tumor, including the gyrus parahippocampalis, splenium corporis callosi, and thalamus. The structure of the cortex was accompanied with a perifocal edema with an 8 mm midline shift. A glioblastoma multiforme grade 4 was diagnosed. The patient immediately underwent image-guided resection. After the operation and his stay at the ICU, headache and the visual disturbances suspend.

30.4 Summary of the Case

A 53-year-old male with recurrent visual and unilateral sensory disturbances, occurring up to 5–7 times a day, was primarily diagnosed as aura without migraine. However, within days a throbbing headache with nausea followed, during and after sensory symptoms. Headache symptoms were sufficiently treated with acetylsalicylic acid, however, with no influence on the visual and sensory disturbances. In the neurological examination, a mild hemihypesthesia at the left side of the face, as well as the left forearm, was found. Since these were the first signs and symptoms of headache and the neurological examination was abnormal, an MR scan of the brain was performed and showed a contrast-enhancing temporo-occipital tumor, including the gyrus parahippocampalis, splenium corporis callosi, and thalamus (Fig. 30.1). The structure of the neoplasm and the fact of a perifocal edema lead to the suspected diagnosis of a glioblastoma multiforme grade 4. Image-guided resection was performed.

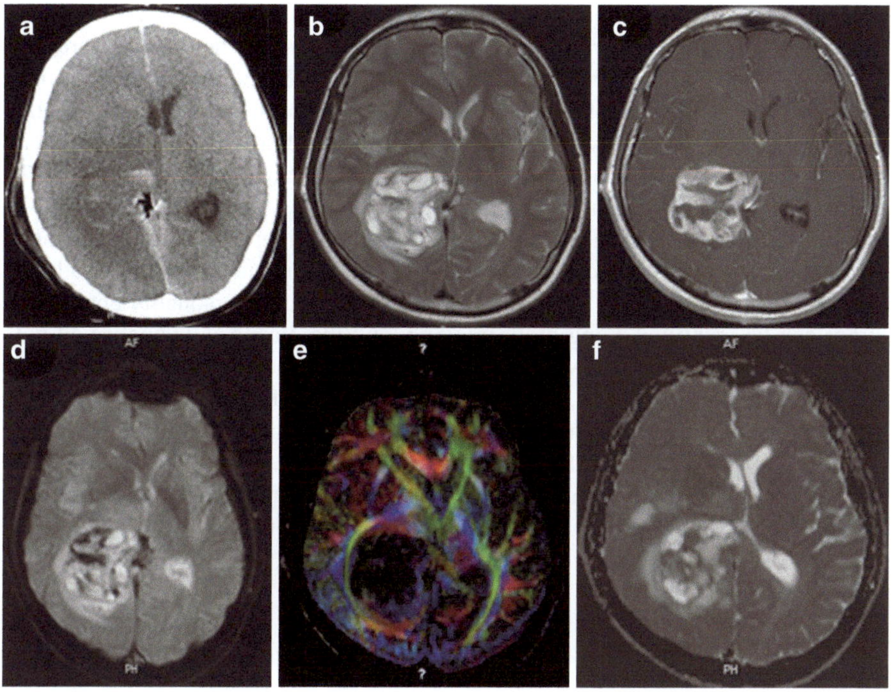

Fig. 30.1 Images of a patient with new onset of aura symptoms and headache: *top row* (**a–c**) shows CT scan unenhanced (**a**), T2-weighted MR image (**b**), and T1-weighted contrast-enhanced MR image (**c**); *bottom row* (**d–f**) shows diffusion and perfusion-weighted MR image (rCBV) and ADC image. Perfusion-weighted image demonstrates rCBV elevation indicative of high-grade glioma. ADC values in more solid temporo-occipital parts are lower than in normal brain tissue, indicating higher cellularity. Final diagnosis was glioblastoma multiforme WHO IV

30.5 Brief General Information

Headache has been recognized as a common symptom of brain tumors for many years. In the 1940s, a series of classic papers described the clinical characteristics and mechanisms of brain tumor-associated headache. With improved neuroimaging and the resultant earlier diagnosis, the spectrum of tumor-associated headache has expanded beyond these classical descriptions. Headache attributed to intracranial neoplasm can be caused by increased intracranial pressure or hydrocephalus caused by neoplasm or attributed directly to neoplasm. However, the associated headache characteristics vary and there is no "typical" brain tumor-associated headache. Migraine features are described in about 15 %; tension-type headaches were seen up to 30 %. Headache pain varies from a dull to a pressure or a throbbing pain. Headache lateralization does not always predict tumor location. There are also other headache syndromes as a symptom of brain tumors such as short-lasting unilateral neuralgiform headache attacks with conjunctival injection and tearing (SUNCT), cluster headache, and primary stabbing headache.

The most common primary malignant brain tumor is glioblastoma multiforme and accounts for 2 % of all cancers. Typical symptoms include persistent headache, seizures, nausea, vomiting, neurocognitive symptoms, and personality changes. A tumor can be identified using brain imaging, and the diagnosis is confirmed with histopathology. Any patient with chronic, persistent headache in association with protracted nausea, vomiting, seizures, change in headache pattern, neurologic symptoms, or positional worsening should be evaluated for a brain tumor. Magnetic resonance imaging is the preferred initial imaging study. Surgical resection of the tumor is the mainstay of therapy. Postoperative radiation and chemotherapy have improved survival in patients with high-grade brain tumors.

Suggested Reading

1. Chandana SR, Movva S, Arora M, Singh T (2008) Primary brain tumors in adults. Am Fam Physician 77(10):1423–1430
2. Forsyth PA, Posner JB (1993) Headaches in patients with brain tumors: a study of 111 patients. Neurology 43(9):1678–1683
3. Kunkle EC, Ray BS, Wolff HG (1942) Studies on headache: the mechanisms and significance of the headache associated with brain tumor. Bull N Y Acad Med 18(6):400–422
4. Schankin CJ, Ferrari U, Reinisch VM, Birnbaum T, Goldbrunner R, Straube A (2007) Characteristics of brain tumour-associated headache. Cephalalgia 27(8):904–911
5. Headache Classification Committee of the International Headache Society (IHS). The international classification of headache disorders, 3rd edition (beta version) (2013) Cephalalgia 33(9):719–721
6. Valentinis L, Tuniz F, Valent F, Mucchiut M, Little D, Skrap M, Bergonzi P, Zanchin G (2010) Headache attributed to intracranial tumours: a prospective cohort study. Cephalalgia 30(4):389–398

Chapter 31
Migraine in the Emergency Department

Justin M. DeLange and Jerry W. Swanson

31.1 Case Description

A 36-year-old woman comes to the emergency department because of acute throbbing headache that began 12 h previously and is associated with nausea and vomiting. She has a past history of migraine headaches with visual aura dating to age 14.

For this attack, she has taken eletriptan 40 mg, ketoprofen 75 mg, and promethazine 25 mg; she developed nausea and vomiting which has persisted. Further, she noted typical, gradual progression of her pain after her visual aura symptoms were present for 20 minutes. She has presented to the emergency department twice in the last 3 years with similar attacks. The patient is currently on topiramate 100 mg every evening for migraine prevention. On examination, her vital signs show a blood pressure of 132/76 with a pulse of 76 bpm. Her skin shows some mild pallor with reduced skin turgor and delayed capillary refill. The remainder of her general and neurological examination is unremarkable.

31.2 Diagnostic Considerations and Testing

Upon first seeing a headache patient in the emergency department, a history regarding the current headache and any prior headaches should be obtained. "Red flags" which suggest a secondary headache disorder should be sought. These include thunderclap headache, systemic signs or symptoms (i.e., fever or weight loss), associated medical comorbidities such as cancer or HIV, neurologic signs or symptoms such as unilateral weakness, new-onset headache in an older patient, changes in the typical headache characteristic or progression, and precipitants including coughing,

J.M. DeLange, DO • J.W. Swanson, MD (✉)
Department of Neurology, Mayo Clinic, 200 First Street SW, Rochester, MN 55905, USA
e-mail: delange.justin@mayo.edu; jwswanson@mayo.edu

A. Siva, C. Lampl (eds.), *Case-Based Diagnosis and Management of Headache Disorders*, Headache, DOI 10.1007/978-3-319-06886-2_31

sneezing, or Valsalva. However, once these "red flags" have been excluded, then treatment for the primary headache disorder, which will most often represent migraine, can then ensue.

The International Headache Society has delineated the diagnostic criteria for migraine headache in the latest edition (ICHD-3 beta). The criteria for migraine without aura require at least five attacks lasting 4–72 h with nausea/vomiting or photophobia/phonophobia. At least two of the following must also be present: unilateral location, pulsating quality, moderate to severe pain intensity, or worsening of pain with physical activity. Migraine with aura shares similar requirements but also includes reversible focal neurologic symptoms that appear gradually and last for 5–60 min. If aura is present, it generally precedes or presents with the headache.

Evidence-based recommendations state that imaging should not be performed if the patient's headache presentation lacks "red flag" features and is consistent with migraine headache. Other laboratory tests that may be considered are CBC, BUN, creatinine, electrolytes, and liver enzymes. This is especially important if there are other medical comorbidities, profound nausea/vomiting with inherent volume status changes, and potential electrolyte abnormalities. ECG testing should also be considered if antiemetics or other agents that can be associated with QT prolongation are to be utilized. Further, if the patient is a woman with childbearing potential, a urine pregnancy test should also be considered as some migraine medications are contraindicated. Likewise, a careful review of the patient's medical history is a must as some acute migraine medications may be contraindicated in certain patients. For example, triptans or dihydroergotamine should not be used in any patient with coronary artery disease or cerebrovascular disease given the vasoconstrictive properties of those medications.

31.2.1 Diagnostic Testing and Further Management in Our Case

Routine laboratory tests including a CBC with differential, electrolytes, BUN, and creatinine were performed and were unremarkable. A urine pregnancy test was performed and was negative. Neuroimaging was not performed since there were no features to suggest a secondary headache and the presentation was typical of her history of migraine. The patient received 1 L of D5 ½ NS intravenously for rehydration. The patient was also given a combination of metoclopramide 10 mg IV with diphenhydramine 25 mg IV which ameliorated her nausea, but her headache did not remit after 1 h. Therefore, the emergency department consulted neurology for further treatment suggestions.

31.3 Management and Treatment

When treating a patient with a migraine headache in the emergency department, a multitude of factors need to be considered. In these circumstances, severe pain and the associated symptoms of photophobia, phonophobia, and nausea and/or vomiting

Table 31.1 Migraine-specific treatments in the emergency department

Class	Treatment	Side effect
Triptans	*Sumatriptan 6 mg SC (max 12 mg/24 h)*	Injection site reaction, paresthesias, hot/cold sensation, chest pressure/pain/tightness, dizziness, flushing, limb pain, vasoconstriction, and nausea
Ergotamine derivatives	*Dihydroergotamine mesylate (DHE) 0.5 mg–1 mg IV. Can repeat q 1 h as needed (max 2 mg/24 h)*	Paresthesias, dizziness, flushing, nausea/vomiting, diarrhea, dyspnea, rash, diaphoresis, elevated blood pressure, anxiety, and vasoconstriction

are often present. Overall, the treatment principles should focus on: (1) treatment of pain with parenteral medications at therapeutic doses; (2) treatment of nausea and/or vomiting; (3) management of fluid status/balance in the event of prolonged or severe vomiting; (4) placement of the patient in a quiet, darkened room; (5) avoidance of medications that are likely to induce rebound, abuse, or intractability; and (6) provision of reassurance for the patient.

Prior to the administration of medications, it may be beneficial to ask the patient what has been effective for treatment of their migraine headaches previously and what was ineffective. Further, it is important to determine what medications have been used prior to coming into the emergency department as this may preclude the use of some medications. For example, a patient that has taken a triptan at home should not receive dihydroergotamine for 24 h since both are potent vasoconstrictors. In the absence of vascular risk factors, migraine-specific medications such as triptans or dihydroergotamine should be considered first given their efficacy. However, other medications may be considered as well. See Tables 31.1 and 31.2 for a list of some medications that may be utilized in the emergency department for migraine.

31.3.1 Triptans (5-HT $_{1B\text{-}1D}$ Agonists)

Triptans are often the treatment of choice in acute migraine headache. The triptan class is an acute medication which specifically targets the 5-HT $_{1B\text{-}1D}$ receptors present in the trigeminovascular system. Triptans should not be used within 24 h of a different triptan agent or dihydroergotamine. Triptans are contraindicated in the setting of coronary artery disease, cerebrovascular disease, peripheral vascular disease, uncontrolled hypertension, severe hepatic disease, hemiplegic migraine, migraine with brain-stem aura (dysarthria, ataxia, decreased consciousness, diplopia, etc.), and pregnancy. Triptans work well not only for pain but may also treat other associated symptoms such as photophobia, phonophobia, and nausea. If triptans are to be used in the emergency department, it is preferential to treat a patient with the subcutaneous formulation of sumatriptan as these patients typically have significant nausea and need rapid relief.

Table 31.2 Nonspecific migraine treatments in the emergency department

Class	Treatment	Side effect
Antiemetics (D2 antagonists)	*Chlorpromazine 12.5–25 mg IV/IM* *Prochlorperazine 10 mg IV/IM* *Promethazine 25 mg IM* *Haloperidol 5 mg IV in 500 ml normal saline over 20 min* *Droperidol 2.5 mg IV*[a] *Metoclopramide 10 mg IV/IM*	Drowsiness, dizziness, blurred vision, akathisia, dystonia, parkinsonism, fluid retention (metoclopramide), QT prolongation (droperidol has black box warning due to risk of QT prolongation), neuroleptic malignant syndrome, hypotension (especially chlorpromazine)
Antiepileptics	*Valproate sodium 300–1,200 mg IV*	Drowsiness, asthenia, nausea/vomiting, injection site reaction, dizziness, hepatotoxicity, hyperammonemia, pancreatitis
NSAIDs	*Ketorolac 30 mg IV/IM* *Acetylsalicylic acid 1 g IV (difficult to obtain in the United States)* *Diclofenac 75 mg IM*	GI bleeding, GI ulceration, dyspepsia, abdominal pain, nausea, vomiting, injection site reaction, bleeding, rashes, nephrotoxicity, cardiovascular risk, anaphylaxis
Corticosteroids	*Dexamethasone 10–25 mg IV (prevents recurrence)*	Nausea, vomiting, dyspepsia, dizziness, mood swing, insomnia, anxiety, hypertension, hyperglycemia, avascular necrosis of bone (rare)
Other	*Magnesium sulfate 1–2 g IV*	Hypotension, flushing, drowsiness

Courtesy of Mayo Foundation. Mayo Foundation retains ownership on original material
[a]*Continuous ECG monitoring should be initiated prior to administration and continued for 2–3 h after dosing*

31.3.2 Dihydroergotamine (DHE)

This medication comprises another migraine-specific option. While DHE does have activity at the 5-HT $_{1B\text{-}1D}$ receptors, it also exerts effects through interaction with serotonergic, adrenergic, and dopaminergic receptors. Similar to triptans, it should not be used in patients with vascular disease (peripheral, coronary, or stroke), uncontrolled hypertension, hemiplegic migraine, migraine with brain-stem aura, hepatic disease, pregnancy, or previous ergot or triptan use in the preceding 24 h. DHE can be used in a one-time fashion but can also be used repetitively for up to 2–5 days. Pretreatment with a D2 antagonist such as metoclopramide should be employed to prevent side effects of nausea that may be common with DHE when it is administered intravenously.

31.3.3 D2 Antagonists

Antiemetics are a valuable tool in the emergency department. Most come in IV and/or IM forms and are useful not only for migraine-related nausea/vomiting but are also beneficial in treating the headache itself. This is thought to be due to the implication of dopaminergic hyperexcitability in some migraine patients. Antiemetic treatment in the emergency department is especially important given that uncontrolled nausea/vomiting may lead to dehydration. D2 antagonists may be used solely or with other drugs such as triptans, DHE, or NSAIDs. Extrapyramidal reactions such as dystonia or akathisia may occur with administration of these agents, and pretreatment with benztropine 1 mg IV/IM or diphenhydramine 25 mg IV/IM should be considered. Further, it is advisable to obtain an ECG prior to the administration of intravenous D2 antagonists as QT prolongation is a possibly fatal albeit rare side effect of this group of medications.

31.3.4 Nonsteroidal Anti-inflammatory Drugs (NSAIDs)

This class contains a large number of medications. In the emergency department, NSAIDs such as ketorolac are typically given utilizing an intravenous route (or intramuscular route if no intravenous access) given that these patients are often in need of fast-acting pain relief and often have nausea limiting oral intake. This class may be used as a rescue in the emergency department when other modalities have failed or may be used in conjunction with other medications such as sumatriptan. NSAIDs should not be used in patients with a history of gastrointestinal bleeding or ulceration and should be used cautiously in patients with a history of cardiovascular disease or renal insufficiency.

31.3.5 Valproate Sodium

This agent is another parenteral option in the emergency department either as monotherapy or combined with other medications such as triptans. It may be useful in patients with cardiovascular disease as a safe alternative to DHE. Further, it tends to not be as sedating as D2 antagonists or DHE. It should not be used in pregnant patients or patients with liver disease. If chosen for a female migraineur of childbearing potential, a urine pregnancy test should be performed prior to administration of this agent.

31.3.6 Corticosteroids

Corticosteroids such as dexamethasone may be employed in the emergency department as an adjunctive agent. Dexamethasone has been shown to prevent headache recurrence in this acute setting but does not affect acute pain. Therefore, dexamethasone may be a good option in conjunction with triptans (or DHE), NSAIDs, or D2 antagonists.

31.3.7 Magnesium Sulfate

Magnesium sulfate is another agent that may be used in the emergency department. While evidence regarding efficacy is mixed, some studies suggest that it is most effective in patients with migraine with aura or in patients with photophobia and/or phonophobia. Given its favorable risk profile, it may be safely used in pregnancy.

31.3.8 Opioids/Opiates

Opioids are not drugs of choice in migraine because of their adverse side effect profile including dependency, medication overuse headache, and absence of studies supporting efficacy. This class should generally be avoided or reserved as a last line of therapy in select patients. Unfortunately, it is often utilized first in many emergency departments. Therefore, other options should be sought prior to use.

31.3.9 Admission Versus Discharge

A number of factors should be assessed when deciding whether to admit an acute migraineur from the emergency department. If a migraineur is severely dehydrated, then that patient may need admission for fluid resuscitation. Significant medical comorbidities should also be examined as this may complicate the acute process (e.g., renal failure, diabetes mellitus) and may necessitate inpatient admission. Patients who have presented to the emergency department with multiple attacks in the same day should also be considered for admission.

31.3.10 Pregnant Migraineur

Special situations that may require modification to any migraine treatment paradigm include pregnant patients. Ergots, including DHE, are contraindicated in pregnancy. Further, NSAIDs are contraindicated in the last trimester as patent ductus arteriosus closure may ensue and are also contraindicated in the first trimester due to risk of abortion. It is very important to determine the stage of pregnancy when considering medication choices. Therefore, it is often useful to confer with the obstetrician regarding the management of migraine in a pregnant patient. Acetaminophen may be a safe alternative (with or without caffeine) that can be offered. Magnesium sulfate is also another safe medication that may be tried. Opiates are relatively safe in pregnancy but again should not typically be drugs of first choice. Based on registry data, sumatriptan may also be safe in pregnancy but given possible vasoconstrictive effects on placental blood vessels should only be used when other interventions have proven ineffective. The control of nausea with first-line agents such as meclizine or promethazine is preferred. Metoclopramide, prochlorperazine, or ondansetron may also be helpful; however, there is a risk of acute dystonic reactions in the mother with metoclopramide and prochlorperazine.

31.3.11 Treatment and Further Management in Our Case

The patient continued to have headache after metoclopramide, and she already had triptans earlier that day; therefore, the patient was treated with valproate sodium 1,000 mg IV and ketorolac 30 mg IV. She also received dexamethasone 10 mg IV. She noted improvement in her headache pain and photophobia. Her nausea was also improved, and she was adequately maintaining her oral hydration at that point. She was discharged with instructions to increase her topiramate to 150 mg and follow up with her neurologist to review additional options for acute and preventive treatment of her migraine attacks.

Suggested Reading

1. Colman I, Friedman BW et al (2008) Parenteral dexamethasone for acute severe migraine headache: meta-analysis of randomised controlled trials for preventing recurrence. BMJ 336(7657):1359–1361
2. Diener HC (1999) Efficacy and safety of intravenous acetylsalicylic acid lysinate compared to subcutaneous sumatriptan and parenteral placebo in the acute treatment of migraine. A double-blind, double-dummy, randomized, multicenter, parallel group study. The ASASUMAMIG Study Group. Cephalalgia 19(6):581–588; discussion 542
3. Dodick DW (2003) Diagnosing headache: clinical clues and clinical rules. Adv Stud Med 3(2):87–92
4. Gelfand AA, Goadsby PJ (2012) A neurologist's guide to acute migraine therapy in the emergency room. Neurohospitalist 2(2):51–59
5. Jakubowski M, Levy D et al (2005) Terminating migraine with allodynia and ongoing central sensitization using parenteral administration of COX1/COX2 inhibitors. Headache 45(7):850–861
6. Loder E, Weizenbaum E et al (2013) Choosing wisely in headache medicine: the American Headache Society's list of five things physicians and patients should question. Headache 53(10):1651–1659

7. Macgregor EA (2014) Headache in pregnancy. Continuum 20(1 Neurology of Pregnancy): 128–147
8. Robertson CE, Black DF et al (2010) Management of migraine headache in the emergency department. Semin Neurol 30(2):201–211
9. Sumamo Schellenberg E, Dryden DM et al (2012) Acute migraine treatment in emergency settings. Agency for Healthcare Research and Quality, Rockville
10. The international classification of headache disorders, 3rd edition (beta version) (2013). Cephalalgia 33(9):629–808

Chapter 32
Headache Attributed to Nontraumatic Subarachnoid Hemorrhage (SAH)

Aksel Siva and Sabahattin Saip

32.1 Case Description

A 55-year-old housewife who was the mother of one of my MS patients calls me on the phone sometime ago. I first thought she was calling for her daughter, but she said that she was calling this time for herself because she had a very severe headache. When asked to give information on the onset and other details of this headache, she described it as a sudden-onset very severe headache reaching its maximum intensity within minutes about three days ago. She had initially nausea and had vomited a few times and was admitted to a nearby hospital. At that hospital, her physical and neurological exams were noted as being normal, but the examining physician decided to refer her for a cranial CT scan, and in the meantime, she was given symptomatic analgesic therapy. However, she could receive a radiology appointment only for the following week! Then as her headache did not get any better, she decided to call me three days after the onset of her continuing severe headache. She replies of still having occasional nausea and some mild photophobia when asked, and despite feeling uncomfortable when standing still, she avoids moving around as her pain gets much worse then.

She describes her headache as being the worst headache of her life and does not recall any trigger that can be correlated with the onset of this headache. She is not known to have migraine headaches, but describes occasional mild to moderate headaches likely to be consistent with episodic tension-type headache and responsive to simple analgesics.

A. Siva (✉) • S. Saip
Department of Neurology, Cerrahpaşa School of Medicine,
Istanbul University, Istanbul, Turkey
e-mail: akselsiva@gmail.com

A. Siva, C. Lampl (eds.), *Case-Based Diagnosis and Management of Headache Disorders*, Headache, DOI 10.1007/978-3-319-06886-2_32

I tell her on the phone to come to the emergency room of our hospital and arrange an emergency CT scan of the brain for her before she arrives. At the emergency room, she is seen by the neurology consultant who finds her neurological and neuro-ophthalmologic exams to be normal, including normal fundi. Her physical exam is also insignificant and her blood pressure is found to be 130/80 mmHg.

Her past medical and neurological histories are insignificant with the exception of surgery for benign fibrocystic breast disease 9 years ago and a few measurements of upper borderline levels of arterial blood pressure recently. She has no known allergies.

Her mother is alive and relatively well. She is treated for high blood pressure and mild type II diabetes; her father had died at age 61 because of ischemic heart disease – MI. She is the second of four siblings, all others being well and alive. She has one daughter who has MS and one son who is alive and well.

32.2 Differential Diagnosis and How to Work Up This Kind of Patient

When a patient is admitted with nontraumatic sudden-onset very severe headache for the "first time in life" reaching its highest intensity within seconds to minutes, the consulting physician needs to rule out the probability of "a life-threatening disorder" such as subarachnoid hemorrhage (SAH), arteriovenous malformations, dural arteriovenous fistula, pituitary apoplexy, cervico-cephalic arterial dissection, cerebral venous thrombosis, reversible cerebral vasoconstriction syndrome, colloid cyst of the third ventricle, spontaneous intracranial hypotension, perimesencephalic (benign) hemorrhage and some other intracranial pathologies. The description of this type of headache is consistent with the so-called thunderclap headache which can be either primary or secondary to underlying serious intracranial conditions that were listed above.

Individuals who develop such a severe sudden-onset headache are more likely to be admitted to the emergency room (ER). When there are signs on physical and/or neurological examinations such as such high blood pressure, any change of consciousness, neck stiffness, neuro-ophthalmologic findings, lateralizing signs, or any other findings, the probability of finding a craniocervical pathology is extremely high, and the patient should be referred for an emergency imaging study, once it is confirmed that the vital signs are stable. On the other hand, in a large number of individuals, who are seen in the ER because of the "worst headache of their life," the physical and neurological examination will be unremarkable. However, this should not make the consulting physician to feel comfortable, and these patients should also be referred for an emergency cranial CT study as well.

Some of the patients with SAH may report only a mild-intensity headache, but many of such individuals will have other warning signs such as seizures, isolated oculomotor nerve palsies, and other focal neurological symptoms and/or agitation, confusion, and obtundation at admission, and some may even disclose EKG abnormalities mimicking myocardial infarction.

The initial imaging modality should be a non-enhancing computerized tomography not only because it is easier and more cost-effective to carry out in the emergency setting but also because it is comparable to or even more sensitive than MRI in showing SAH.

Once the differential diagnosis includes the suspicion of SAH or other life-threatening pathologies, the workup of such a patient should be extended until these diagnostic possibilities are ruled out. In an individual in whom SAH remains a potential diagnosis, a normal imaging study should be followed by a spinal tap. (Some of the other diagnostic probabilities of "ER headaches" and their workup are discussed in other chapters.)

The opening cerebrospinal fluid pressure, its color, and appearance; the presence, type, and number of cells; and the biochemistry of the CSF and when indicated microbiology should be studied. A complete CSF study that is found to be normal following a normal imaging study will enable the physician to rule out most of the major critical diagnostic probabilities. However, it should be kept in mind that there can be always exceptions!

CBC, ESR, hsCRP, and standard biochemistry including thyroid functions is part of the routine ER workup.

32.3 Diagnostic Workup of the Case

She is admitted for a CT scan (Fig. 32.1) which shows hemorrhage within the anterior interhemispheric fissure and bilateral sylvian cisterns more prominent on the left. This image is consistent with subarachnoid hemorrhage (SAH), and the distribution and asymmetry of the blood within the subarachnoid space are suggestive of anterior circulation aneurysm rupture, most likely an anterior communicating artery aneurysm. The patient then undergoes a digital subtraction arteriography (DSA) which shows three aneurysms. The bleeding one is the left anterior communicating artery aneurysm, and secondary arterial vasospasm is clearly seen on the DSA (Fig. 32.2). There are also two other unruptured aneurysms, one at the bifurcation of the left middle cerebral artery and the other at the tip of the basilar artery.

The patient was then referred to the department of neurosurgery, and two of the aneurysms, the one that bled at the left anterior communicating artery and the unruptured one at the bifurcation of the left middle cerebral artery, are clipped. She makes a complete recovery, and after a few weeks, she undergoes an endovascular closure of the aneurysm at the tip of the basilar artery with coiling.

32.4 Summary of the Case

A 55-year-old housewife with a sudden onset of "the worst headache of her life" is admitted to the ER after 3 days of the onset of her severe headache as it was not improving. She was first seen in another hospital soon after the onset but was told

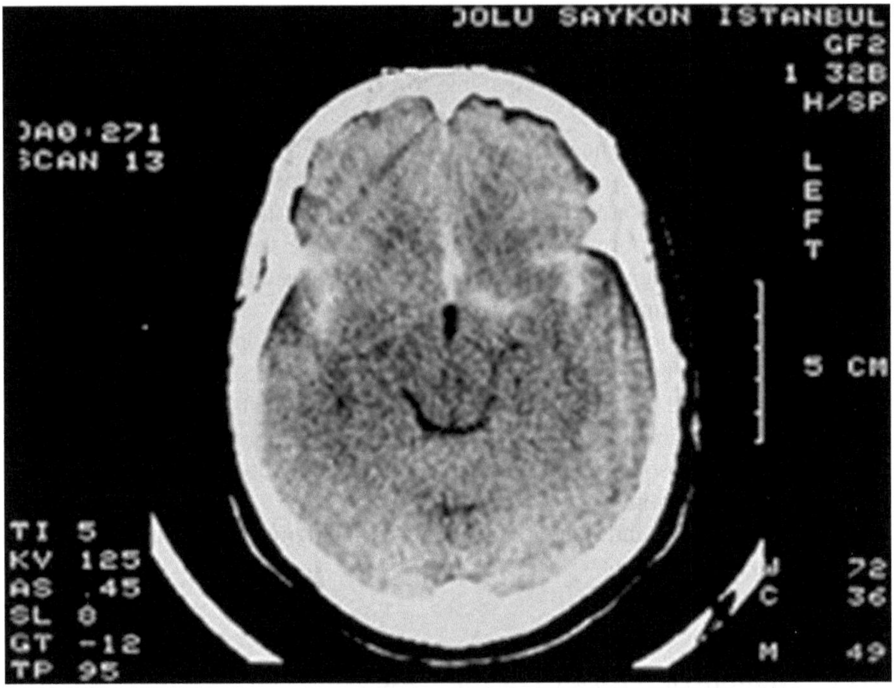

Fig. 32.1 CT scan done on the third day of sudden-onset severe headache which shows hemorrhage within the anterior interhemispheric fissure and bilateral sylvian cisterns more prominent on the left

that her examination was normal and then was referred for a cranial CT scan. However, instead of having an emergency scan, she was given a late appointment. As she was not getting better then, she was readmitted to our ER. Her neurological and physical exams were insignificant, and there was no neck stiffness. Based on the features of her headache history which was consistent with an abrupt-onset head pain that reached its peak intensity within seconds to minutes and was accompanied with nausea and vomiting raised the suspicion of SAH or other diagnostic probabilities of either primary or secondary thunderclap headache types. Therefore, she was referred for an emergency CT scan which disclosed SAH. Following a DSA study that confirmed a ruptured aneurysm, as well as two others, she was treated first by surgery and later by an endovascular coiling procedure of which she made an uneventful recovery.

32.5 Definition of Subarachnoid Hemorrhage

According to "The International Classification of Headache Disorders, 3rd edition (beta version)" [*Cephalalgia* 2013; 33(9) 629–808], the definition of "headache attributed to nontraumatic subarachnoid hemorrhage (SAH)" is described as typically severe and sudden, peaking in seconds (thunderclap headache) or minutes.

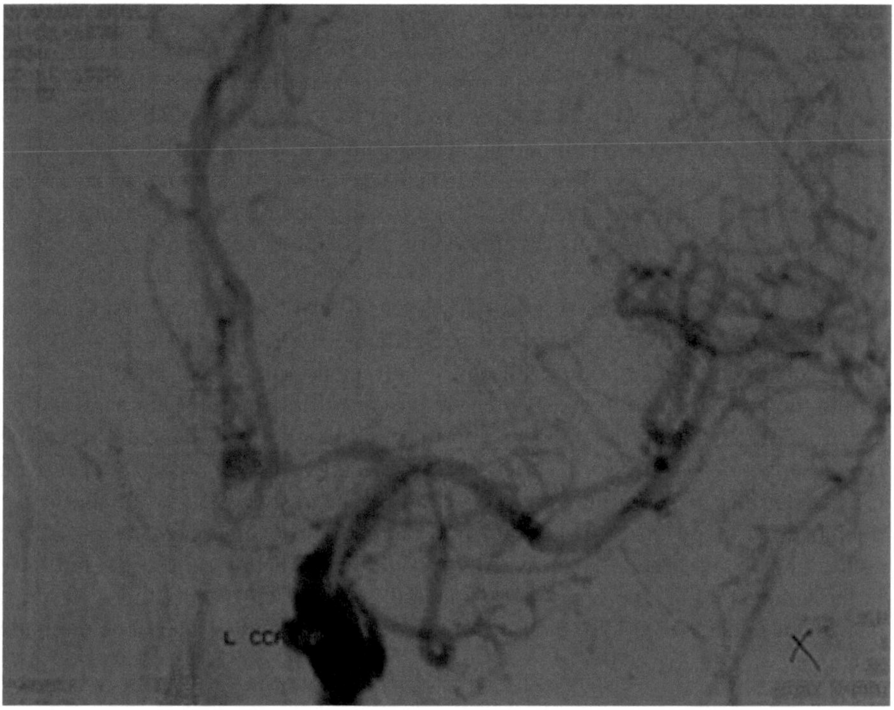

Fig. 32.2 Digital subtraction arteriography showing the left anterior communicating artery aneurysm and secondary arterial vasospasm

This headache may be the sole symptom of SAH, and the diagnostic criteria will include the absence of head trauma supported with the demonstration that the development of headache was in close temporal relation to other symptoms and clinical signs of SAH and then improved in parallel with stabilization or improvement of other symptoms or clinical or paraclinical signs of SAH.

As expected with all other set of criteria, this headache should not be better explained by any other ICHD-3 diagnosis.

32.6 Brief General Information

SAH is a diagnosis which should not be missed as the mortality rate can be as high as 50 %. Depending on the severity of the bleeding, 10–20 % of patients may die before arriving at the hospital. Besides, a significant number of patients with SAH are left disabled. There is a risk of rebleeding which is 3–4 % during the first 24 h, about 1 % per day during the first month, and 3 % per year long-term risk after 3 months in unrepaired aneurysms. Other risks in a patient with SAH are vasospasm with delayed cerebral ischemia, hydrocephalus, elevated intracranial pressure, seizures, and hyponatremia. Approximately 85 % of SAHs are secondary to a ruptured intracranial saccular aneurysm, 10 % are caused by the benign perimesencephalic syndrome, and the remainder are caused by arteriovenous anomalies and other rare conditions. Most SAH headaches last days to weeks and initially nausea and vomiting occurs as well. Photophobia is also common. The probability of SAH is very low if the intensity of the severe headache develops over minutes to hours and the pain lasts less than one hour. The presence of any neurologic sign or impairment of consciousness increases the likelihood of an SAH or other underlying serious conditions.

The noncontrast-enhanced CT scan has a sensitivity of 98 % in the first 12 h after onset of the SAH, which drops to 93 % at 24 h and 50 % at 7 days. A CSF study will reveal xanthochromia in almost all cases with aneurysmal SAH when it is done within the first 12 h and 2 weeks after the onset of the symptoms and analyzed by spectrophotometry, but it should be kept in mind that in some patients, when the lumbar puncture (LP) is done very early, the bleeding may be missed. Recently, a CT-angiography (CTA) following a CT scan has been suggested as an alternative diagnostic strategy instead of performing an LP. However, there are also some concerns with this strategy, such as risks of additional radiation exposure (especially in the young!), time, and costs and comparability between LP and CTA. Besides, one of the other concerns is how to manage when incidental and asymptomatic aneurysms are discovered.

Key Points for Patients Who Are Admitted with "Sudden-Onset Very Severe Headaches"

- Limited clinical data suggest that headaches requiring more than several minutes to peak in intensity are low risk for SAH.
- However, although that abrupt onset of headache is always of concern for SAH, one study showed that this occurred only half of the time in patients with SAH.
- Sudden-onset HA is seen more often in patients with benign causes of thunderclap headaches.
- Nearly half of patients with SAH have headaches that deviate from the "classical" description.
- No characteristic location has been determined; neck pain is common, but neck pain is also common in migraine.
- In a large series of SAH, 34 % of headaches occurred during nonstrenuous activity and 12 % developed during sleep.
- A past history of recurrent headaches, including their frequency and site and whether they were migrainous or not, was found not to be associated with the risk of SAH.

Key Points Regarding How to Work Up Patients Who Are Admitted with "Sudden-Onset Very Severe Headaches" and Suspected to Have Subarachnoid Hemorrhage

A sudden-onset "first or worst" nontraumatic headache, which reaches its maximal intensity within seconds to a few minutes and which lasts at least more than one hour, whether associated with any neurologic sign or not, should raise the probability of subarachnoid hemorrhage or other underlying life-threatening neurologic diseases.

To rule out subarachnoid hemorrhage:

- A noncontrast cranial CT (if found normal) followed by a lumbar puncture is recommended.

Alternatively:

- CT followed by CT-angiography may be a reasonable diagnostic strategy with comparable sensitivity to a CT followed by LP in these patients with a relatively less margin of suspicion!

Other alternatives may be:

- A combination of Susceptibility weighted imaging (SWI) and Fluid attenuated inversion recovery FLAIR-MRI which was recently shown to yield a higher detection rate for SAH than CT alone and then can be supplemented by MRA (currently a more sophisticated approach limited to some centers).
- Repeat angiography should be performed, particularly in patients who have a non-perimesencephalic SAH pattern, for detection of initially unrecognized ruptured aneurysms.

Key Epidemiological Data Regarding Unruptured Intracranial Aneurysms

- The overall rupture risk of unruptured intracranial aneurysms in the 50–65-year-old age group has been reported to remain below 1 % (0.87 %) per year in a recent large community study from Norway.
- Although that the vast majority of intracranial aneurysms do not rupture, it is important to identify those who are likely to be at highest risk for rupture as such an outcome carries very high morbidity and mortality rates. The most important factors predicting rupture are aneurysm size (≥5 mm) and site (posterior circulation aneurysms). Although nondefinite, morphology, enlargement over time, age (>50 years), gender (women), and a positive family history of intracranial aneurysms with SAH are some other potential risk factors.

Suggested Reading

1. Bederson JB, Connolly ES Jr, Batjer HH et al (2009) Guidelines for the management of aneurysmal subarachnoid hemorrhage: a statement for healthcare professionals from a special writing group of the Stroke Council, American Heart Association. Stroke 40:994–1025
2. Broderick J, Connolly S, Feldmann E et al (2007) Guidelines for the management of spontaneous intracerebral hemorrhage in adults: 2007 update: a guideline from the American Heart Association/American Stroke Association Stroke Council, High Blood Pressure Research Council, and the Quality of Care and Outcomes in Research Interdisciplinary Working Group. Stroke 38:2001–2023
3. Carter KN, Anderson N, Jamrozik K et al (2005) Migraine and risk of subarachnoid haemorrhage: a population-based case-control study. J Clin Neurosci 12:534–537
4. Chappell ET, Moure FC, Good MC (2003) Comparison of computed tomographic angiography with digital subtraction angiography in the diagnosis of cerebral aneurysms: a meta-analysis. Neurosurgery 52:624–631
5. Cianfoni A, Pravatà E, De Blasi R, Tschuor CS, Bonaldi G. Clinical presentation of cerebral aneurysms. Eur J Radiol. 2013;82(10):1618–22. doi:10.1016/j.ejrad.2012.11.019. [Epub 2012 Dec 10]
6. Davenport R (2002) Acute headache in the emergency department. J Neurol Neurosurg Psychiatry 72:ii33–ii37
7. Friedman L (2011) Headache in the emergency department. Curr Pain Headache Rep 15:302–307
8. Frontera JA, Levine SR (2011) Subarachnoid hemorrhage. In: Greenamyre JT (ed) MedLink neurology. MedLink Corporation, San Diego. Available at www.medlink.com. Last updated: 24 Aug 2011
9. Laligam N, Sekhar LN, Ramanathan D, Hallam DK et al (2011) What is the correct approach to aneurysm management in 2011? World Neurosurg 75:409–411
10. Linn FHH, Rinkel GJE, Algra A et al (1998) Headache characteristics in subarachnoid haemorrhage and benign thunderclap headache. J Neurol Neurosurg Psychiatry 65:791–793
11. Loewenstein JE, Gayle SC, Duffis EJ et al (2012) Thenaturalhistoryandtreatmentoptionsforunrupturedintracranialaneurysms. Int J Vasc Med Article ID 898052
12. Lummel N, Schoepf V, Burke M et al (2011) 3D fluid-attenuated inversion recovery imaging: reduced CSF artifacts and enhanced sensitivity and specificity for subarachnoid hemorrhage. AJNR Am J Neuroradiol 32:2054–2060
13. Mark W, Green MW (2012) Secondary headaches. Contin Lifelong Learn Neurol 18:783–795
14. McCormack RF, Hutson A (2010) Can computed tomography angiography of the brain replace lumbar puncture in the evaluation of acute-onset headache after a negative noncontrast cranial computed tomography scan? Acad Emerg Med 17:444–51
15. Müller TB, Sandvei MS, Kvistad KA et al (2013) Unruptured intracranial aneurysms in the Norwegian Nord-Trøndelag Health Study (HUNT): risk of rupture calculated from data in a population-based Cohort study. Neurosurgery 73:256–261
16. Naidech AM, Janjua N, Kreiter KT et al (2005) Predictors and impact of aneurysm rebleeding after subarachnoid hemorrhage. Arch Neurol 62:410–416
17. Schievink WI, Karemaker JM, Hageman LM et al (1989) Circumstances surrounding aneurysmal subarachnoid hemorrhage. Surg Neurol 32(4):266–272
18. The international classification of headache disorders, 3rd edition (beta version) (2013). Cephalalgia 33:629–808
19. van Gelder JM (2003) Computed tomographic angiography for detecting cerebral aneurysms: implications of aneurysm size distribution for the sensitivity, specificity, and likelihood ratios. Neurosurgery 53:597–605
20. Verma RK, Kottke R, Andereggen L et al (2013) Detecting subarachnoid hemorrhage: comparison of combined FLAIR/SWI versus CT. Eur J Radiol 82:1539–1545
21. Vlak HMM, Algra A, Brandenburg R et al (2011) Prevalence of unruptured intracranial aneurysms, with emphasis on sex, age, comorbidity, country, and time period: a systematic review and meta-analysis. Lancet Neurol 10:626–636

Chapter 33
Headache in Systemic Diseases

Dimos D. Mitsikostas and Christina I. Deligianni

33.1 Case Description

A right-hand 47-year-old man, officer at the Hellenic Navy, has been presented at the outpatient headache clinic complaining of new-onset headaches. Headaches started 3–4 months ago gradually; they were mild to severe (rated 5–8/10), located within the entire head, pressing, lasting from 30 min to 2 h and worsening by physical activity but not associated with nausea, vomiting, phonophobia, photophobia or osmophobia. Headache attacks were more frequent during the morning and responded to paracetamol 500 mg in the beginning but later on did not any more. Two months ago he had visited the emergency room at the Athens Naval Hospital to report those headaches. Physical and neurological examination was normal at that time. He had a brain CT scan that did not show any abnormality. He was advised to keep a headache diary, treat the headache attacks with naproxen 500 mg and schedule appointment with the headache clinic. In the diary, headaches followed the pattern the patient reported in the emergency room, responded to naproxen, but slowly the intensity and frequency increased. Headaches became pulsating and accompanying with face flush. When the pain was severe, it was accompanied with nausea but not vomiting. He reported no photophobia or phonophobia. Physical activity typically triggered headaches, and during the attack, pain severity did not change by body position. The mean frequency was 25 days with headache per month. He reported no recent or previous trauma. His wife, who was present at the interview, did not mention snoring. Sleep was normal as usual and he reported no anxiety or depressive symptoms. Recent blood tests in the context of the annual check-up were normal. He described no recent surgical or dental procedure or regional or general anaesthesia. At the time of interview, the Hamilton rating scales

D.D. Mitsikostas, MD, PhD (✉) • C.I. Deligianni, MD
Neurology Department, Athens Naval Hospital, Athens, Greece
e-mail: dimosmitsikostas@me.com

A. Siva, C. Lampl (eds.), *Case-Based Diagnosis and Management of Headache Disorders*, Headache, DOI 10.1007/978-3-319-06886-2_33

for anxiety and depression scores were 12 and 8 (normal values). No medication overuse was noted in the headache diary nor reported by the patient. His wife agreed on this.

He could recall only infrequent, mild headaches associated with flu syndromes or alcohol consumption previously. Personal medical history was negative for neurological or systemic disease, acute or chronic. He was a smoker for 15 years (10 cigarettes per day approximately) and social drinker. Family history was negative for any chronic neurological disorder nor for primary or secondary headaches. His father was suffering from metabolic syndrome and his mother from hypothyroidism. He was married with two kids, and he could recall no recent stressful event in his personal, family or professional life.

The interview was semi-structured and included the Hamilton scales as standard interview with any patient at the Athens Naval Headache Clinic.

Neurological and physical examination was normal. Blood pressure was 150 mmHg systolic and 90 mmHg diastolic. Cardiac rate was 75 p/min. BMI = 31.

33.2 Differential Diagnosis, Workup and Follow-Up

This is a case of a new-onset, non-traumatic, almost morning headache with mild progressive features and neurological and physical examination of a middle-aged healthy man without a previous medical history who did not report psychiatric symptoms. He had already had a normal brain CT scan. Only blood pressure was elevated, but he had no other blood pressure measurement before. This data did not indicate a life-threatening situation and no emergency evaluation was required. In the contrary, the criteria for probable new daily persistent headache (NDPH) were fulfilled. NDPH is a disorder evolving from frequent episodic tension-type headache (TTH), with daily or very frequent episodes of headache, typically bilateral, pressing or tightening in quality and of mild to moderate intensity, lasting hours to days or unremitting. The pain did not worsen with routine physical activity (this was the only criterion not fulfilled by the patient's headache characteristics), but may be associated with mild nausea, photophobia or phonophobia, International Headache Classification of Headache Disorders-IIIbeta edition (ICHD-IIIb). Differential diagnosis includes other primary headache disorders, mainly chronic TTH. It is a matter of time to put this diagnosis in this case, however. Along with the headache diagnosis, there were some red flags in this case: the recent onset of headache, the crescendo of severity and intensity and the abnormal arterial blood pressure. Because of these considerations, the patient was advised to undergo a brain MRI, to keep an arterial blood pressure diary (three times per day for at least 10 days) along with the headache diary. Amitriptyline 25 mg in one evening dose was given as preventive treatment. The reason to order MRI scan was to exclude any intracranial space-occupying abnormality that could cause this headache type, since the previous CT scan was performed without contrast.

The patient underwent MRI and kept both diaries and 10 days later returned with the results. The MRI showed T2/FLAIR (Fluid Attenuated Inversion Recovery images) lesions in the white matter, a common finding and common clinical problem in daily

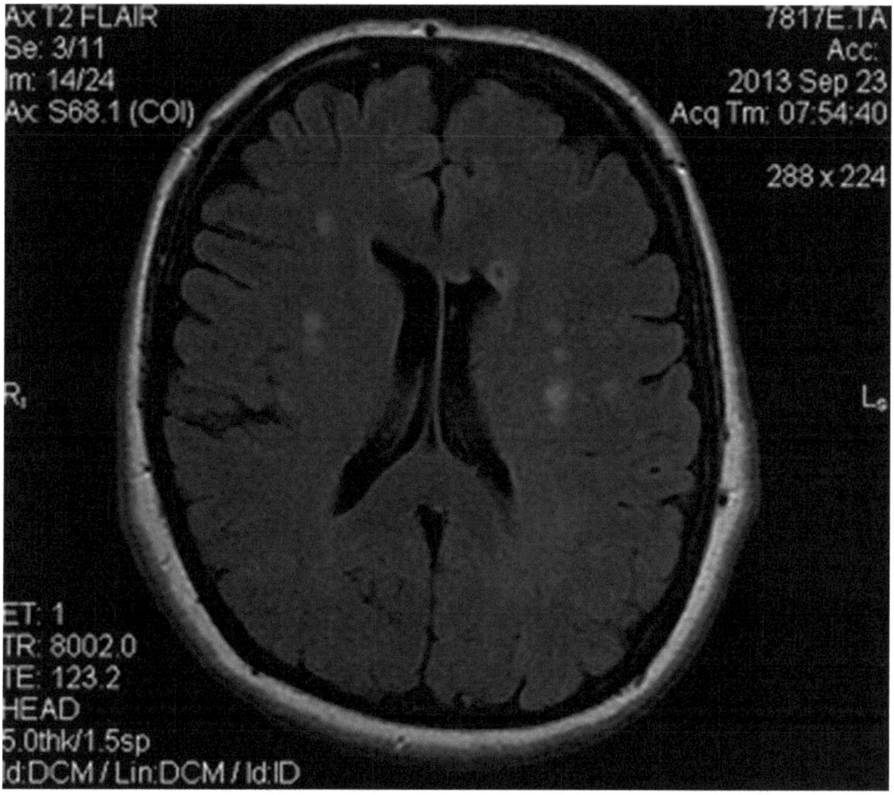

Fig. 33.1 MRI showing T2/FLAIR lesions in the white matter

practice (Fig. 33.1). The topography and morphological characteristics of T2 lesions refer to several conditions, including small vessel disease and demyelination mainly, or atypical T2 lesions, not relevant clinically. Headaches, although present, became mild and did not require acute treatment already. But the arterial blood pressure diary showed several abnormal measurements (up to 210 mmHg systolic and 130 mmHg diastolic). The patient referred to cardiology department for consultation. After evaluation (ECG and echocardiogram), the diagnosis was idiopathic arterial blood pressure, and the patient started treatment with atenolol 50 mg. White matter lesions were considered as lacunes due to hypertension, and low-dose aspirin (100 mg) was added. For symptomatic treatment of headaches, paracetamol 1 g was offered. He was advised to avoid nonsteroidal anti-inflammatory drugs (NSAIDs) because of the hypertension risk.

Three months later the patient had a scheduled follow-up. Headaches worsened both in severity and intensity. Blood pressure did not respond to treatment and add-on treatment was given (nifedipine 30 mg daily). He reported episodic anxiety-like symptoms with face flushes together with headache and high blood pressure. Headaches did not respond to acute treatment. At that point, differential diagnosis of headaches changed and other disorders included, such as arteriovenous fistula, cerebral venous thrombosis, intracranial hypertension and headache attributed to arterial hypertension. Intracranial abnormalities were excluded however by brain MRI. Of note, physical and neurological examination remained normal. It seemed that headache attributed to arterial hypertension was the most likely diagnosis. According to ICHD-IIIb, this headache subtype is usually bilateral and pulsating, caused by arterial hypertension, during an acute rise in systolic (to 180 mmHg) and/or diastolic (to 120 mmHg) blood pressure and remits after normalisation of blood pressure, like in the patient. Another similar identity was headache attributed to hypertensive encephalopathy, but the patient had no confusion, lethargy, visual disturbances or seizures. Neither the observed MRI lesions could match with this diagnosis. If the patient was female pregnant, pre-eclampsia and eclampsia should also be included in the differential diagnosis. No other disorder could explain all the signs and features of the patient with one exception – phaeochromocytoma, a rare systemic disorder that only needs measuring of catecholamines' levels in the blood and urine without any invasive procedure. Cushing's syndrome could also mimic this situation.

33.3 Diagnosis

Plasma metanephrine, 24-h urine creatinine, total catecholamines, vanillylmandelic acid and metanephrines were all elevated (>two times above the normal values). Full screening of the pituitary axis did not reveal any other abnormality. MRI of the abdomen revealed a small paraganglioma in the left adrenal gland. The tumour was removed surgically, the headaches were resolved, and blood pressure was normalised confirming the diagnosis of headache attributed to phaeochromocytoma. Biopsy revealed non-malignant tissue with zellballen pattern, typical for phaeochromocytoma. Brain T2 lesions were considered as lacunes due to hypertension or non-specific T2 lesions. The patient had another brain MRI after surgery that did not show changes. Aspirin was withdrawn.

33.4 General Information Related to the Case

Phaeochromocytoma (pheo-chroma means dark colour in Greek) is a rare catecholamine-secreting tumour derived from chromaffin cells. Only 0.2 % of hypertensive individuals have this condition that may be asymptomatic in several cases. Phaeochromocytomas may occur in certain familial syndromes, including multiple endocrine neoplasia (MEN) 2A and 2B, neurofibromatosis and von Hippel-Lindau (VHL) disease. About 10 % of cases are malignant however. Phaeochromocytoma causes headache, epigastric pain, tremor, nausea, weakness, weight loss, palpitations, anxiety and constipation, but explosive headache remains the most often presenting symptom. Delay in diagnosis is common. Subarachnoid haemorrhage and reversible cerebral vasoconstriction syndrome are potential life-threatening complications. Seizures, stroke and delirium may also occur. Arterial hypertension may cause headache, often bilateral and pulsating, usually during an acute rise in systolic (to 180 mmHg) and/or diastolic (to 120 mmHg) blood pressure that is remitting after blood pressure normalisation. Notably, mild (140–159/90–99 mmHg) or moderate (160–179/100–109 mmHg) chronic arterial hypertension does not appear to cause headache. Headache should be developed in temporal relation to the onset of hypertension, worsened in parallel with worsening hypertension and significantly improved with improvement in hypertension. Whether moderate hypertension predisposes to headache at all remains controversial, but there is some evidence that it does. Ambulatory blood pressure monitoring in patients with mild and moderate hypertension has shown no convincing relationship between blood pressure fluctuations over a 24-h period and presence or absence of headache. Hypertensive encephalopathy presents with persistent elevation of blood pressure to 180/120 mmHg and at least two of confusion, reduced level of consciousness, visual disturbances including blindness and seizures. It is thought to occur when compensatory cerebrovascular vasoconstriction can no longer prevent cerebral hyperperfusion as blood pressure rises. As normal cerebral autoregulation of blood flow is overwhelmed, endothelial permeability increases and cerebral oedema occurs. On MRI, this is often most prominent in the parieto-occipital white matter. Headache in hypertensive encephalopathy is a presenting symptom, and it is usually bilateral and pulsating, and it improves after normalisation of blood pressure. Headache, with the same characteristics, also occurs in women during pregnancy or the immediate puerperium with pre-eclampsia or eclampsia. It remits after resolution of the pre-eclampsia or eclampsia. The posterior reversible encephalopathy syndrome (PRES) characterised by headache, visual disorders, seizures, altered mentation, consciousness disturbances and focal neurological signs was initially described in these patients. Whether breakdown or activation of cerebral autoregulatory system results in fluid leakage remains debatable. Headache attributed to phaeochromocytoma occurs as a paroxysmal headache in most (51–80 %) of patients with phaeochromocytoma. It is often severe, frontal or occipital and usually described as either pulsating or constant in quality. Headache is typically short lasting (<15 min in 50 % and < 1 h in 70 % of patients). Associated features include apprehension and/or anxiety, often with a sense of impending death, tremor, visual disturbances, abdominal or chest pain, nausea, vomiting and occasionally paraesthesia. The face can blanch or flush during the attack.

Throbbing severe headache, with sudden onset, occurs in patients with spinal cord injury and autonomic dysreflexia. It may be a life-threatening condition that manifests as a paroxysmal rise in blood pressure among other symptoms and clinical signs. It is often triggered by bladder or bowel irritation (by infection, distension or impaction) or other noxious stimuli. The time to onset of autonomic dysreflexia after spinal cord injury is variable and has been reported from 4 days to 15 years. Apparently, prompt recognition of the condition and adequate management are critical.

Arterial hypotension may cause headache too. In this case, headache and pain, mostly at the back of the neck but sometimes spreading upwards to the occipital region ('coat hanger' distribution), are attributed to postural hypotension and developing only in upright posture. Headache spontaneously improves in horizontal posture. When specifically asked, 75 % of patients with orthostatic hypotension reported neck pain.

Key Points: What Does This Case Tell Us?

- Comorbidity of probable NDPH and idiopathic arterial hypertension in a 47-year-old man, with a BMI of 31, seems very likely undoubtedly. Causative rare conditions may be underlying, however.
- When a comorbid condition starts with headaches simultaneously, a causative relation is always probable.
- Treating a patient by different physicians increases the risk to misdiagnose rare conditions when both situations are common; thus, close collaboration is needed.
- Everyday findings in brain MRI in headache sufferers may confuse and misdirect the diagnosis, while clinical data are obvious towards other situations.

Suggesting Reading

1. Anderson NE, Chung K, Willoughby E et al (2013) Neurological manifestations of phaeochromocytomas and secretory paragangliomas: a reappraisal. J Neurol Neurosurg Psychiatry 84:452–457
2. Balasubramanian G, Nellaiappan V (2014) Functional paraganglioma. BMJ Case Rep doi: 10.1136/bcr-2013-203425
3. Gipponi S, Venturelli E, Rao R et al (2010) Hypertension is a factor associated with chronic daily headache. Neurol Sci 31(Suppl 1):171–173
4. Kantorovich V, Pacak K (2010) Pheochromocytoma and paraganglioma. Prog Brain Res 182:343–373
5. Lance JW, Hinterberger H (1976) Symptom of pheochromocytoma with particular reference to headache, correlated with catecholamine production. Arch Neurol 33:281–288
6. Marra A, Vargas M, Striano P et al (2014) Posterior reversible encephalopathy syndrome: the endothelial hypotheses. Med Hypotheses 82:619–622

Chapter 34
Headaches in Patients with Idiopathic Intracranial Hypertension

Fabio Antonaci, Cristina Voiticovschi-Iosob, and Giorgio Bono

34.1 Case Description

A 39-year-old North African housewife without any previous health problems came to our headache centre with a 4-week history of sudden-onset, bilateral (mainly right side), severe headache. Pain was continuous and fluctuating in severity, with associated photo- and phonophobia, not worsened by physical activity or exercise and not disabling with partial benefit from NSAIDs. Primarily, she was referred by her family doctor to the ENT specialist for evaluation. In the absence of clinical abnormalities, a cerumen plug from the left ear (suspecting a sinus headache) was removed without any other indication. A few days later, she also started experiencing fluctuating then permanent horizontal diplopia, so that she was referred to the local headache centre.

At first observation she denied fever, nausea, vomiting and any other sensorimotor symptoms with the exception of diplopia. The general examination (BMI 24.8),

F. Antonaci (✉)
Department of Neurological and Behavioral Sciences, Headache Center,
C. Mondino National Institute of Neurology Foundation, IRCCS, University of Pavia,
Via Mondino 2, Pavia 27100, Italy
e-mail: fabio.antonaci@unipv.it

C. Voiticovschi-Iosob
Department of Neurology, State Medical and Pharmaceutical University "Nicolae Testemitanu", Republic of Moldova, 165 Stefan cel Mare Street, Chisinau 2004, Republic of Moldova

University of Pavia, Pavia, Italy
e-mail: nicolae@mededu.moldline.net

G. Bono
Department of Biotechnology and Life Science, University of Insubria,
Via Dunant 1, Varese 21100, Italy
e-mail: giorgio.bono@uninsubria.it

A. Siva, C. Lampl (eds.), *Case-Based Diagnosis and Management of Headache Disorders*, Headache, DOI 10.1007/978-3-319-06886-2_34

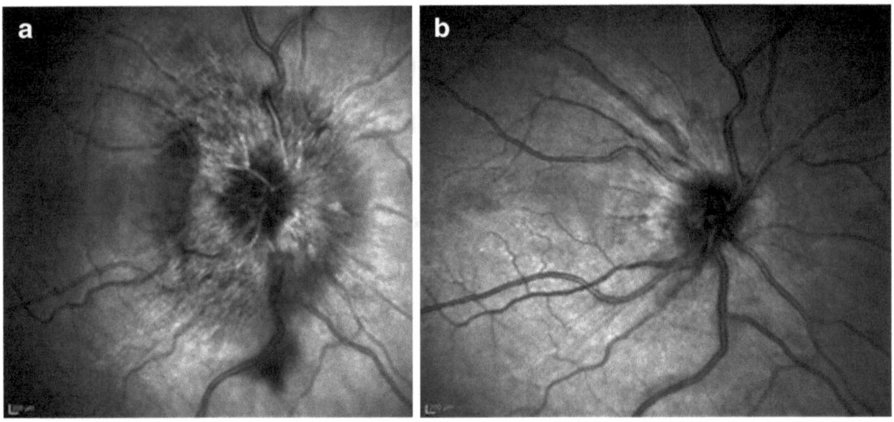

Fig. 34.1 Fundus phlebography: bilateral papilloedema with peripapillary haemorrhages ((**a**) right eye on admission, (**b**) right eye after treatment)

blood pressure, heart rate, respiration rates and body temperature were normal. Visual acuities were 10/10 in both eyes, with normal confrontation visual fields and pupillary responses. A 6th right side nerve palsy was noticed. The intraocular pressure (10 mmHg) was normal. Pain was increased with light pressure on the right eye ocular bulb. Nonetheless, the fundus oculi examination showed bilateral papilloedema with peripapillary haemorrhages without spontaneous venous pulsations (Fig. 34.1 left side, right eye). No exophthalmos was noticed. Other findings regarding the neurologic examination were normal, and there was no clinical sign of meningeal irritation.

The re-evaluation of clinical history neither showed evidence of recent cranial/extracranial infection nor ongoing pharmacological treatment (oral contraceptives). There was no history of tick bites, joint pains or target rash. Her past medical, neurological, surgical, travel and family history was unremarkable. She had no known allergies. There was no evidence of neuroinflammatory or general immunological disorders in her family history. Her mother and her father were in good health, the patient being the first of three healthy sisters. She has a 10-year-old healthy child.

34.2 Differential Diagnosis and How to Work Up This Kind of a Patient

Considering the de novo headache with slowly increasing severity, with a partial and temporary response to the treatment and with subsequent onset of horizontal diplopia, a situation of increased intracranial pressure could be a first working hypothesis.

In the presence of headache with increasing severity after weeks, followed by diplopia without other neurologic signs in a young, slightly overweight woman, the differential diagnosis versus other categories of secondary headache should be considered with a thorough workup.

Certain patients may face a sudden, somewhat severe, headache, hours/up to weeks preceding rupture of an intracranial aneurysm. This is generally referred as 'sentinel headache', which is usually short lasting, isolated or associated with general or focal neurologic symptoms/signs. In our case, considering a relatively long-lasting de novo headache, the search for an intracranial aneurysm is mandatory, headache symptoms being attributable to possible small bleeding from aneurysm and diplopia to direct compression of cranial oculomotor nerves. However, our patient did not have symptoms/signs of even minor meningeal irritation from SAH. However, inflammatory, infectious and neoplastic meningitis may eventually be present with isolated headache and diplopia (without other neurologic deficits and meningitis). But more frequently systemic symptoms and focal or general neurologic deficits (other cranial nerve palsies, cognitive/behavioural arousal dysfunction, etc.) became evident with time.

Once a dangerous secondary headache is excluded from aneurysm or other arterial malformations, other intravascular causes of persisting headache and diplopia should be considered, such as cerebral venous thrombosis, extracranial dissection and cranial arteritis. Most of these conditions should be ruled out by appropriate neuroimaging (standard plus neurovascular study) and lumbar puncture (neurosarcoidosis, neuroborreliosis, etc.).

Furthermore, local inflammatory causes should be ruled out such as orbital cellulitis/myositis and ENT complications, such as tumours or fungal infections of the anterior skull base.

On the other hand, the cause of severe persisting headache, possibly complicated by diplopia, dizziness and other minor symptoms, may be consistent with the diagnosis of idiopathic intracranial hypotension (IIH). This condition strictly is characterised by a typical orthostatic headache, being generated exclusively during the vertical position. Orthostatic headache in the presence of low CSF pressure (either spontaneous or secondary), or CSF leakage (spontaneous or secondary), is usually accompanied by neck pain, tinnitus, changes in hearing, photophobia and/or nausea. It remits after normalisation of CSF pressure or successful sealing of the CSF leakage (blood patch).

In our case, however, CSF pressure was increased (280 mm H_2O).

Systemic disease as SLE, Behcet's disease, uraemia, iron deficiency anaemia, Addison's disease, hypothyroidism and polycystic ovarian disease might be associated with intracranial hypertension. The same goes for medications such as tetracycline, oral contraceptive pill, lithium, progesterone, growth hormone and steroid withdrawal.

Finally, ophthalmoplegic migraine has not included in the differential diagnosis, because it is not included in the ICHD-III beta version.

34.3 Topics for Analysis

34.3.1 How Do the Examinations Aid to Manage the Workup?

Bilateral optic disc swelling in the presence of normal optic nerve function is consistent with an increased intracranial pressure. Diagnosis of IIH is focused on symptoms only attributable to intracranial hypertension, ruling out vascular lesions, mass, or ventriculomegaly on neuroimaging, and other aetiology of intracranial hypertension established (Fig. 34.1).

Still, further causes of intracranial hypertension should be taken into account: inflammatory, infectious and malignant disorders involving the meninges, brain tumour and a venous sinus thrombosis.

A markedly elevated blood pressure (malignant hypertension) can also give rise to disc swelling in addition to headache, with a clinical picture different from the present case.

Any de novo continuous headache should be investigated with neuroimaging focusing on parenchymas, arterial/venous circulation and meninges.

In patients with evidence of papilloedema, neuroimaging should be performed prior to lumbar puncture, to exclude the risk of herniation and to search for any secondary cause of intracranial hypertension. CT or MR venography is requested to exclude cerebral venous sinus thrombosis.

If the neuroimaging does not show a mass lesion, obstructive hydrocephalus, or evidence of cerebral venous thrombosis, a lumbar puncture should follow to confirm the diagnosis of suspected 'benign' intracranial hypertension and to rule out malignant, infectious or inflammatory disorders simulating IIH symptoms and sign (Fig. 34.2).

The CSF examination should include cytology, bacteriology, full viral test (PCR and viral and syphilis markers) and serology for parasites and fungi. In some patients, especially children, an opening pressure of up to 280 mm CSF is normal, but, for most of the cases, an opening pressure above 280 mm CSF should be considered elevated.

Patients should also undergo blood tests including complete blood counts, erythrocyte sedimentation rate, coagulation, and electrolytes and tests for syphilis, thyroid function tests and electrophoresis.

In our patient, blood tests included complete blood counts, routine chemistry, erythrocyte sedimentation rate, C-reactive protein, coagulation panel, thyroid function tests, rheumatoid factor, antinuclear antibody, anti-ds-DNA antibody and antineutrophil cytoplasmic antibodies, which were all normal with the exception of positive ANA Ab (homogenous pattern 1:640).

Basal brain MRI was normal (Fig. 34.1a). Venous angiography showed no abnormality (Fig. 34.1b).

Lumbar puncture showed a slightly elevated opening pressure (i.e.>250 mm H_2O) with normal laboratory profile (no white blood cell, 19 mg/dL of protein, 85 mg/dL of glucose, absence of oligoclonal banding).

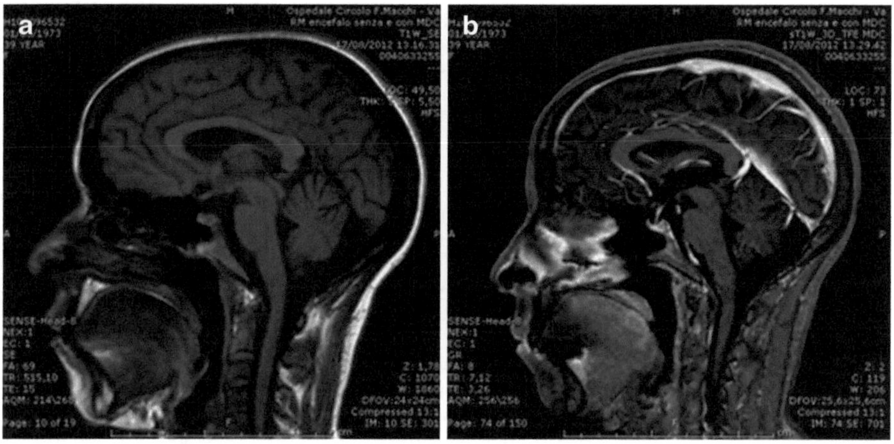

Fig. 34.2 (**a**) Basal brain MRI; (**b**) venous angio-MRI with gadolinium

34.4 Topics for Discussion

34.4.1 Which Is the Diagnosis? Which Is the Treatment for Our Patient?

Given the specific symptoms of headache and diplopia in a young slightly overweight female, associated with raised CSF pressure with normal CSF profiles, papilloedema and normal neuroimaging without other causes of intracranial hypertension, a diagnosis of IIH can be given.

The first aim of treatment is to relieve symptoms and preserve vision from optic atrophy by restoring normal CSF pressure values. The medical treatments for IIH include diuretics, particularly carbonic anhydrase inhibitors (acetazolamide) and topiramate, which may also help patients to reduce weight. Systemic corticosteroids may be used in cases undergoing progressive visual loss. Weight loss should be advised for patients with obesity, since weight reduction may relieve optic disc swelling. The surgical option is indicated when patients have severe papilloedema and are at risk of visual loss or when the medical treatments fail to control papilloedema. CSF diversion and shunting (lumboperitoneal or ventriculoperitoneal) are the main choices. Optic nerve sheath fenestration may be indicated when papilloedema persists over time despite the recovery from raised intracranial pressure.

CSF diversion surgery usually results in prompt normalisation of intracerebral pressure and resolution of papilloedema. Complications of surgery may be a shunt obstruction that requires revision, CNS infection, shunt migration and low CSF pressure headache eventually complicated by subdural hematoma.

Our patient underwent the procedure of lumboperitoneal shunting, and her headache promptly improved; diplopia disappeared over the following several days even

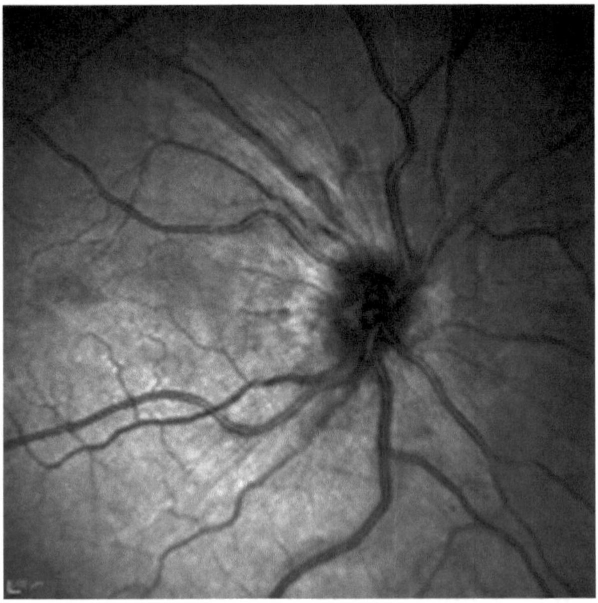

Fig. 34.3 Improved papilloedema 4 weeks later after lumboperitoneal shunt

though papilloedema and peripapillary haemorrhages persisted (Fig. 34.3). She was discharged home with a 1-month corticosteroid therapy prescription and close ophthalmological follow-up. After surgical procedure 4 weeks later, a marked resolution of papilloedema on follow-up funduscopy was observed (Fig. 34.3).

Absence of papilloedema has been reported in case series of patients with IIH, but its absence may be more suggestive of an alternative aetiology for headache and vision loss. The percentage of IIH patients without papilloedema among refractory chronic/transformed migraine patients is reported ranging from 5 to 14 % in a small series of patients.

The result of untreated cases of IIH might be a permanent visual loss (severe in 10 %); relapses may occur in 40 % of cases in long-term follow-up.

34.5 Summary of the Case

A 39-year-old North African housewife with sudden onset of severe headache is admitted to the headache centre after 4 weeks from the beginning of symptoms. Ten days later she presented binocular horizontal diplopia (6th nerve palsy) in precedence of continuing headache. On hospital admission, her physical and neurologic examinations were normal. Given the acute onset and continuous severe headache, followed by horizontal diplopia without other focal neurologic signs in a young overweight woman, the hypothesis of IIH should be investigated. Accordingly, in the present case, fundus oculi examination showed papilloedema with bilateral peripapillary haemorrhages; brain MRI with contrast was normal also excluding meningeal dural enhancement and vascular pathologies (MRI angiography). LP showed opening CSF pressure over the normal range, thus confirming the diagnosis of headache attributed to IIH (ICHD-III beta: 7.1.1). Surgical treatment (lumboperitoneal shunting) followed by short-term corticosteroid therapy allowed full recovery from symptoms and resolution of bilateral papilloedema.

34.6 Definition of Idiopathic Intracranial Hypertension

According to 'The International Classification of Headache Disorders, 3rd edition (beta version)' [14], headache attributed to idiopathic intracranial hypertension (IIH) is described as typically frontal, retro-orbital, 'pressure-like' or explosive caused by idiopathic intracranial hypertension, usually accompanied by other symptoms of IIH with remission after normalisation of cerebrospinal fluid pressure.

IIH is typically a disorder of obese women. The male/female ratio is 1/4–15. Typical symptoms include headache, papilloedema, transient visual loss, diplopia and tinnitus. Headache is continuous and may be worse in the morning or increased by Valsalva manoeuvres, and it may last hours; nausea is common but not vomiting. Other headache syndromes frequently coexist such as rebound headache from analgesics or caffeine overuse. Transient visual obscuration is explained by transient ischaemia of the optic nerve head by papilloedema. Diplopia is usually horizontal resulting from abducens nerve palsy. Unilateral or bilateral pulsatile tinnitus may be explained by flow disturbances in the cerebral venous system. With progression of disease, ischaemic optic neuropathy may occur, producing irreversible impairments of central vision in 1/3 of the cases, but most visual defects in IIH are reversible if intracranial pressure is well controlled.

More unusual is the absence of papilloedema with raised ICP. Such cases are considered rare; however, because clinicians do not routinely do lumbar punctures on patients without papilloedema, the true incidence of this presentation is likely underestimated. Many patients with IIH also show intracranial hypertension several years after onset of the disease. Accordingly, IIH may be a chronic condition, warranting long-term follow-up.

34.7 Brief General Information

IIH is a disorder of elevated cerebrospinal fluid pressure of unidentified cause and classically presents with headache and, frequently, vision changes in women with obesity of childbearing age. The incidence was estimated at 0.9/100 000 cases with 8.6/100 000 cases of prevalence. The female/male ratio ranges are between 4.3:1.0 and 15:1. IIH generally occurs in obese women in the fertile period of life. Obesity is present in more than 70 % of adult IIH patients. The patient has no localising neurologic findings, and there is no obstruction or deformity of the ventricular system. Neurologic examination is normal except for enhanced CSF pressure (>200 mm of H_2O in nonobese and > 250 mm of H_2O in obese patient), and no secondary cause of intracranial hypertension can be found. The CSF pressure should be measured with the patient in the lateral decubitus position and the legs as relaxed as possible.

Headache is the most common symptom associated with IIH which leads the patients to seek the physician. Headache attributed to IIH is a daily-occurring diffuse headache aggravated by physical activity and may be associated with nausea. The other symptoms of increased intracranial pressure may be pulsatile tinnitus, transient visual obscurations and visual loss, papilloedema and diplopia. Vision loss is the most feared sequel of IIH, but most vision loss is transient and occurs in 68–85 % of patients. Brain MRI is performed to exclude secondary causes of elevated intracranial pressure and to identify the associated IIH signs, which include partially or totally empty sella turcica, deformities of the pituitary gland/decreased pituitary height, distension and enhancement of the optic nerve (optic nerve sheath) and enlarged perioptic subarachnoid space, posterior globe flattening and tortuosity of the optic nerve, intraocular protrusion of optic nerve head and slitlike ventricles.

In conclusion we may summarise as follows: (a) benign intracranial hypertension is not benign; (b) IIH is not always idiopathic; (c) an early diagnosis is critical; (d) early and intensive treatment plan is critical; and (e) treatment consists of acetazolamide, diuretics, weight loss and eventual shunting.

A systematic, multidisciplinary strategy and frequent, long-term follow-up are needed.

Key Points for Patients Who Are Admitted with Suspected IIH Headache

- The IIH diagnosis is based on the criteria of The International Classification of Headache Disorders, 3rd edition (beta version).
- Headache is the most common symptom in IIH and papilloedema is the major clinical finding.
- IIH remains a diagnosis of exclusion, when it does not occur in overweight women, and it is mandatory looking for a secondary cause (e.g. an organic stenosis of the lateral sinus).
- The upper limit of the opening pressure of the CSF was established at 250 mm H_2O for adults and 280 mm H_2O for children, but in practice, this limit is not very accurate.
- The factors of poor prognosis must be recognised in order to adjust the therapeutic strategy.
- Fulminant IIH is a very rare condition of idiopathic intracranial hypertension, and it is characterised by an acute onset and by a rapid deterioration of visual function.
- The IIH treatment depends on the severity of ocular signs and surgical therapies such as CSF diversion procedures, and fenestration of the optic nerve may be necessary in some cases with persistent symptoms or progressive visual deterioration.
- The patients who had IIH should be followed by a neurologist and by an ophthalmologist, and repeated visual fields are required.

Suggested Reading

1. Ball AK, Clarke CE (2006) Idiopathic intracranial hypertension. Lancet Neurol 5:433–442
2. Brodsky MC, Vaphiades M (1998) Magnetic resonance imaging in pseudotumor cerebri. Ophthalmology 105:1686–1693
3. Burde RM, Savino PJ, Trobe JD (eds) (2002) Clinical Decisions in Neuro-ophthalmology, 3rd edn. Mosby, St. Louis
4. Corbett JJ, Savino PJ, Thompson HS et al (1982) Visual loss in pseudotumor cerebri. Follow-up of 57 patients from five to 41 years and a profile of 14 patients with permanent severe visual loss. Arch Neurol 39:461–474
5. Corbett JJ, Thompson HS (1989) The rational management of idiopathic intracranial hypertension. Arch Neurol 46:1049–1051
6. Degnan AJ, Levy LM (2011) Pseudotumor cerebri: brief review of clinical syndrome and imaging findings. AJNR Am J Neuroradiol 32(11):1986–1993
7. Dunghana S, Sharrack B, Woodroofe N (2010) Idiopathic intracranial hypertension. Acta Neurol Scand 121:71–82
8. Friedman DI (2004) Pseudotumor cerebri. Neurol Clin 22:99–131
9. Korsmorsky GS (2014) Idiopathic intracranial hypertension: pseudotumor cerebri Current clinical review. Headache 54(2):389–393
10. Mathews MK, Sergott RC, Savino PJ (2003) Pseudotumor cerebri. Curr Opin Ophthalmol 14:364–370
11. Shah VA, Kardon RH, Lee AG, Corbett JJ, Wall M (2008) Long-term follow-up of idiopathic intracranial hypertension. The Iowa experience. Neurology 70:634–640
12. Skau M, Brennum J, Gjerris F, Jensen R (2005) What is new about idiopathic intracranial hypertension? An updated review of mechanism and treatment. Cephalalgia 26:384–399
13. Szewka AJ, Bruce BB, Newman NJ, Biousse V (2013) Idiopathic intracranial hypertension: relation between obesity and visual outcomes. J Neuroophthalmol 33(1):4–8
14. Headache Classification Committee of the International Headache Society (IHS). The International Classification of Headache Disorders, 3rd edition (beta version) (2013) Cephalalgia 33(9):629–808
15. Wall M, George D (1991) Idiopathic intracranial hypertension: a prospective study of 50 patients. Brain 114:155–180

Chapter 35
Headache in Patients with Intracranial Pressure Changes: Intracranial Hypotension Headache

Wouter I. Schievink and Constance R. Deline

35.1 Case Description

A 67-year-old man noted the acute onset of an exquisitely orthostatic, occipital pressure-type headache associated with nausea and auditory echoing. His symptoms resolved spontaneously over a 2-week period. Two months later, his wife noted the insidious onset of marked behavioral changes that started with poor decision-making and progressed over the next month to include a deterioration in his driving skills and behaviors such as leaving doors open and spilling food and beverages on himself without noticing. He was occasionally mute and hypersomnolent. The initial diagnosis was dementia due to Alzheimer's disease.

35.2 Differential Diagnosis and How to Work Up This Sort of Patient

Acute headache that is worse when upright and improved with recumbency is recognized as resulting from low intracranial pressure when it occurs following a lumbar puncture, following spinal surgery, or in a patient with an over-draining CSF shunt. Inadvertent dural punctures following epidural injections and posttraumatic spinal CSF leaks may or may not be recognized promptly. When an orthostatic

W.I. Schievink, MD (✉)
Department of Neurosurgery, Cedars-Sinai Medical Center, Los Angeles, CA 90048, USA
e-mail: schievinkw@cshs.org

C.R. Deline, MD
Harrisburg, PA 17109, USA
e-mail: connie.deline@verizon.net

A. Siva, C. Lampl (eds.), *Case-Based Diagnosis and Management of Headache Disorders*, Headache, DOI 10.1007/978-3-319-06886-2_35

headache occurs spontaneously, the diagnosis of intracranial hypotension from single or multiple spontaneous spinal CSF leaks is more often delayed or missed.

The headache is usually but not always orthostatic, ranges from mild to severe, typically has an onset over minutes to hours, and is most often occipital or suboccipital but may be diffuse, frontal, or temporal. The headache may occasionally be absent or resolve despite persistence of other signs and symptoms. Common associated symptoms include neck stiffness or pain, nausea with or without vomiting, hearing changes, photophobia, interscapular pain, upper limb radicular symptoms, sense of imbalance, and subtle cognitive dysfunction. Less common symptoms or signs include visual changes, various cranial nerve palsies, Parkinsonism, ataxia, cerebellar hemorrhage, dementia, stupor and coma, stroke, and even death. Clinical stigmata of heritable disorders of connective tissue may be noted.

Because the headache may be relatively acute in onset with associated symptoms that include stiff neck, photophobia, phonophobia, nausea, and vomiting, cranial CT is done in many cases to rule out subarachnoid hemorrhage. While generally less helpful than cranial MRI in the diagnosis of intracranial hypotension, subdural fluid collections or obliteration of subarachnoid cisterns and ventricular collapse may be found.

Following a negative cranial CT, a lumbar puncture may be performed to rule out meningitis or subarachnoid hemorrhage below the detection of cranial CT. Most commonly, the opening pressure will be less than 60 (reference 65–195 mm H_2O) and can be unmeasurable or subatmospheric; however, normal pressures do not rule out a spinal CSF leak. Analysis of the CSF may show xanthochromia, normal or elevated protein, normal glucose, lymphocytic pleocytosis, and normal or high erythrocyte count. A lumbar puncture is not required to make the diagnosis: when clinical suspicion of spinal CSF leak is high, several imaging studies are helpful.

Cranial MRI is abnormal in 80 % and has 5 main findings, remembered by the mnemonic SEEPS:

1. Subdural fluid collections
2. Enhancement of pachymeninges
3. Engorgement of venous structures
4. Pituitary hyperemia
5. Sagging of the brain

Subdural hematomas are not uncommon and can often be managed without surgical evacuation but rather by treating the underlying spinal CSF leak. Sagging of the brain may be evident from ventricular collapse, effacement of the perichiasmatic cisterns with bowing of the optic chiasm over the pituitary fossa, effacement of the prepontine cistern with flattening of the pons against the clivus, and descent of the cerebellar tonsils mimicking a Chiari I malformation.

Findings on spinal MRI include meningeal enhancement, meningeal diverticula, extrathecal fluid collections, and dilated epidural or intradural veins. Myelographic sequencing obviates the need for a dural puncture to instill intrathecal contrast; however, intrathecal gadolinium contrast is occasionally used off-label for MR myelography.

CT myelography can define the location and extent of a CSF leak. Meningeal diverticula or nerve root sleeve dilatations may also be visualized. Dynamic CT myelography is usually used to detect rapid leaks.

Digital subtraction myelography is helpful in visualizing rapid and/or extensive leaks seen on other imaging without precise localization, leaks that are anterior to the spinal cord, and more recently recognized CSF-venous fistula leaks that drain directly from the intrathecal space into the epidural veins.

Radioisotope cisternography may confirm the presence of CSF leaking by virtue of early accumulation of tracer in the kidneys and bladder and a paucity of tracer activity over the cerebral convexities but is insensitive in localizing leaks.

Patients are often misdiagnosed with various primary headache disorders such as migraine or tension headaches, nonspecific new daily persistent headache, or headache secondary to viral meningitis. There is limited published data to suggest that patients with headache attributed to chronic whiplash may have a traumatic spinal CSF leak. Delayed diagnoses are primarily due to the lack of familiarity by treating physicians; however, over the last decade, awareness of spontaneous spinal CSF leaks appears to be improving.

Not all orthostatic headaches are caused by spinal CSF leaks. Postural orthostatic tachycardia syndrome (POTS) may present with prominent positional headache. In practice, this may be difficult to sort out since patients with spinal CSF leaks may have positional tachycardia to compensate physiologically for intracranial hypotension, may have preexisting POTS, or can develop secondary POTS. Headaches may also be positional in diabetes insipidus and cervicogenic headaches and in patients that are post decompression surgery for Chiari malformation without CSF leak.

35.3 Diagnostic Workup of the Case

Cranial MRI done as part of the diagnostic workup for dementia showed severe sagging of the brain and meningeal enhancement, diagnostic of spontaneous intracranial hypotension. CT myelography showed a low opening pressure of 20 mm H_2O and a large ventral extrathecal fluid collection.

35.4 Summary of the Case

While this patient initially presented with orthostatic headache, it resolved while increasing symptoms of cognitive dysfunction developed. It was not until cranial MRI revealed findings typical of intracranial hypotension that the correct diagnosis was made.

The patient underwent a series of eight lumbar and thoracic epidural blood patches. After each epidural blood patch, he improved remarkably; however, his pre-procedure clinical state relapsed after 1–2 weeks each time.

Because his leak was ventral and extensive and multiple EBPs did not result in durable improvement, digital subtraction myelography was carried out. This revealed a ventral CSF leak at the level of the thoracic 2–3 disc space. The patient underwent an uneventful thoracic laminectomy with transdural repair of a ventral dural rent. Postoperatively, the patient's symptoms gradually resolved over a 2-day period, and he has remained symptom-free during 1 year of follow-up.

35.5 Definition of Headache Attributed to Low Cerebrospinal Fluid Pressure

The International Classification of Headache Disorders, 3rd edition, beta version [Cephalalgia 2013; 33:629–808] describes "headache attributed to low cerebrospinal fluid pressure" under categories of those occurring following a lumbar dural puncture, after iatrogenic or traumatic event, or those occurring spontaneously. In each of these categories, the hallmark of headache that changes with position is noted. The criteria refer to low CSF pressure of <60 mm H_2O or imaging evidence of CSF leak in spontaneous or traumatic cases as well as iatrogenic cases other than the post-LP situation.

Proposed *diagnostic criteria* for headache due to *spontaneous* intracranial hypotension published in 2011 consist of:

A. Orthostatic headache
B. The presence of *at least one* of the following:

   Low opening pressure ($\leq$60 mm H_2O)
   Sustained improvement of symptoms after epidural blood patching
   Demonstration of an active spinal cerebrospinal fluid leak
   Cranial magnetic resonance imaging changes of intracranial hypotension (e.g., brain sagging or pachymeningeal enhancement)

C. No recent history of dural puncture
D. Not attributable to another disorder

35.6 Brief General Information

Intracranial hypotension from spontaneous spinal CSF leaking is an important cause of headache that can result in significant disability. The prevalence has not been well studied; however, a retrospective study of an urban emergency room found this diagnosis at half the frequency as subarachnoid hemorrhage. The diagnosis should be considered on the basis of clinical presentation. An underlying weakness of the spinal dura is often found, with a significant proportion of patients meeting diagnostic criteria for heritable disorders of connective tissue. A subset of these patients is at risk of vascular complications as well.

Cranial MRI will reveal one or more of the typical findings in 80 % of cases. CT myelography, MR myelography, and digital subtraction myelography are the imaging modalities of choice to identify the spinal CSF leak.

Treatments for spinal CSF leaking vary from conservative to surgical procedures. The specific situation will dictate the course of action.

Conservative care includes bed rest, oral and IV hydration, oral and IV caffeine, and use of an abdominal binder. Steroids are not recommended despite some reports of short-term benefit.

Epidural blood patching (EBP) with autologous blood is the standard initial procedure for most patients seeking treatment. This can be directed at the level of leaking or nondirected (placed at lumbar or thoracolumbar locations) when leak site has not yet been localized or for diagnostic purposes. Volumes range from small (10 mL) to large (100 mL), but usually a small volume of 10–20 mL is used for the first EBP. In patients that do not respond or respond but have relapsing symptoms, a larger-volume EBP is recommended. We usually perform larger-volume patching at 2 levels: both the thoracolumbar junction and lower lumbar level. The volume of blood varies based on the patient's anatomy and is limited mainly by local pain or radicular pain. Some patients require several EBPs.

Epidural patching with fibrin sealant is usually X-ray or occasionally CT guided to specific confirmed or suspected leak location(s).

In patients who have failed repeated EBPs and the leak has not been localized, an infusion of saline into the epidural space may offer symptomatic benefit. We have a small cohort of patients who have an implanted epidural PORT-A-CATH for regular infusions of saline.

Surgical repairs are used when simpler measures fail and symptom severity warrants intervention. Because the anatomy and location of spinal CSF leaks may not be simple, they are not always technically straightforward to repair. The specific procedure is tailored to the individual.

Complications of intracranial hypotension include subdural hematomas; cerebral venous sinus thrombosis, as well as a range of cranial nerve palsies; and more rarely cerebellar infarction, dementia, stupor and coma, and death. Patients with ongoing spinal CSF leaking for months or years can develop neuroendocrine dysfunction which would be expected to correct with successful treatment, although this has not been well studied to date. Secondary POTS may develop.

Rebound intracranial hypertension following successful treatment is not uncommon but is usually self-limited. CSF production appears to be upregulated in response to intracranial hypotension; this may take some time to normalize after treatment. It may require treatment for a period of weeks or months, most commonly with acetazolamide.

Prognosis is generally favorable; however, the subset of patients with normal cranial MRI at diagnosis tends to have a poorer prognosis. In those with successful treatment, recurrences in both the short term and long term do occur.

Key Points About Headache Due to Intracranial Hypotension

- Intracranial hypotension may be iatrogenic, traumatic, or spontaneous.
- Headache is usually but not always orthostatic; the orthostatic nature of the headache often diminishes with time; headache may even be absent.
- Headache may be the first presenting symptom of a heritable disorder of connective tissue; a subset of patients may have vascular involvement.
- Misdiagnosis and delayed diagnosis are common.
- Negative cranial or spinal imaging does not rule out spinal CSF leaking.
- Degree of disability is often underestimated.
- Intracranial hypotension results from cranial CSF leaks only rarely.

Key Points About Imaging

Cranial MRI findings – *mnemonic SEEPS* – findings evident in 80 %:

*S*ubdural fluid collections
*E*nhancement of pachymeninges
*E*ngorgement of venous structures
*P*ituitary hyperemia
*S*agging of the brain

Spinal MRI with/without myelographic sequencing – findings:

- Meningeal enhancement
- Meningeal diverticula
- Extrathecal fluid collections
- Dilated epidural or intradural veins

CT myelography (dynamic, early, or delayed) – findings:

- Meningeal diverticula
- Nerve root sleeve dilatations
- Extrathecal contrast

Digital subtraction myelography – helpful in visualizing leaks in three situations:

- Rapid and/or extensive leaks seen on other imaging but without precise localization
- Leaks that are anterior to the spinal cord
- CSF-Venous Fistula leaks that drain from the thecal sac into epidural veins

Connective Tissue Spectrum Abnormalities Associated with Spinal CSF Leaks

Reported heritable disorders of connective tissue (HDCT):

- Marfan syndrome
- Ehlers-Danlos, joint hypermobility type
- Ehlers-Danlos, classic type
- Unclassified heritable disorders of connective tissue

Other associated diagnoses:

- Autosomal dominant polycystic kidney disease
- Meningeal diverticula (as isolated finding)

Clinical stigmata of heritable disorders of connective tissue:

Joint hypermobility, joint dislocations, degenerative joint disease, tall stature, arachnodactyly, high-arched palate, skin hyperelasticity, soft/thin/transparent skin, easy bruising, slow wound healing, widened/thin scars, blue/gray sclera, lens dislocation (personal or family history), retinal detachment, scoliosis, flat feet, aortic or other arterial aneurysms (personal or family history), bicuspid aortic valve, mitral valve prolapse, spontaneous pneumothorax

Suggested Reading

1. Hoxworth JM, Trentman TL, Kotsenas AL, Thielen KR, Nelson KD, Dodick DW (2012) The role of digital subtraction myelography in the diagnosis and localization of spontaneous spinal CSF leaks. Am J Roentgenol 199:649–653
2. Mokri B (2014) Spontaneous CSF leaks: low CSF volume syndromes. Neurol clin 32:397–422
3. Schievink WI, Moser FG, Maya MM (2014) CSF-Venous fistula in spontaneous intracranial hypotension. Neurology 20 [Epub ahead of print]
4. Luetmer PH, Schwartz KM, Eckel LJ, Hunt CH, Carter RE, Diehn FE (2012) When should I do dynamic CT myelography? Predicting fast spinal CSF leaks in patients with spontaneous intracranial hypotension. AJNR Am J Neuroradiol 33:690–694
5. Mokri B (2013) Spontaneous Low pressure, Low CSF volume headaches: spontaneous CSF leaks. Headache 53:1034–1053
6. Mokri B, Low PA (2003) Orthostatic headaches without CSF leak in postural orthostatic tachycardia syndrome. Neurology 61:980–982
7. Reinstein E, Pariani M, Bannykh S, Rimoin DL, Schievink WI (2013) Connective tissue spectrum abnormalities associated with spontaneous cerebrospinal fluid leaks: a prospective study. Eur J Hum Genet 21:386–390
8. Schievink WI (2006) Spontaneous spinal cerebrospinal fluid leaks and intracranial hypotension. JAMA 295:2284–2296

9. Schievink WI (2013) Novel neuroimaging modalities in the evaluation of spontaneous cerebrospinal fluid leaks. Curr Neurol Neurosci Rep 13:358
10. Schievink WI, Dodick DW, Mokri B, Silberstein S, Bousser MG, Goadsby PJ (2011) Diagnostic criteria for headache due to spontaneous intracranial hypotension: a perspective. Headache 51:1442–1444
11. Schievink WI, Maya MM, Louy C (2005) Cranial MRI predicts outcome of spontaneous intracranial hypotension. Neurology 64:1282–1284
12. Schievink WI, Maya MM, Louy C, Moser FG, Tourje J (2008) Diagnostic criteria for spontaneous spinal CSF leaks and intracranial hypotension. AJNR Am J Neuroradiol 29:853–856
13. Schievink WI, Maya MM, Moser F, Tourje J, Torbati S (2007) Frequency of spontaneous intracranial hypotension in the emergency department. J Headache Pain 8(6):325–328
14. Schievink WI, Schwartz MS, Maya MM, Moser FG, Rozen TD (2012) Lack of causal association between spontaneous intracranial hypotension and cranial cerebrospinal fluid leaks. J Neurosurg 116:749–754
15. Chazen JL, Talbott JF, Lantos JE, Dillon WP (2014) MR Myelography for Identification of Spinal CSF Leak in Spontaneous Intracranial Hypotension. AJNR Am J Neuroradiol 22 [Epub ahead of print]

Chapter 36
Headache Attributed to Psychiatric Disorders

Maurice B. Vincent and Flávio Alheira

36.1 Case Description

A 14-year-old girl came to the office because of permanent and refractory headaches. She was symptom-free until the age of 12, when she started suffering from occasional headache attacks, some of them preceded by syncope. The first spell occurred at an airport toilet just prior to a family trip, during which no abnormality was present. However, attacks increased to 4–5 per week right after returning to town, precluding her from attending school. The present frequency of faints is around twice a month.

The headache was described as extremely intense, holocranial and pulsating, accompanied by nausea, photophobia and phonophobia. Short-lasting photopsias consisting of tiny flashing bright spots scattered throughout the entire visual field may be present on rare attacks, as well as paraesthesia at the right arm and motor aphasia. The headache frequency was initially low but became continuous 1 year ago. Symptoms included paroxysmal tremor in both legs, gait instability, hair loss, distractibility, fatigue, dysuria and diarrhoea (twice a month). She could not identify any trigger or aggravating factors. Menarche and thelarche occurred at the age of 11. Menses were all accompanied by excruciatingly severe dysmenorrhoea. She denied having sexual intercourses and drug abuse of any kind, except for prescribed medicines. Her mother referred occasional unilateral headaches, her grandmother had a history of depression, and an uncle from the father's side was crack and cannabis addicted.

Regardless the innumerable physicians she visited including neurologists, dentists, ophthalmologists and otorhinolaryngologists, the disease progressed all the same.

M.B. Vincent, MD, PhD (✉) • F. Alheira
Faculdade de Medicina, Hospital Universitário Clementino Fraga Filho,
Universidade Federal do Rio de Janeiro, Rio de Janeiro, Brazil
e-mail: vincent@ufrj.br

A. Siva, C. Lampl (eds.), *Case-Based Diagnosis and Management of Headache Disorders*, Headache, DOI 10.1007/978-3-319-06886-2_36

Several MRI and CT scans, a lumbar puncture, tilt-table testing, ECG and blood samples were normal. She missed school for 6 months because of the pain and was admitted on several occasions to different hospitals for up to once a week. Her parents showed a list of 32 medicines used either alone or in combination to reduce pain. For the last 6 months, she was under 1,000 mg divalproate together with 10 mg atenolol, 40 mg amitriptyline, 2.5 mg tizaninide, 5 mg flunarizine, 20 mg pyridoxine, 20 mg riboflavin, 100 mg tryptophan, 100 mg coenzyme Q_{10} and 150 mg feverfew on a daily basis, with a combination of naratriptan, domperidone and celecoxib as acute medicines. Her general and neurological examinations were normal. The blood pressure was 100/70 mmHg and the heart rate was 72 bpm.

Despite the fact that she considered her life miserable, the pain unbearable and the medications hopeless, she was particularly unconcerned during the interview. It became obvious that the triviality in her speech and behaviour were completely incompatible with the seriousness of her disease. In a second interview she admitted that, simultaneously with the beginning of her symptoms, the family was "forced" to move due to an accident suffered by her father. "Because of that, he could no longer take care of a house with a backyard and garden", she said. Since she loved her house, school, friends and the neighbourhood, she "became enraged but had no courage to tell anyone". When asked why she did not share her feelings with her family, she answered, "it was not fair with my father, it was not his fault after all". She then tried to deliberately boycott the school but "did not succeed having marks low enough to get held back". However, because of the excessive nonattendances, she had to change to a new school. During holidays the symptoms always tend to decrease almost completely, the maximum severity occurring at the start of a new school term.

36.2 Differential Diagnosis and How to Work Up Such a Patient

The case history represents the most relevant source of information for headache diagnosis, and this patient is no exception. First, distinguishing between a primary and a secondary disorder is mandatory. The age of onset, normal physical examination, innocuous previous neuroimaging and lack of red flags are the four elements that strongly indicate the presence of a primary headache in this case. Second, the clinical profile must be analysed for a proper diagnosis. Are there features that suggest a particular primary headache? The diagnoses of migraine without aura, migraine with aura and chronic migraine are possible, but a headache diagnosis does not rule out other concomitant disorders.

Considering the faints, signs and symptoms allowing the distinction between seizure, vertigo and vestibular dysfunctions must be investigated. The clinical picture usually suffices for the diagnosis. Seizures may involve suddenness, jerks, postictal confusion, incontinence, lateral tongue bites and slow recovery. Vertigo is characterized by a feeling that surroundings are turning or spinning, which tends to aggravate with head movements. Syncope has a more gradual onset as compared with seizure, tends to last less and has a quicker recovery and may occur at upright position, not infrequently at the bathroom. The physical examination must include blood pressure and heart rate in supine, sitting and standing positions and careful examination of eye movements and eyelids, vestibuloocular reflexes and vestibulospinal reflexes. A tilt-table test, an ECG and a cardiological workup are necessary. The possibility of psychogenic syncope is considered if no cause is found. Some migraine patients are particularly prone to syncope without any other precipitating factor.

Her absolute lack of concern was clearly out of proportion considering the impact of her disease. In addition, symptoms did not occur during holidays and became apparent after her father's accident. She deliberately tried to fail at school and admitted she could not cope with the new life. This psychological context allows the possibility of a somatization disorder.

To address possible psychological aspects in a headache case, three points must be investigated in particular:

1. Circumstances during the disease onset: are there external elements (familial, academic, professional, environmental, emotional) that could play a role in the case?
2. Situations clearly related with both aggravation and amelioration of the symptoms: does the clinical picture vary with psychological influences to a great extent?
3. Patient's behaviour, expectations and concerns: are they compatible with the impact produced by the disease?

In the ancient "somatization" hypothesis, a mental disorder would manifest as somatic symptoms, a concept that seems to be too simplistic. Diagnoses should not be considered mutually exclusive; on the contrary, the presence of migraine in this case does not rule out a concomitant psychogenic headache.

Formally considered as *somatic symptom disorder, with predominant pain* according to the DSM-5, this diagnosis depends on clinical suspicion, as no biomarker is available. The question remains as whether there is a superimposed somatic disorder or the headache is entirely migrainous in nature but with a significant psychological influence, as in the DSM-5 *psychological factors affecting other medical conditions*. Although the close association between the psychological factors and the change in the course of the known migraine condition supports the second possibility, in favour of the first is the presence of other somatic symptoms.

36.3 Diagnostic Workup of the Case

This patient underwent a series of unnecessary MRI and CT scans. In somatoform disorders, repetitive diagnostic testing is common. In a similar case, the ultimate procedure will always be the clinical exam. Not infrequently, collecting a comprehensive history at a second moment, as we did, will provide the essential information required for the diagnosis.

The three most relevant aspects in this case were the following:

1. The change in her environment and the accident suffered by her father were concomitant with the headache onset. She admitted great discomfort with her new life.
2. The clinical picture varied in close relation with her academic activities, disappearing during holidays and increasing at the beginning of a new term.
3. Her behaviour was out of proportion considering the constant migraine and its impact on her life.

The lack of a proper psychological diagnosis leads to the excess of medicines and procedures undertaken by such patients. In refractory headaches, changing or combining medicines just because they had not been tried have very little chance to be beneficial. Treatments must be chosen based on logical decisions motivated by the diagnosis, previous medical records and personal restrictions. This patient was prescribed escitalopram and recommended to psychotherapy.

36.4 Summary of the Case

A 14-year-old girl with a refractory migrainous headache came to the office with a 1-year history of continuous headache, syncope-like episodes, tremor in both legs, excruciating menstrual cramps, lack of concentration, fatigue, dysuria, diarrhoea and dysmenorrhoea. The clinical examination was normal, so were the neuroimaging and other supplementary exams. The headache was absolutely irresponsive to all treatments tried so far. The interview disclosed three aspects suggesting a clear psychogenic motivation for the development/ worsening of the headache. First, the symptoms started in close relation with a moving to a new neighbourhood and school. Second, the headache would not occur during holidays. Third, her absolute neutrality during the interview was not in agreement with the seriousness of her disease. The plethora of concomitant symptoms, the impossibility of dealing with her personal emotions and the normality of the clinical investigations led to the diagnosis of psychogenic headache.

36.5 Definition of Psychogenic Headache

Apart from migraine, according to the International Classification of Headache Disorders (ICHD-3), the possible diagnosis for this patient is listed in item 12.1, *headache attributed to somatization disorder*. When a pre-existing headache becomes chronic or worse in close temporal relation to a psychiatric disorder, both the initial headache diagnosis and a diagnosis of headache attributed to psychiatric disorder should be given. For a headache attributed to somatization disorder, evidence of causation must be demonstrated by at least one of the following:

(a) The headache parallels the development of other somatic symptoms attributed to somatization disorder.
(b) There is constant or remitting headache that parallels the fluctuation of other somatic symptoms attributed to somatization disorder.
(c) The headache vanishes in parallel with remission of the other somatic symptoms.

For the somatization disorder, both the following items are required according to the International Headache Society (IHS):

1. Multiple physical symptoms with onset before age 30 years not fully explained by a known medical condition or in excess of what would be expected for that medical condition
2. Four or more pain symptoms from four different sites or functions; at least two gastrointestinal symptoms other than pain; at least one sexual symptom other than pain; and a pseudoneurological symptom not limited to pain such as impaired balance, incoordination, weakness, aphonia, etc.

36.6 Brief General Information

Identifying and classifying psychogenic headaches is not an easy task. The influence of psychological factors in headache practice should not be overlooked and may be far more important than generally suspected. First, the diagnosis depends mostly on clinical judgement and is therefore subjective to some extent. Second, the epidemiology, pathophysiology and comorbidities of primary headaches are not completely understood. The simple coexistence of headache and psychiatric disorders such as depression and anxiety is no proof of a causal relationship. Third, the neurobiology of somatic symptom disorders and its implications on the realm of primary headaches is open for future research. SPECT studies have shown hypoperfusion in the frontal, prefrontal, temporoparietal and cerebellar areas in somatization disorders. As a general rule for the attending physician, the best position to deal with headaches is to always examine the subject with great interest in the person who has a disease and not only in the disease that the person has.

Suggested Reading

1. Borkum JM (2010) Chronic headaches and the neurobiology of somatization. Curr Pain Headache Rep 14(1):55–61
2. Curfman D, Chilungu M, Daroff RB, Alshekhlee A, Chelimsky G, Chelimsky TC (2012) Syncopal migraine. Clin Auton Res 22(1):17–23

3. Dimsdale JE, Levenson J (2013) What's next for somatic symptom disorder? Am J Psychiatry 170(12):1393–1395
4. Gambini O, Islam L, Demartini B, Scarone S (2010) Psychiatric issues in patients with headaches. Neurol Sci 31(Suppl 1):S111–S113
5. Garcia-Campayo J, Fayed N, Serrano-Blanco A, Roca M (2009) Brain dysfunction behind functional symptoms: neuroimaging and somatoform, conversive, and dissociative disorders. Curr Opin Psychiatry 22(2):224–231
6. Golferini F, Facchin P, Cavinato M, Lovison L, Pitassi I, Battistella PA (1988) Diagnostic factors in pediatric primary headache. J Clin Epidemiol 41(1):27–33
7. Mayou R, Kirmayer LJ, Simon G, Kroenke K, Sharpe M (2005) Somatoform disorders: time for a new approach in DSM-V. Am J Psychiatry 162(5):847–855
8. Radat F, Milowska D, Valade D (2011) Headaches secondary to psychiatric disorders (HSPD): a retrospective study of 87 patients. Headache 51(5):789–795
9. Stone J, Evans RW (2011) Functional/psychogenic neurological symptoms and headache. Headache 51(5):781–788

Chapter 37
Headache Attributed to Somatization Disorders: Is It Tension-Type Headache, Is It "Somatization Headache," or Both?

Ugur Uygunoglu and Aksel Siva

37.1 Case Description

A 51-year-old woman working as a financial consultant was admitted to our headache outpatient clinic with a complaint of continuous headache for 2 years. She described the characteristics of her headache as a heavy sensation and pressure involving the whole head. The severity was mild to moderate and she did not describe worsening with physical activity. When said there were no accompanying symptoms such as nausea, vomiting, and/or photo-phonophobia. She was taking painkiller pills containing metamizole sodium 500 mg 4–6 times per month, each time one or two tablets without any significant benefit.

Before admission to our center, she visited many neurologists, by most of whom she was told to have some kind of a tension-type headache. Also a number of other physicians came up with several other diagnoses. Several antidepressants, mostly selective serotonin reuptake inhibitors, were prescribed as preventive treatment. However, most of these drugs had either caused side effects, preventing her to continue the treatment, or were ineffective. Consequently, she discontinued all long-term preventive treatments for her headache.

She emphasized that the onset of her headache was associated with a lawsuit while she had been working as a manager in a foundation company, and the severity of her headache increased in every inquiry. She also mentioned that her headache starts when she considers that she could not adequately express herself. Interestingly, abdominal, chest, and back pain also accompanies the headache simultaneously.

Her past history was significant for either headache or back pain or both since university years, worsening or improving at different times in her life. She received different diagnoses for this painful syndrome. However, over the years despite

U. Uygunoglu, MD (✉) • A. Siva, MD
Department of Neurology, Cerrahpasa School of Medicine,
Istanbul University, Istanbul, Turkey
e-mail: akselsiva@gmail.com

A. Siva, C. Lampl (eds.), *Case-Based Diagnosis and Management of Headache Disorders*, Headache, DOI 10.1007/978-3-319-06886-2_37

extensive investigations, no associated underlying organic disorder or disease could be found. She was also referred to internal medicine because of gastrointestinal symptoms such as abdominal pain, nausea, and dyspepsia. She received a diagnosis of gastritis, but endoscopic study did not reveal any significant abnormality. Her neurological examination was normal. Cranial magnetic resonance imaging did not reveal any abnormality. She was on valsartan hydrochlorothiazide and amlodipine treatment for hypertension and insulin and oral antidiabetics for diabetes mellitus. She has no known allergies. She is the second of five siblings, and there is no remarkable medical history in others with the exception of an elder brother who recently had an episode consistent with transient global amnesia. Her mother died because of breast cancer, and she reported dying of her father at old age. She does not smoke and does not use alcohol regularly.

In her physical examination, there was tenderness bilaterally in the regions of the great occipital nerve, upon which we performed bilateral great occipital nerve blockade with methylprednisolone and lidocaine 2 %. The patient's headache did not improve after this procedure.

We referred the patient for a psychological evaluation because of the strong relationship between the onset and worsening of her headache with stressful events. The psychiatrist's impression was that she had a somatoform disorder and passive aggressive behavior disorder according to DSM-IV criteria. He suggested behavioral psychotherapy for treatment. Currently she continues her psychotherapy and her headaches improved greatly.

Key Points

- Headache can present as a somatic symptom of depression and/or generalized anxiety disorder. The features of headache may be suggestive of tension-type headache (TTH), and when the psychiatric background is not explored, the patient may receive a diagnosis of primary TTH – and the underlying psychiatric disorder, of which the headache is only one of its somatic symptoms, may be easily missed!
- Considering that the criteria for "TTH" consist of a non-throbbing, nonsevere headache with no lateralization, which shows no worsening with physical activity and not accompanied by nausea or vomiting and finally none or one of photophobia and phonophobia, then most nonmigraine headaches of long duration may be easily diagnosed as TTH.
- Although that a headache, which may be related to "a somatoform disorder," may have features of migraine and/or tension-type headache, it will not be consistent with the full criteria of episodic migraine or episodic TT. However, it may be difficult to differentiate it from the primary headache disorder when it may be a comorbid problem occurring in the setting of chronic migraine or chronic TTH.

- According to ICHD-3 beta, when a preexisting headache with the characteristics of a primary headache disorder such as migraine or TTH becomes chronic or worsens significantly in close temporal relation to a psychiatric disorder, both the initial primary headache diagnosis and a diagnosis of "12. Headache attributed to psychiatric disorder" should be coded once the causal relationship can be confirmed.
- Epidemiological data are suggestive that headache and psychiatric disorders occur together at frequencies higher than would be expected by chance.

37.2 Definition of Somatization Disorder

According to the DSM-IV criteria, which is currently accepted by ICHD-3, *somatization disorder* is defined as a chronic disorder characterized by a history of many physical complaints beginning before age 30 years that occur over a period of several years and result in treatment being sought or significant impairment of functioning. Physical symptoms must include 4 pain symptoms, 2 gastrointestinal symptoms, 1 sexual symptom, and 1 pseudo-neurological symptom, and these symptoms should not to be attributed to any medical condition. However, in the DSM-V, the new DSM version which was published in 2013, diagnoses of somatization disorder, hypochondriasis, pain disorder, and undifferentiated somatoform disorder were deleted, and "somatoform disorders" are now called *somatic symptom and related disorders*.

Somatic symptoms include stomach pain, back pain, extremity pain, menstrual problems (female), sexual problems, headaches, chest pain, dizziness, fainting, palpitations, dyspnea, bowel problems, nausea, indigestion, fatigue, and insomnia. The occurrence of these somatic symptoms tends to increase by chronification of headache regardless of the type of headache, and also patients who have frequent severe attacks have more somatic symptoms than patients with infrequent attacks. Besides these observations, it has been emphasized that psychiatric comorbidity shows a significant impact on the occurrence of somatic complaints.

It is still controversial whether *headache attributed to somatization disorder* is due to a psychiatric disorder or as a result of bioorganic cause. The interaction of cognitive and perceptual processes with behavioral, affective, and biological changes has been considered as the main factor of somatic symptoms by authors arguing biological process. Based on signal-filtering model, somatoform disorders can be understood as disorders in the perception of bodily signals. These (mis)perceptions may be explained by this model. In signal-filtering model of somatoform disorders, possible psychobiological and psychological influences are grouped to signal amplifying (over-arousal, distress, chronic hypothalamic-pituitary-adrenal axis, physical deconditioning, sensitization) and signal filtering (selective attention, infections, anxiety, depressive mood, lacking distraction). In addition to signal-filtering model, although there is still lack of adequate evidence, the endocrine system, immunological system, monamino acid neurotransmitters and the involvement of the nucleus caudatus have been suggested to play a role in developing somatoform symptoms.

Pennebaker's model revealed the relationship between intensity of physiological signals and severity of somatoform symptoms through the method of distractibility, which was also supported with showing the reduced activation of pain-relevant cerebral structures by functional magnetic resonance imaging. These findings may explain the benefit of exercise, biofeedback, relaxation, and cognitive-behavioral treatments in somatization disorder.

37.3 When to Suspect "Somatization Headache" (or "Headache Attributed to Psychiatric Disorders")?

- When the headache is closely related to stressful life events, onset and/or worsening under psychogenic influence.
- When headache is the main and presenting symptom and cannot be attributed to an either primary or secondary headache disorder other than a primary psychiatric disorder, of which a causal relationship is clear.
- When facial impression and mimics are suggestive of apprehensiveness.
- At least one of the following of other bodily symptoms is present, such as back and other nonspecific (nonorganic) pain disorders (including myofascial pain syndrome?), and/or gastrointestinal symptoms of long duration without underlying clear-cut GI disease.
- When asked, the patient reveals sexual dysfunction/dissatisfaction.
- Keep in mind that although "somatization headache" may be by itself the whole story (!), most of the time it will appear as comorbid "headache" type and/or will cause a worsening of the underlying primary headache disorder, mostly migraine or TTH. Not uncommonly there may be coexistent "depressive disorders" or "anxiety disorders," also another cause for considering a plus-diagnosis, once noticed.
- When a diagnosis of "depressive disorders" or "anxiety disorders" according to DSM-IV (or preferably by the new DSM-V criteria) is made as the primary psychiatric disorder, the presence of headache may be attributed to "coded as ICHD-3 beta – A12 Headache attributed to psychiatric disorders" as listed in ICHD-3 beta and in its appendix section, once all other primary and secondary headache disorders are excluded.
- However, not all individuals with headaches, which may be diagnosed as "headache attributed to somatization disorder," may have all the bodily symptoms of somatization. This should not force the physician to exclude that diagnosis in daily clinical practice.

37.4 A Critical Comment on What TTH Is and What It Is Not: ICHD Criteria?

What is TTH?

A headache with at least two of the following four elements:

- Non-throbbing
- Nonsevere
- Nonlateralizing
- Not worsening with physical activity and one of these two criteria:
  - Not accompanied by nausea or vomiting
  - None or one of photophobia and phonophobia

Practically according to the TTH criteria, when read the other way around, TTH is based on a number of "no" answers as above, which in turn may be interpreted as all primary headaches that are not migraine (and cluster and trigeminal autonomic cephalalgias (TACs)) are likely to be diagnosed as (erroneously) TTH.

Not all episodic/chronic TTH are primary – in many other conditions and disorders, the features of the headache may be suggestive of TTH. It should be kept in mind that in many psychiatric disorders, "headache" may be in fact one of the somatic symptoms of the underlying problem, hence being "secondary episodic (or chronic) TTH."

37.5 Treatment of Somatization Disorders

Most of the patients with somatoform disorders have multiple and persistent complaints causing difficulties for treatment. Predisposing, precipitating, and maintaining factors for somatoform pains have to be well determined before starting treatment. Treatment strategies in somatoform pain consist in pharmacological and non-pharmacological approaches. Antidepressants including tricyclics particularly constitute pharmacological treatment. Cognitive and behavioral approaches are the mainstay of non-pharmacological therapies and show superiority to pharmacological treatment. Early recognition of somatoform pain and starting treatment immediately prevent the chronification of disease and provide prominent efficacy.

37.6 Comments

Although headache attributed to somatization disorder was classified in ICHD-2 and ICHD-3 (beta version) as a distinct entity, it is difficult to differentiate the type of headache in patients not fulfilling whole criteria of somatoform pain with comorbid psychiatric disorders. International Headache Society (IHS would probably add new diagnoses such as anxiety disorder or depression in "headache attributed to psychiatric disorders" to avoid confusion regarding with headache attributed to somatization disorder.

Another diagnosis associated with a psychiatric condition which can be found in the ICHD-3 beta version is "A12.2 Headache attributed to psychotic disorder." This headache is described when headache is considered as a manifestation of a delusion whose content involves a mechanism that the patient believes explains the headache, such as headache being the result of a device implanted in the head by aliens.

Key Points on Somatization

- Expression of intrapsychic conflicts or emotional problems with bodily symptoms or signs.
- Somatization is a coping behavior.
- We all somatize, to a certain extent. It is not the rule for somatization to be always associated with a psychiatric disorder.
- Common neurological somatoform symptoms:
  - Headache
  - Atypical facial pain
  - Low back pain
  - Dizziness
  - Paresthesias

37.7 What About Other Psychiatric Disorders and Headache?

The association between headaches and a number of various psychiatric disorders (listed below) is discussed in the appendix section of ICHD-3 beta. As the evidence of a causal relationship is considered relatively weak for most of these listed psychiatric disorders, it is emphasized that a special caution should be paid before a diagnosis of headache attributed to any of them is made. In order to reach such a diagnosis, a causal relationship between the headache and the psychiatric disorder in question (as listed below) should be confirmed either by showing that the headache onset occurs simultaneously with that psychiatric disorder or the headache clearly worsens after the psychiatric condition becomes evident. One other diagnostic criterion is that the headache should not be attributed to any other ICHD-3 diagnosis.

List of other headaches that may be attributed to other psychiatric disorders – ICHD-3 beta addendum:

A12 Headache attributed to psychiatric disorder
A12.3 Headache attributed to depressive disorder
A12.4 Headache attributed to separation anxiety disorder
A12.5 Headache attributed to panic disorder
A12.6 Headache attributed to specific phobia
A12.7 Headache attributed to social anxiety disorder (social phobia)
A12.8 Headache attributed to generalized anxiety disorder
A12.9 Headache attributed to posttraumatic stress disorder
A12.10 Headache attributed to acute stress disorder

37.8 What About Fibromyalgia Syndrome and Somatization Disorders?

One other differential diagnosis to be considered in individuals with probable somatization disorder is "fibromyalgia," another disorder in question. Depending on the diagnostic criteria used, the prevalence of fibromyalgia is up to 8 % of the population. According to the American College of Rheumatology, the original diagnostic criteria for fibromyalgia syndrome (FMS) depended on the presence of chronic widespread pain with a number of demonstrable tender points (1990). However, in a more recent revised version, six self-reported symptoms such as impaired sleep, fatigue, poor cognition, headaches, depression, and abdominal pain were included. Although pain with palpation is the main symptom in FMS, headache, fatigue, disturbed sleep, anxiety, depression, irritable bowel syndrome, concentration or memory problems, and numbness/tingling sensations may be seen, and most of these symptoms overlap with the symptoms of somatization disorder. Emotional factors are the most relevant factor of worsening of symptoms alike to somatization disorder.

Whether FMS is a centralized pain state as a result of pain amplification of central nervous system origin is not clear. On the other hand, psychological, behavioral, and social issues as well as genetic factors all have been implicated to contribute to the pathogenesis of fibromyalgia.

Patients developing fibromyalgia commonly have lifelong histories of chronic pain throughout their body, including headache and regional pain syndromes. These individuals are more likely to have psychiatric disorders, including depression, anxiety, obsessive-compulsive disorder, and posttraumatic stress disorder, necessitating to obtain a careful and detailed history in order not to miss comorbid problems. As rheumatologic disorders also have been reported to be seen in 10–30 % of people who complies with the criteria of FMS, these disorders also should be ruled out when a diagnosis of FMS is considered.

In conclusion, FMS is a purely clinical diagnosis that should also be included in patients with headache who report widespread chronic pain and somatoform symptoms.

Suggested Reading

1. American Psychiatric Association (1994) Diagnostic and statistical manual of mental disorders: DSM-IV, 4th edn. American Psychiatric Association, Washington, DC
2. American Psychiatric Association (2013) Diagnostic and statistical manual of mental disorders: DSM-V, 5th edn. American Psychiatric Association, Washington, DC
3. Bantick SJ, Wise RG, Ploghaus A, Clare S, Smith SM, Tracey I (2002) Imaging how attention modulates pain in humans using functional MRI. Brain 125(Pt 2):310–319
4. Clauw JD (2014) Fibromyalgia: a clinical review. JAMA 311(15):1547–1555
5. Headache Classification Committee of the International Headache Society (IHS) (2013) The international classification of headache disorders, 3rd. Edition (beta version). Cephalalgia 33:627–808
6. Henningsen P, Zipfel S, Herzog W (2007) Management of functional somatic syndromes. Lancet 369(9565):946–955
7. Maizels M, Burchette R (2004) Somatic symptoms in headache patients: the influence of headache diagnosis, frequency, and comorbidity. Headache 44(10):983–993
8. Pennebaker JW, Gonder-Frederick L, Stewart H, Elfman L, Skelton JA (1982) Physical symptoms associated with blood pressure. Psychophysiology 19(2):201–210
9. Rief W, Barsky AJ (2005) Psychobiological perspectives on somatoform disorders. Psychoneuroendocrinology 30(10):996–1002
10. Wolfe F, Clauw DJ, Fitzcharles MA et al (2011) Fibromyalgia criteria and severity scales for clinical and epidemiological studies: a modification of the ACR preliminary diagnostic criteria for fibromyalgia. J Rheumatol 38(6):1113–1122

Chapter 38
Trigeminal Neuralgia

Ivan Milanov and Vesselina Grozeva

38.1 Case Description

A 45-year-old woman was referred to our clinic with a 5-year history of intermittent trigeminal neuralgic pain in the area of the right ophthalmic branch (V1) of the fifth cranial nerve. The pain had started suddenly one afternoon without any reasonable explanation. The patient experienced severe, sharp, sometimes shock-like, electrical, right-sided orbital/periorbital pain, coming in brief episodes of 2–4 s. The pain occurred spontaneously, sometimes 40–50 times a day but could be triggered also by touching the forehead and by wind across the face. She was completely pain-free between the episodes. There were no autonomic symptoms associated with the attacks. The intensity of her pain was 7–8/10, according to the visual analog scale (VAS).

She could differentiate bouts lasting from 5 to 9 months and remission periods of 3–5 months.

She did not have any past medical history. A differential diagnosis including diseases such as multiple sclerosis, vasculitis, hypertension, diabetes, stroke, head trauma, or other pain disorders was ruled out. Family history was negative for neurological disorders or vasculopathy. Carbamazepine 600 mg/daily was the only medicine she was taking. It was controlling the pain well for the past 4 years, without any side effects.

Nevertheless, the characteristic of her attacks changed during the last year, which was the reason why she was referred to our department. She started experiencing attacks with higher pain intensity (9–10/10 VAS), some of them accompanied by tearing of the right eye. No other additional autonomic symptoms such as eye redness,

I. Milanov, MD, PhD, DSc (✉) • V. Grozeva, MD
Department of Neurology, Medical University – Sofia, Sofia, Bulgaria

Headache Department, University Neurological Hospital "St. Naum" 1, Lyuben Russev Str., Sofia 1113, Bulgaria
e-mail: milanovivan54@gmail.com

A. Siva, C. Lampl (eds.), *Case-Based Diagnosis and Management of Headache Disorders*, Headache, DOI 10.1007/978-3-319-06886-2_38

ptosis, edema of the eyelid, or sweating of the forehead were reported. She did not have any pain-free periods during the last 12 months. General and neurological examination showed no deficits. Laboratory investigations revealed no abnormalities. Cranial magnetic resonance imaging (MRI) with and without contrast and arterial and venous MR angiography were normal.

38.2 Differential Diagnosis and How to Work Up This Kind of Patient

After excluding all the secondary causes for trigeminal neuralgia (TN) by neurological examination, brain imaging, and MR angiography, the next step was to make sure this was indeed a "classical" TN. The major differential diagnosis with the first branch of TN, especially when presenting with lacrimation, is the group of the trigeminal autonomic cephalalgias (TACs) (see Chap. 34) and the short-lasting unilateral neuralgiform headache attacks with conjunctival injection and tearing (SUNCT) in particular.

SUNCT syndrome resembles V1 trigeminal neuralgia in unilaterality of pain, triggering mechanisms, brevity, and frequency of attacks. Contrary to SUNCT, TN is slightly female predominant. TN occurs between 50 and 70 years, while the mean age of onset of SUNCT is 50, and our patient was 45. The pain in both disorders can have the same distribution, but the presence of accompanying ipsilateral vasomotor phenomena is not typical for TN. They both have a very short attack duration although V1-TN attacks are much shorter than those of SUNCT. TN attacks could last up to 30 s, but the attacks lasting 5 s or less predominate. SUNCT attacks last 10–20 s, and they present with full-blown autonomic features 1–2 s after onset of pain. In comparison to SUNCT, in V1-TN attacks, autonomic signs either appear occasionally or are present to a minor extent. In SUNCT, there is a lack of a therapeutic effect of carbamazepine, which is not the case with our patient.

The differential doubt arose with the change of clinical symptoms, when tearing accompanying some of the attacks with higher pain intensity had started. The following question was asked: "Should the lacrimation be considered as a part of our patient's V1-TN or a transformation of TN to SUNCT might have occurred?"

V1-N patients may report mild autonomic signs (usually lacrimation) that tend to appear during severe attacks and after suffering for years from headache, whereas SUNCT attacks are characterized by both conjunctival injection and lacrimation appearing in a dramatic and abrupt way from the onset of symptoms. We have not observed conjunctival injection, neither any other autonomic symptom such as nasal stuffiness, rhinorrhea, changes in pupil size, or palpebral width. Therefore, could we suggest that the V1 TN was following its natural course? According to some authors, V1 trigeminal neuralgia and SUNCT seem to represent two different disorders. Although, there are several reports that TN and a TAC may occur simultaneously or independently, always at the same side of the head. A large dispute exists whether or not these conditions are pathogenically distinct. Many cases of TN with lacrimation are described in the literature.

Table 38.1 Medicaments used for treatment of TN

Drug	Dosage	Adverse effects
Carbamazepine	200–1,200 mg daily (divided doses)	Nausea, drowsiness, fatigue, dizziness, memory problems, diplopia, nystagmus, liver dysfunction, hematosuppression
Oxcarbazepine	300–1,800 mg daily (2 divided doses)	Decreased blood sodium level, dizziness, fatigue, headache, tremor, drowsiness, diminished concentration, diplopia
Phenytoin	300–500 mg daily	Nystagmus, ataxia, slurred speech, decreased coordination, mental confusion
Lamotrigine	100–150 mg daily (2 divided doses; starting dose, 25 mg every other day for 6–8 days, dose is increased by 25–50 mg every 1–2 weeks)	Drowsiness, dizziness, headache, vertigo, rash, Stevens-Johnson syndrome
Gabapentin	1,200–3,600 mg daily (3 or 4 divided doses)	Fatigue, somnolence, dizziness, ataxia, nystagmus, and tremor
Topiramate	200–300 mg daily (2 divided doses)	Fatigue, nervousness, tremor, weight loss, difficulty with concentration/attention
Baclofen	5–80 mg daily (3 divided doses)	Transient drowsiness, dizziness, weakness, and fatigue

According to Goadsby, et al. 2001, TN and SUNCT should not be classified separately, because modest cranial parasympathetic activation can occur in any form of first division nociceptive activation, whether primary, such as in migraine, or secondary, such as experimental head pain or trigeminal neuralgia.

Based on the previous discussion, we accepted the primary diagnosis, “classical” TN. Carbamazepine was changed with oxcarbazepine 1,800 mg/daily. The patient responded well in the beginning, resulting in lowering the frequency of crises, diminishing their pain intensity and frequency of lacrimation. Our aim was to reduce pain and achieve symptomatic relief, for which carbamazepine and oxcarbazepine are shown to be the best option and first-line therapy. Effective treatment can be achieved also with other antiepileptic drugs (Table 38.1). We followed up the patient in the next 4 months in order to see if the course of the disease would change. It stayed more or less the same during this short period. Unfortunately, we lost contact with the patient afterwards.

38.3 Diagnostic Workup

The diagnosis of idiopathic or “classical” TN is based mainly on the clinical history of pain attacks according to the International Classification of Headache Disorders [ICHD, 3rd edition (beta version)] criteria, together with a neurological exam and imaging studies. Symptomatic or secondary TN has to be excluded on the first place. Thorough head and neck examination should be performed, ruling out any dysfunction of the cranial nerves. A special attention deserves not only the trigeminal nerve (V) but also the facial (VII) and vestibulocochlear nerve (VIII), which lie adjacent to the trigeminal nerve in the cerebellopontine angle (CPA). If a symptomatic TN with involvement of the CPA is present, a subtle facial weakness and hearing loss on that side will be found. Hemifacial spasm may also occur.

Diagnostic brain imaging should be part of the initial diagnostic algorithm of any patient with TN symptoms. Landmarks around the trigeminal ganglion and the CPA are visualized. Although a routine brain computer tomography (CT) scan is usually sufficient for screening for a CPA tumor, it may not show small tumors, and the examination carries an appreciable dose of ionizing radiation. MRI has better sensitivity in the detection of intracranial lesions and improved definition and avoids ionizing radiation. Some authors recommend MRI of patients with trigeminal neuralgia as a routine consideration during their assessment. MRI imaging often demonstrates MS plaques better and the anatomic relationships of the trigeminal root.

38.4 Summary of the Case

We describe a clinical case of a 45-year-old woman, presenting initially with a typical first branch trigeminal neuralgia, who after 4 years of onset, started experiencing lacrimation on the affected side during the most severe attacks. No other accompanying autonomic symptoms were observed. Neurological, laboratory, and imaging exams were all normal before and after lacrimation had occurred. She did not have any past medical history, neither positive family history for multiple sclerosis, vasculitis, hypertension, etc. Carbamazepine 600 mg/daily was controlling well the symptoms until the clinical presentation of her TN changed. The primary diagnosis of "classical" TN was questioned because of the appearance of autonomic features, typical for TACs. Finally, we accepted the fact that our patient's V1 TN was following its natural course, because mild autonomic signs like lacrimation may appear during severe attacks and after suffering for years from this disorder.

38.5 Definition According to the ICHD

TN causes sudden, usually unilateral, severe brief, sharp electric-shock type recurrent pains in the distribution of one or more branches of the trigeminal nerve. Pain attacks start and terminate abruptly, and they can be evoked by trivial stimuli. Around 60 % of the patients with TN have the mandibular division of the trigeminal nerve involved, V3-TN. Only 30 % of the patients present with V2-maxillary division involvement. And less than 5 % of the patients experience involvement of V1-ophthalmic branch.

38.6 Brief General Information

TN has an incidence of approximately 4/100,000. Although familial cases are reported, the majority of cases occur spontaneously, and TN does not appear to be more common in any ethnic group, geographic region, or climate. TN occurs in both genders, with a slight female predominance. TN is most common over the age of 50. TN may be idiopathic, "classical" (the majority of patients), or "symptomatic," secondary to another disease process affecting the trigeminal system. Although the underlying mechanism of TN remains partially unknown, the effects of direct stimulation by closely located blood vessels are the most common related abnormalities. Benign tumors and vascular anomalies that compress the trigeminal nerve root can produce symptoms clinically indistinguishable from classical TN. Injury to the nerve root is a suggested initiating factor in the disease. It has been reported that TN in younger patients can be due to MS (demyelination in the root entry zone, the pontine tract, or the nuclei), tumors, aneurysms, angiomas, or vascular malformations. Diabetes mellitus is also proven to be a causative factor for TN, for which family history and blood sugar levels should be examined. TN may result also from infarction of the root entry zone of the trigeminal nerve and pons.

Key Points

- V1 in involvement of the trigeminal nerve is the least common presentation of all types of classical TN.
- If TN is present with any autonomic symptom or with atypical duration of the attacks, it should be differentiated from TACs, especially SUNCT.
- Lacrimation, and less commonly conjunctival injection, can be observed during the most severe attacks in some patients with long history of TN.
- MRI should be performed to rule out all secondary causes, before setting the diagnosis "classical TN."
- Carbamazepine or oxcarbazepine response can be also useful as a diagnostic treatment test.

Suggested Reading

1. Bederson JB, Wilson CB (1989) Evaluation of microvascular decompression and partial sensory rhizotomy in 252 cases of trigeminal neuralgia. J Neurosurg 71:359–367
2. Benoliel R, Sharav Y (1998) Trigeminal neuralgia with lacrimation or SUNCT syndrome? Cephalalgia 18:85–90
3. Bracale C, Graziussi G, Avella F (1982) Familial essential trigeminal neuralgia. Riv Neurobiol 28:299–302
4. Braga FM, Bonatelli AP, Suriano I et al (1986) Familial trigeminal neuralgia. Surg Neurol 26:405–408

5. Coffey RJ, Fromm GH (1991) Familial trigeminal neuralgia and Charcot-Marie-Tooth neuropathy. Report of two families and review. Surg Neurol 35:49–53
6. Collier J (1922) Diseases of the nervous system. In: Price FW (ed) A textbook of the practice of medicine, 1st edn. Hodder and Stoughton, London
7. Dandy WE (1934) Concerning cause of trigeminal neuralgia. Am J Surg 24:447–455
8. Delitala A, Brunori A, Chiappetta F (1999) Trigeminal neuralgia resulting from infarction of the root entry zone of the trigeminal nerve: case report. Neurosurgery 45(1):202
9. Devor M, Amir R, Rappaport ZH (2002) Pathophysiology of trigeminal neuralgia: the ignition hypothesis. Clin J Pain 18:4–13
10. Fothergill J (1776) Of a painful affection of the face. Medical Society of London, London
11. Goadsby PJ, Matharu MS, Boes CJ (2001) SUNCT syndrome or trigeminal neuralgia with lacrimation. Cephalalgia 21(2):82–83
12. Goru SJ, Pemberton MN (2009) Trigeminal neuralgia: the role of magnetic resonance imaging. Br J Oral Maxillofac Surg 47(3):228–229. doi:10.1016/j.bjoms.2008.08.006, Epub 2008 Oct 19
13. Hannerz J (1993) Trigeminal neuralgia with chronic paroxysmal hemicrania: the CPH-tic syndrome. Cephalalgia 13:361–364
14. Kim JB, Yu S (2013) Neurological picture. Trigeminal neuralgia after pontine infarction affecting the ipsilateral trigeminal nerve. J Neurol Neurosurg Psychiatry 84(8):881–882. doi:10.1136/jnnp-2013-305024, Epub 2013 Mar 26
15. Lynch MA, Brightman VJ, Greenberg MS (1994) Chronic oral sensory disorders: pain and abnormalities of taste. In: Cohen GS, Brightman VJ (eds) Burket's oral medicine: diagnosis and treatment, 9th edn. Wilkins, Philadelphia, p 334
16. Mazoni GC, Torelli P (2005) Epidemiology of typical and atypical craniofacial neuralgias. Neurol Sci 26:65–67
17. Metzer WS (1991) Trigeminal neuralgia secondary to tumor with normal exam, responsive to carbamazepine. Headache 31:164–166
18. Moller AR (1991) The cranial nerve vascular compression syndrome: II. A review of pathophysiology. Acta Neurochir (Wien) 113:24–30
19. Okeson JP (2005) Neuralgias of the orofacial region. In: Harmon L (ed) Bell's orofacial pains: the clinical management of orofacial pain, 6th edn. Quintessence Publishing Co Inc, Illinois, p 114
20. Pareja JA, Barón M, Gili P et al (2002) Objective assessment of autonomic signs during triggered first division trigeminal neuralgia. Cephalalgia 22(4):251–255
21. Pareja JA, Cuadrado ML, Caminero AB et al (2005) Duration of attacks of first division trigeminal neuralgia. Cephalalgia 25(4):305–308
22. Pareja JA, Sjaastad O (1997) SUNCT syndrome. A clinical review. Headache 37:195–202
23. Puca A, Meglio M (1993) Typical trigeminal neuralgia associated with posterior cranial fossa tumors. Ital J Neurol Sci 14:549–552
24. Ransohoff J (1969) Surgical treatment of trigeminal neuralgia current status (in memory of Byron Stookey, MD). Headache 9:20–26
25. Sjaastad O, Kruszewski P (1992) Trigeminal neuralgia and 'SUNCT' syndrome: similarities and differences in the clinical pictures. An overview. Funct Neurol 7:103–107
26. Sjaastad O, Pareja JA, Zukerman E et al (1997) Trigeminal neuralgia. Clinical manifestations of first division involvement. Headache 37:346–357
27. Sjaastad O, Saunte C, Salvesen R et al (1989) Shortlasting unilateral neuralgiform headache attacks with conjunctival injection, tearing, sweating, and rhinorrhea. Cephalalgia 9:147–156
28. Sjaastad O, Zhao JM, Kruszewski P et al (1991) Short-lasting unilateral neuralgiform headache attacks with conjunctival injection, tearing, etc. (SUNCT): 111. Another Norwegian case. Headache 31:175–177

29. Headache Classification Committee of the International Headache Society (IHS). The International Classification of Headache Disorders, 3rd edition (beta version) (2013) Cephalalgia 33:629–808
30. Toda K (2007) Trigeminal neuralgia—symptom, diagnosis, classification, and related disorders. Oral Sci Int 4:1–9
31. Vassilakis D, Phylaktakis M, Selviaridis P et al (1988) Symptomatic trigeminal neuralgia. J Neurosurg Sci 32:117–120
32. Watson P, Evans R (1985) Cluster-tic syndrome. Headache 25:123–126
33. Zakrzewska JM (1997) Trigeminal neuralgia. Prim Dent Care 4:17–19

Chapter 39
Central Neuropathic Pain: Multiple Sclerosis-Related Headaches

Robert Charlson, Ilya Kister, and Richard Lipton

39.1 Case Description

A 32-year-old man presents to his neurologist with a history of new-onset right-sided occipital head and neck pain. His medical history is significant for clinically isolated syndrome, anxiety, and frequent migraine headaches since his early twenties. His migraine headaches occur about three times per month and are heralded by typical visual aura half the time. The pain is unilateral usually on the left, pulsatile, and severe. Headaches are associated with prominent nausea and sensitivity to light. Three years ago, he had an episode of right leg weakness, blurry vision in his left eye, difficulty with depth perception, and pain on lateral eye movements that lasted several weeks. On the basis of his symptoms, neurologic deficits, and imaging, clinically isolated syndrome was suspected at the time and he received a course of IV Solu-Medrol with resolution of his symptoms.

He now presents with new "pain and strange feelings" in the right occiput and neck. The pain was described as sharp and shooting with an "electric shock" sensation on the right side of his neck. The pain occurs several times per week, lasts seconds, and then subsides. Between episodes of pain, he notes sensitivity to touch in the right occiput. The pain occasionally radiates to the front of the head and may worsen with head movement. He denies any new weakness or sensory changes.

On examination, the patient has a slight decrease in vision in the left eye not corrected with a pinhole and mild left optic nerve pallor. His right iliopsoas is

R. Charlson, MD • R. Lipton, MD
Department of Neurology, Albert Einstein College of Medicine, Bronx, NY, USA

I. Kister, MD (✉)
Department of Neurology, Multiple Sclerosis Center, New York University School of Medicine, New York, NY 10026, USA
e-mail: ilya.kister@nyuml.org

A. Siva, C. Lampl (eds.), *Case-Based Diagnosis and Management of Headache Disorders*, Headache, DOI 10.1007/978-3-319-06886-2_39

slightly weak (4+/5), and he has diffuse hyperreflexia, more pronounced on the right side. He has mild sensory loss to touch and pin prick in the C1-C2 distribution and experiences touch as painful in that region. His gait is mildly hemiparetic, and he has difficulty with tandem walking. The rest of his examination is normal, including a negative Lhermitte's sign and Spurling's test.

39.2 Differential Diagnosis and How to Work Up This Kind of Patient

Our patient presents with typical migraine with aura as well as signs and symptoms of a second pain disorder suggestive of occipital neuralgia. Consistent with the definition set out in the International Classification of Headache Disorders, third edition (ICHD-3), our patient has pain in the distribution of the greater or lesser occipital nerve with recurrent paroxysmal attacks of severe, sometimes shooting pain lasting seconds to minutes. In addition, he has the requisite dysesthesia or allodynia with tenderness over the branches of the nerve. At this point, we do not yet know if he would respond to occipital nerve blocks. Finally, ICHD-3 requires that the clinical picture is not better explained by another disorder.

Occipital neuralgia-like symptoms can arise in both the peripheral and central nervous systems. Given patient's history, the present symptoms suggest the onset of a central pain syndrome, most likely attributable to multiple sclerosis (MS). Once thought to be relatively rare in the MS population, central pain syndromes, including occipital and trigeminal neuralgia, are increasingly recognized as highly prevalent and clinically significant. MS patients will frequently present with atypical or nonspecific pains, and in evaluating any new complaints, the clinician must keep in mind a broad differential.

Occipital neuralgia is most often idiopathic but can arise from injury to the nerve at peripheral locations along the path from the C1 and C2 nerve roots to the distal branches of the greater or lesser occipital nerves. Potential etiologies along this path include trauma, repetitive flexion and extension, bone tumors, and vascular lesions. Within the central nervous system, diseases affecting the dorsal root entry zone, extramedullary and intramedullary spinal cord disease, and lesions in the region of the trigeminal nucleus caudalis may give rise to occipital neuralgia. Multiple sclerosis and other inflammatory disorders of spinal cord (i.e., neuromyelitis optica, idiopathic myelitis) can cause occipital neuralgia, usually in context of other cord symptoms and signs. In an MS patient, "electric" type of pain radiating down the neck could be due to "Lhermitte's sign." This pain syndrome has been linked to cervical lesions in MS but can occur with other cervical pathologies. In MS, Lhermitte's sign is typically provoked by neck flexion, radiates to the back or lower legs, but is highly variable in location and duration of pain.

The differential diagnosis of occipital neuralgia also includes a number of more common causes of occipital and neck pain, including symptoms due to cervical spondylosis and muscular or tendinous causes. Other more rare causes of pain that can mimic occipital neuralgia include vascular lesions such as cavernous angioma and a dural arteriovenous fistula at the cervical level, as well as neoplastic ones such as intramedullary tumors, schwannoma of the craniocervical junction, lymphoma, or an osteolytic lesion of the cranium. Herpes is always in differential of pain in radicular distribution, even in the absence of rash, which may antecede pain or be absent altogether (herpes sine herpes).

In a patient with MS, occipital neuralgia is likely related to the underlying diagnosis, but it is prudent to obtain cervical, gadolinium-enhanced MRI to exclude rarer secondary causes and to assess for the presence of a culprit demyelinating lesion.

39.3 Diagnostic Workup of the Case

Our patient received an MRI of the brain and cervical spine (Figs. 39.1 and 39.2). The cervical spine MRI reveals several lesions, most notably, in the region of C2 (Fig. 39.1a, b), which could account for the occipital neuralgia features. There are also lesions in the right C2 lateral fasciculus, right lateral central cord at C2-C3, and the right anterolateral cord at C4-C5. MRI of the brain shows, most notably, the large Dawson's finger on sagittal image (Fig. 39.2a) and the several periventricular and juxtacortical lesions on the axial FLAIR images (Fig. 39.2b).

After the workup, the patient underwent an occipital nerve block with xylocaine and immediately achieved a significant (80 %) reduction in his pain intensity. He was then started on carbamazepine, which was increased to 400 mg twice daily with good control of his symptoms.

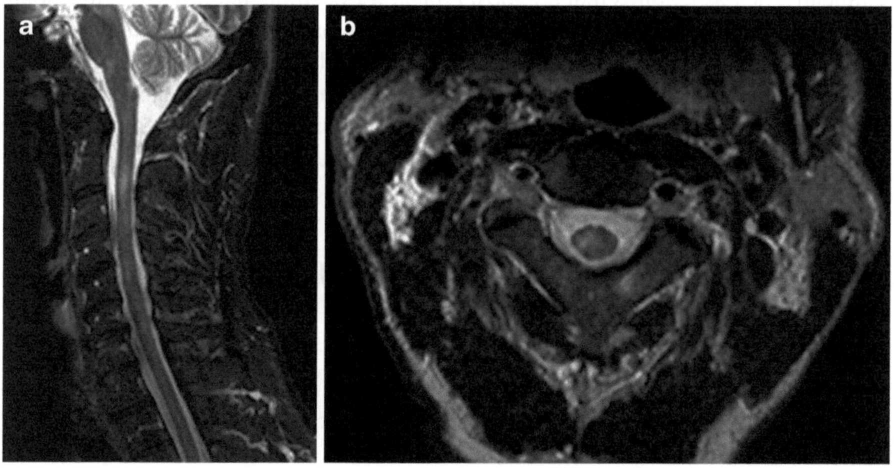

Fig. 39.1 (**a**, **b**) Multiple cervical lesions noted on MRI spine consistent with multiple sclerosis

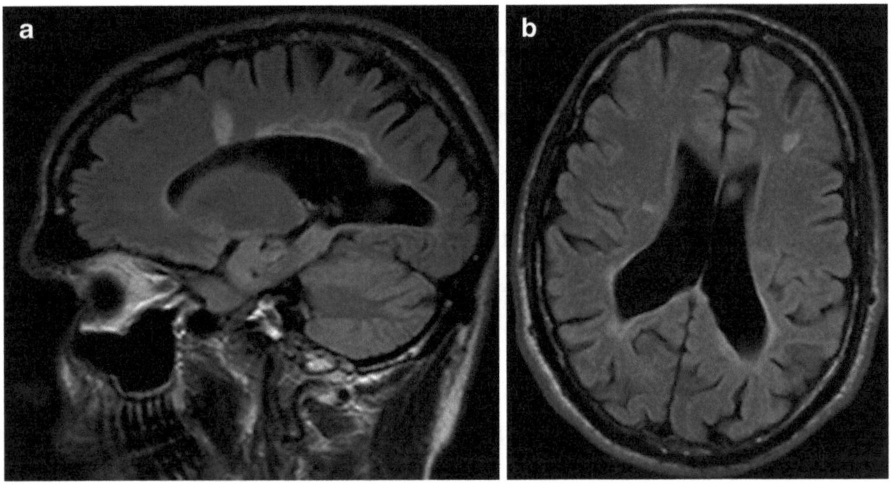

Fig. 39.2 (**a**, **b**) Periventricular and juxtacortical lesions on MRI brain

39.4 Summary of the Case

Our patient presented for evaluation for new paroxysmal occipital pain in the setting of relapsing remitting MS and a long-standing history of migraine with visual aura. His occipital symptoms are described as stabbing, sharp, and intermittent, with pain around the posterior scalp on the left with allodynia in that area. Pain radiated to the front of the head, a finding explained by convergent input to the trigeminal nucleus caudalis from the upper cervical roots and the first division of the trigeminal nerve. Clinically, he has features that are most typical for occipital neuralgia, though some aspects are reminiscent of Lhermitte's sign, which may share a common pathogenesis in some cases (i.e., lesions in the upper cervical spine) of occipital neuralgia. His workup confirmed the presence of a lesion in the upper cervical spine consistent with a probable demyelinating etiology. Such localization has been noted in case series of MS patients with occipital neuralgia-type pain.

39.5 Definition of Central Neuropathic Pain Attributable to Multiple Sclerosis

The International Association for the Study of Pain (IASP) in its Taxonomy, revised in 2011, defined central pain as "pain initiated or caused by a primary lesion or dysfunction in the central nervous system." This was distinguished from peripheral neuropathic pain (i.e., caused by damage to the peripheral somatosensory nervous system, such as peripheral neuropathy or radiculopathy) as well as from nociceptive pain (i.e., from damage to nonneural tissue attributed then to activation of nociceptors, such as damage to muscles, joints, viscera, etc.). The International Headache Society criteria define the syndrome of central neuropathic pain attributable to MS as involving unilateral or bilateral craniocervical pain with a range of clinical symptoms. Sensory symptoms, if present, should be attributable to demyelination of the central nervous system, though precise localization is often difficult. Silent lesions and unexplained symptoms are common.

39.6 Brief General Information

Central pain syndromes in MS are both common and clinically significant. A range of recent data has found that the large percentage of MS patients experience neuropathic pain and many will present with multiple pain complaints. Central pain in MS may manifest as dysesthetic limb pain, trigeminal neuralgia (TN), occipital neuralgia, Lhermitte's sign, and painful tonic spasms, among others. Though prevalence estimates vary, most support the idea that dysesthetic limb pain remains the most common form of central pain in MS, followed by Lhermitte's sign, and then the cranial neuralgias. Beyond a single case series, very little evidence regarding occipital neuralgia in MS has been reported. Trigeminal neuralgia, however, has been recognized for some time as a common entity in MS patients. Some cases of TN in MS show well-situated plaques in the trigeminal root zone of the pons, while other patients with similarly placed lesions remain asymptomatic.

Central pain syndromes have been attributed to damage to the spinothalamocortical pathways. However, imaging studies generally show disseminated lesions in both brain and spinal cord, which do not readily correlate to pain symptomatology. Damage to spinal cord nociceptive pathways mediated through loss of GABA inhibitory interneurons has also been proposed as a possible contributing factor. Regardless, pain symptoms in MS are often patchy, highly variable, and typically associated with abnormalities in quantitative sensory testing.

Risk factors for the development of chronic pain in MS patients are inconsistent, with the association between pain syndromes and older age, longer disease duration, and greater disease severity being somewhat controversial. There is good evidence, however, that patients with one pain syndrome appear to be more likely to have another pain syndrome. Chronic pain has also been frequently linked to comorbid depression, anxiety, and several other psychosocial factors including scores on pain coping scales and pain-related catastrophizing.

In our patient, a new central pain syndrome is superimposed on long-standing migraine, reflecting the complicated reality of coexisting pain syndromes in MS. Migraine appears to be associated with MS, and MS patients have been found in a number of studies to be more than twice as likely to report migraine headaches.

Despite case reports of headaches triggered by acute MS lesions, in the majority of cases, the headache symptoms preceded the diagnosis of MS, suggesting a more complex relationship between primary headache disorders and MS than a "single-lesion" theory may imply. Given that most headache disorders precede the diagnosis of MS by several years, recent work has looked at the idea that migraine may predispose patients to developing MS. In particular, our own recent work suggests that migraine constitutes a modest risk factor for the development of MS. Hypothetically, migraine may lead to changes in the permeability in the blood-brain barrier and endothelial damage, thereby lowering the threshold for developing CNS-directed autoimmune process in susceptible individuals.

The relationship between headache and MS disease characteristics remains incompletely understood. Migraine does not appear to be associated with higher disability or lesion burden on MRI, but may be more common in patients of younger age and relapsing form of the disease. There is evidence that MS patients with migraine also have more central pain complaints, including brief shooting pains into the jaw and back of the head, facial pain, temporomandibular joint syndrome, Lhermitte's sign, and painful spasms.

Clinicians who are encountering patients with headache and MS also need to be aware that treatment with interferons-beta (IFNb) can trigger or worsen preexisting headaches. In our experience, the effects of IFNb can be mitigated in most cases by pretreatment with NSAIDs and, sometimes, oral prednisone, as well as ensuring adequate hydration status on days of injection. Interestingly, although natalizumab infusions can cause headache, recent work with patients with known migraine found that only IFNb, but not natalizumab, increased the rate of preexisting migraine.

In conclusion, the coexistence of pain syndromes in MS is the rule rather than the exception, and the framework of central pain includes a diverse group of syndromes and presentations that are clinically significant in the MS population.

Key Points Regarding Central Pain Syndromes in MS

- Central pain syndromes are not only common in MS but are frequently comorbid with other pain complaints including migraine.
- Neuralgia-form pain syndromes can be associated with central nervous system lesions in MS and are often localizable to the cervical spine.
- Central pain syndromes may manifest as dysesthetic limb pain, Lhermitte's sign, occipital and trigeminal neuralgia, and painful tonic spasms, among other disorders.
- Migraine is also associated with MS, and patients with both migraine and MS are at increased risk for a range of other central pain complaints.
- Despite the occasional reports of isolated lesions causing new-onset migraine or other headaches, the relationship between migraine and MS remains complex; preexisting migraine does appear to be a modest risk factor for developing MS.
- IFNbs are well known to trigger or worsen preexisting headaches, but these can be avoided with proper pretreatment.

Suggested Reading

1. D'Amico D, La Mantia L, Rigamonti A et al (2004) Prevalence of primary headaches in people with multiple sclerosis. Cephalalgia 24:980–984
2. De Santi L, Annunziata P (2012) Symptomatic cranial neuralgias in multiple sclerosis: clinical features and treatment. Clin Neurol Neurosurg 114(2):101–107
3. Foley PL, Vesterinen HM, Laird BJ (2013) Prevalence and natural history of pain in adults with multiple sclerosis: systematic review and meta-analysis. Pain 154:632–642
4. Headache classification committee of the International Headache Society (2013) The International Classification of Headache Disorders, 3rd Edition (beta version). Cephalalgia 33(9):777
5. International Association for the Study of Pain: Taxonomy (2011) URL: http://www.iasp-pain.org
6. Kister I, Caminero AB, Monteith TS et al (2010) Migraine is comorbid with multiple sclerosis and associated with a more symptomatic MS course. J Headache Pain 11:417–425
7. Kister I, Munger KL, Herbert J, Ascherio A (2012) Increased risk of multiple sclerosis among women with migraine in the Nurses' Health Study II. Mult Scler 18(1):90–97
8. Lin GY, Wang CW, Chiang TT et al (2013) Multiple sclerosis presenting initially with a worsening of migraine symptoms. J Head Pain 14:70
9. Mohrke J, Kropp P, Uwe ZK (2013) Headaches in multiple sclerosis patients might imply an inflammatorial process. PLoS One 8(8):e69570
10. Moisset X, Ouchchane L, Guy N et al (2013) Migraine headaches and pain with neuropathic characteristics: comorbid conditions in patients with multiple sclerosis. Pain 154:2691–2699
11. Nurmikko TJ, Gupta S, MacIver K (2010) Multiple sclerosis-related central pain disorders. Curr Pain Headache Rep 14:189–195
12. O'Connor AB, Schwid SR, Herrmann DN et al (2008) Pain associated with multiple sclerosis: systemic review and proposed classification. Pain 137:96–111
13. Osterberg A, Boivie J, Thuomas KA (2005) Central pain in multiple sclerosis – prevalence and clinical characteristics. Eur J Pain 9:531–542
14. Truini A, Barbanti P, Pozzilli C, Cruccu G (2013) A mechanism-based classification of pain in multiple sclerosis. J Neurol 260:351–367
15. Villani V, Prosperini L, De Giglio L et al (2012) The impact of interferon beta and natalizumab on comorbid migraine in multiple sclerosis. Headache 52:1130–1135
16. Wasner G (2010) Central pain syndromes. Curr Pain Headache Rep 14:489–496

MIX
Papier aus verantwortungsvollen Quellen
Paper from responsible sources
FSC® C105338

If you have any concerns about our products,
you can contact us on
ProductSafety@springernature.com

In case Publisher is established outside the EU,
the EU authorized representative is:
Springer Nature Customer Service Center GmbH
Europaplatz 3, 69115 Heidelberg, Germany

Printed by Libri Plureos GmbH
in Hamburg, Germany